THE PRACTICE OF M-MODE AND TWO-DIMENSIONAL ECHOCARDIOGRAPHY

DEVELOPMENTS IN CARDIOVASCULAR MEDICINE

VOLUME 23

Other volumes in this series:

THE PRACTICE OF M-MODE AND TWO-DIMENSIONAL ECHOCARDIOGRAPHY

edited by

J. ROELANDT, MD

Thoraxcenter, Erasmus University
Rotterdam

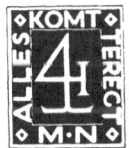

1983

MARTINUS NIJHOFF PUBLISHERS
THE HAGUE / BOSTON / LONDON

Distributors:

for the United States and Canada
Kluwer Boston, Inc.
190 Old Derby Street
Hingham, MA 02043
USA

for all other countries
Kluwer Academic Publishers Group
Distribution Center
P.O.Box 322
3300 AH Dordrecht
The Netherlands

Library of Congress Cataloging in Publication Data

Main entry under title;

The Practice of M-mode and two-dimensional echo-
    cardiography.

    (Developments in cardiovascular medicine ;
v. 23)
    Includes index.
    1. Ultrasonic cardiography. 2. Heart--Diseases
--Diagnosis. I. Roelandt, Jos. II. Series. [DNLM:
1. Echocardiography--Methods. W1 DE997VME v.23 /
WG 141.5.E2 P895]
RC683.5.U5P73 1982   616.1'207543   82-14434

ISBN-13:978-94-009-6792-2   e-ISBN-13:978-94-009-6790-8
DOI: 10.1007/978-94-009-6790-8

CONTENTS

VI. APPLICATION OF M-MODE AND TWO-DIMENSIONAL ECHOCARDIOGRAPHY IN CORONARY ARTERY DISEASE

PREFACE

The extension of conventional M-mode to two-dimensional echocardiography has been a major advance for the evaluation and management of cardiac disease. Their combined use is optimal for a comprehensive analysis of anatomy and structure function and thus best serving the patient.

This book critically examines the validity of the applications of these ultrasound techniques in common cardiac disorders.

In addition to the clinical value of contrast and Doppler echocardiography, several chapters are devoted to problems related to quantitation of both M-mode and two-dimensional echocardiography.

This volume is specifically aimed at the practicing cardiologist and provides an in-depth appreciation of most recent echocardiographic advances.

J. ROELANDT

LIST OF CONTRIBUTORS

Anliker, M., MD, Department of Cardiology, University Hospital Zürich, Rämistrasse 100, 8091 Zürich, SWITZERLAND.

Carroll, J.D., MD, Department of Cardiology, University Hospital of Zürich, Rämistrasse 100, 8091 Zürich, SWITZERLAND.

Cate, F.J. ten, MD, Harbour Hospital, Haringvliet 2, 3011 TD Rotterdam, THE NETHERLANDS.

Cikes, I., MD, Institute of Cardiovascular Disease, School of Medicine, University of Zagreb, Kispaticeva 12, 41000 Zagreb, YUGOSLAVIA.

Domburg, R.T. van, PhD, Thoraxcenter, Academic Hospital Dijkzigt and Erasmus University, P.O. Box 1738, 3000 DR Rotterdam, THE NETHERLANDS.

Ernst, A., MD, Institute of Cardiovascular Disease, School of Medicine, University of Zagreb, Kispaticeva 12, 41000 Zagreb, YUGOSLAVIA.

Hanrath, P., MD, Department of Cardiology, University Hospital Hamburg-Eppendorf, Martinistrasse 52, 2000 Hamburg 20, BRD.

Hess, D.M., MD, Department of Cardiology, University Hospital Zürich, Rämistrasse 100, 8091 Zürich, SWITZERLAND.

Hunter, S., MD, Department of Cardiology, Freeman Hospital, Newcastle-upon-Tyne, GREAT BRITAIN.

Jenni, R., MD, Department of Cardiology, University Hospital Zürich, Rämistrasse 100, 8091 Zürich, SWITZERLAND.

Krayenbühl, H.P., MD, Department of Cardiology, University Hospital Zürich, Rämistrasse 100, 8091 Zürich, SWITZERLAND.

Kremer, P., MD, Department of Cardiology, University Hospital Hamburg- Eppendorf, Martinistrasse 52, 2000 Hamburg 20, BRD.

Langenstein, B.A. MD, Department of Cardiology, University Hospital Hamburg- Eppendorf, Martinistrasse 52, 2000 Hamburg 20, BRD.

Leech, G., PhD, Cardiac Department, Saint George's Hospital, Blackshaw Road, London, SW17 OQT, GREAT BRITAIN.

Lubsen, J., PhD, Thoraxcenter, Academic Hospital Dijkzigt and Erasmus University, P.O. Box 1738, 3000 DR Rotterdam, THE NETHERLANDS.

Meltzer, R.S., MD, Thoraxcenter, Academic Hospital Dijkzigt and Erasmus University, P.O. Box 1738, 3000 DR Rotterdam, THE NETHERLANDS. Present address: Cardiology Division, Mount Sinai Medical Center, New York, NY 10029, USA.

Polster, J., MD, Department of Cardiology, University Hospital Hamburg- Eppendorf, Martinistrasse 52, 2000 Hamburg 20, BRD.

Prasquier, R., MD, Service de Cardiologie, Hôpital Beaujon, 100 Boulevard du Général Leclerc, 92118 Clichy, FRANCE.

Roelandt, J., MD, Thoraxcenter, Academic Hospital Dijkzigt and Erasmus University, P.O. Box 1738, 3000 DR Rotterdam, THE NETHERLANDS.

Rijsterborgh, H., PhD, Thoraxcenter, Academic Hospital Dijkzigt and Erasmus University, P.O. Box 1738, 3000 DR Rotterdam, THE NETHERLANDS.

Schlüter, M., PhD, Department of Cardiology, University Hospital Hamburg- Eppendorf, Martini—strasse 52, 2000 Hamburg 20, BRD.

Schweizer, P., MD, Abteilung Innere Medizin I, Medizinische Fakultät, Rheinisch-Westfälische Technische Hochschule, Goethestrasse 27 – 29, D – 5100 Aachen, BRD.

Souquet, J., PhD, Advanced Technology Laboratories Inc., 13208 Northup Way, Bellevue, Washington 98008 – 0639, USA.

Sutherland, G.R., MD, Department of Cardiology, Freeman Hospital, Newcastle-upon-Tyne, GREAT BRITAIN.

Touche, T., MD, Service de Cardiologie, Hôpital Beaujon, 100 Boulevard du Général Leclerc, 92118 Clichy, FRANCE.

Vervin, P., MD, Service de Cardiologie, Hôpital Beaujon, 100 Boulevard du Général Leclerc, 92118 Clichy, FRANCE.

Vieli, A., MD, Department of Cardiology, University Hospital Zürich, Rämistrasse 100, 8091 Zürich, SWITZERLAND.

I. INSTRUMENTATION AND EXAMINATION TECHNIQUES OF M-MODE AND TWO-DIMENSIONAL ECHOCARDIOGRAPHY

The extension of conventional M-mode to two-dimensional echocardiography has been an important advance and their combined use is optimal for a comprehensive analysis of cardiac disease and thus best serving the patient. The fundamental principles underlying real-time two-dimensional imaging of the heart and how they determine the image quality ultimately achievable are discussed in chapter 1.

It appears that comparative advantages and limitations of commercially available systems are rapidly changing and that their sophistocation is increasing which makes differences between them less pronounced for the practicing cardiologist.

The technique of two-dimensional examination of the heart and great vessels is described in chapter 2. A wealth of diagnostic information is obtained from a multitude of cardiac tomographic views which are imaged from several chest wall transducer positions.

Consequently, recommendations for nomenclature and image orientation standards are necessary to make studies from different laboratories comparable. All these tomographic views have been validated and are extensively discussed and their specific clinical value outlined.

Roelandt, J. (ed.) The practice of M-mode and two-dimensional echocardiography
© *1983, Martinus Nijhoff Publishers. The Hague / Boston / London*
ISBN 978-94-009-6792-2.

1. PERFORMANCE CHARACTERISTICS OF TWO-DIMENSIONAL CARDIAC SCANNERS

GRAHAM J. LEECH

INTRODUCTION

The dramatic advances made in echocardiography have been possible only because of the intensive efforts of the recording equipment manufacturers to keep abreast both of the increasingly sophisticated demands of clinicians and of the available technology, notably in the area of video recording and signal processing. Recognition of the fact that both the clinical and technological aspects of echocardiography are equally important has led to close cooperation between engineering and medical professionals and as a result many cardiologists have acquired a high level of expertise in the technical area.

However, in such a rapidly evolving field, it is difficult even for those closely involved to keep abreast of all the latest developments; this is particularly true of electronic techniques, where recent developments in microelectronics and digital image processing have already been incorporated into the latest generation of two-dimensional (2-D) ultrasound scanners. As a result the machines now available offer a number of features, the potential advantages of which are not understood by many users. It is the purpose of this paper to describe some of these features, and to discuss in general terms some of the factors which influence the quality of the cardiac images.

TOMOGRAPHIC ULTRASOUND SCANNING

Ultrasound images of cross-sectional planes (tomograms) of organs such as the liver have been possible for a number of years using the compound B-scanning technique. An ultrasound transducer is supported by a linkage of mechanical arms, which constrain it so that it is free to move only in a particular plane. Information on its position and the angle at which the ultrasound beam is directed is conveyed to the instrument by means of servo-potentiometers attached to the linkage arms. The transducer is aimed at the organ to be studied and the resulting echoes are displayed on an oscilloscope in B-mode format (a line of dots of light, whose intensities represent the amplitude of echoes). The orientation of the B-mode line corresponds to that of the transducer. The transducer position and

Roelandt, J. (ed.) The practice of M-mode and two-dimensional echocardiography
© *1983, Martinus Nijhoff Publishers. The Hague / Boston / London*
ISBN 978-94-009-6792-2.

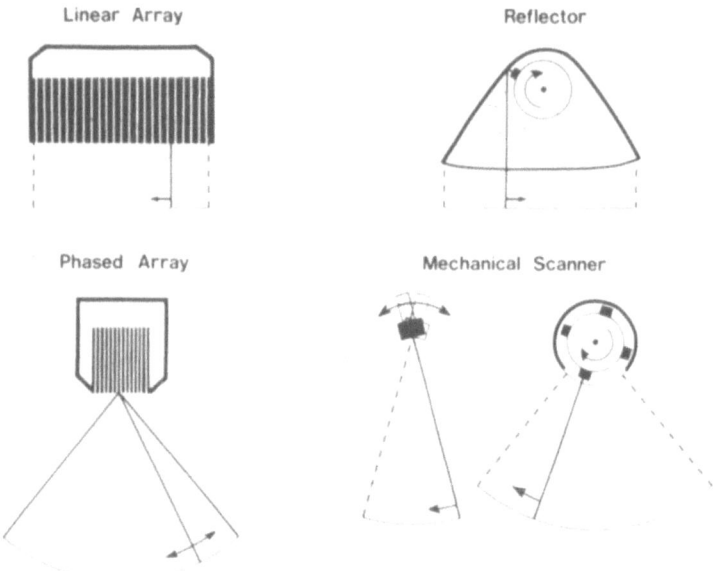

Figure 1. Two-dimensional scanning methods.

beam angle are then changed, and the new B-mode echo pattern, with its corresponding orientation, is displayed alongside the first, a storage oscilloscope being convenient for this purpose. As the operator scans the beam to and fro, a complete image of a cross-section of the selected organ is built up.

This technique can only be used to study organs which do not move significantly during the few seconds it takes to complete the scan. Most organs do not move much, and such movement as there is has no physiological significance. However, the heart not only moves rapidly, but the motion patterns are of great interest. A tomographic heart scanner must therefore complete each scan in 1/25 s or less, in order to 'freeze' the valve leaflet motions, and a succession of images must be made for at least the duration of one cardiac cycle. This cannot be done manually, so some form of mechanically or electronically driven scanner must be used.

A number of systems have been devised for rapid cardiac B-scanning (Figure 1). Broadly, these fall into two classes: those in which a plane is scanned in rectilinear fashion by generating a succession of ultrasound beams which travel along parallel paths and those in which the beam is scanned through an arc, effectively from a point origin, giving an image in the form of a sector of a circle. For either type, the scanning can be accomplished by electro-mechanical or purely electronic means. An important difference between cross-sectional scanners used for abdominal organs and those used for cardiac studies is that for the latter there is no fixed spatial reference point. The beam is steered relative to the transducer assembly, which by convention is shown in a fixed position on the oscilloscope screen (usually at the top).

Rectilinear scanners are generally preferred for abdominal and obstetric scanning and are replacing compound B-scanners in many institutions because they speed the examination, but for cardiac applications they are severely handicapped by the very limited access to the heart permitted by bone and lung tissue, which are essentially impenetrable to ultrasound. In a rectilinear scan, the scan width corresponds to the transducer size, and this means that portions of the image are frequently obscured by rib or lung shadowing. For this reason, almost all commercial cardiac scanners employ the sector scan technique.

SECTOR SCANNING METHODS

The simplest type of sector scanner, which mimics M-mode most closely, contains a single transducer which is oscillated through an angle of up to 90 deg. The angular position of the transducer is detected by a servo potentiometer, which varies the orientation of the B-mode display correspondingly. However, there are some problems associated with an oscillatory motion. The angular velocity of the transducer is not constant, but the ultrasound pulses are transmitted at equal intervals, so the scan lines are more widely spaced at the centre of the sector than at the edges. Also, if the transducer is in contact with the patient's chest, it can cause some discomfort and generates high mechanical stresses which are a potential source of unreliability.

An alternative method uses an assembly of several transducers, which rotate inside a plastic dome filled with liquid. As each element enters the scan arc, it is connected to the pulse generator; when it reaches the end of the scan, the next element takes over, in the same way as the rotating beacon of a lighthouse scans a succession of beams across the sea. Since the angular velocity is constant, registration with the oscilloscope display is easier, and there is no vibration.

The electronically steered sector scanner (often called a 'phased array') generates a similar scan pattern to the mechanical sector scanner, but has no moving parts. It typically comprises 32 transducers, each $10 \times 0,5$ mm, laid side by side to form an assembly having overall dimensions 10×20 mm. Its operation depends on pulsing the individual elements in a rapid and precisely controlled sequence. In Figure 2, a simplified array is shown in which the top element is pulsed first. Because the element is small compared with the ultrasound wavelength, it generates a pressure wave which has a cylindrical profile. When the wave from the top element has travelled only a short distance, the next element is pulsed, and so on. The waves combine to form a single compound wave, which travels in a direction at an angle to the axis of the array. By repeating this sequence, but with different pulsing intervals, it is possible to scan the beam through a wide angle. Although relatively simple in concept, in practice controlling the pulsing sequence to the necessary precision is not easy.

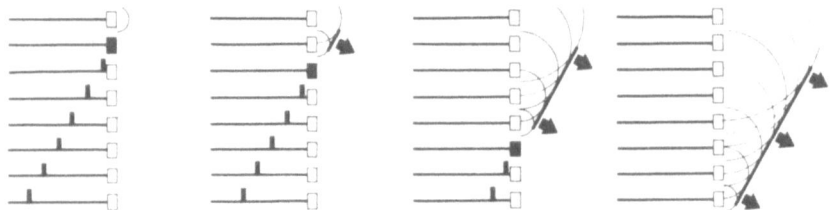

Figure 2. Principle of electronic beam steering.

With a mechanical scanner, detection of echoes is accomplished in the same way as for M-mode, the small amount by which the transducer angle changes during the interval between pulse transmission and arrival of the echoes being of no consequence. In the case of the electronically steered scanner, however, except when the beam direction is along the axis of the transducer array, the returning echo wavefront does not arrive at all elements simultaneously. The sequence of electrical signals generated is thus comparable to that of the original transmission pulses shown in Figure 2, and before they can be added together, they must be synchronised. One way to do this is to pass the signal from each element through a 'delay line', an electronic device which slows it down by a controllable amount. With suitable delay line settings, the signals from all the elements can be aligned temporally, then added together. However, to provide one delay line per element is costly and to adjust them for each transmitted pulse presents considerable technical problems, so other techniques are now being used to achieve the same result.

THE CHARACTERISTICS OF AN ULTRASOUND BEAM

It is convenient to think of the beam of ultrasound pulses as being like a thin pencil of light which illuminates only the very small area of the heart at which it is directed, but in fact this is far from the case and the shape and intensity characteristics of the wave pattern generated by an ultrasound transducer are very complex indeed. Considering the case where the transducer is excited by a continuous sine-wave electrical signal (it is, of course excited by brief pulses, but this complicates the situation even further), the total wave intensity at any point is the sum of the intensities of a large number of wavelets, each arising from an elemental area of the crystal. For any point, the distances to various parts of the crystal are not equal, so the wavelets do not arrive simultaneously. At some points, they tend to reinforce each other, giving high total intensity, but at others they cancel each other out, and the resultant intensity is zero. The characteristics of the resultant beam are roughly as follows (Figure 3).

There is a central 'main beam'. Near to the transducer, its cross-section is approximately the same as that of the crystal; this region is called the 'near field', or

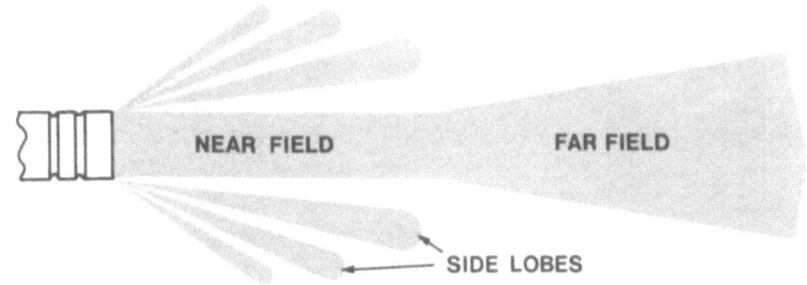

Figure 3. Diagram of an ultrasound beam, with side-lobes.

Fresnel zone. The intensity within the Fresnel zone is very non-uniform: at any cross-section it can be represented as as a series of concentric rings and as the section is moved further from the transducer the number of rings reduces until, at range $d^2/4L$ (where d = crystal diameter and L = wavelength) it enters the far field, or Fraunhofer zone. Here there are no maxima and minima and intensity decreases as the square of the range, and with increasing angle to the beam axis. The main beam diverges at an angle, φ, given by: $\varphi = \sin^{-1}(1.22L/D)$.

Surrounding the main beam are a series of concentric cones called 'side lobes', having a common apex at the centre of the crystal. Each cone represents a region of relatively high intensity, with the spaces between them regions of low intensity. The peak intensity of the inner side lobes is much greater than that of the outer cones. The nominal boundaries of the main beam and side lobes are usually those at which the intensity is 50% (-6dB) of the nominal maximum.

The dimensions of the ultrasound beam are thus determined by the crystal size and the ultrasound wavelength. Although a small crystal gives an initially narrower beam, the Fresnel zone is shorter, with greater angle of divergence in the far field and the side lobe intensities are also greater.

LINE DENSITY IN TWO-DIMENSIONAL IMAGES

Figure 4 shows a single 2-D scan. It comprises a number of radial lines, each displaying echoes in B-mode format. For the image to be accurate, the structures in the scan plane must not move significantly during the time it takes to complete the scan. For a working depth of 20 cm, echoes from the furthest structures take 270 microseconds to return, so the maximum pulse rate is 3750 per second. If each image is to be completed in 1/25 s (a reasonable rate to 'freeze' valve leaflet motions), it can comprise only 150 lines. The line density depends on the scan angle; if this is only 30 deg., 150 lines gives 5 lines/deg., but if the scan angle is increased to 90 deg., line density falls to 1,6 lines/deg. In the sector format inadequate line density is, of course, most noticeable at maximum range.

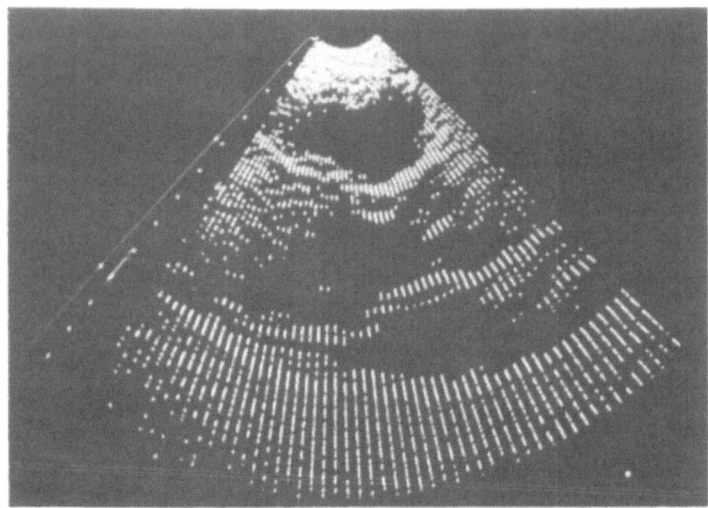

Figure 4. Single frame image showing radial scan lines.

There thus has to be a compromise in any sector scanning system between number of scans per second, scan angle and line density. If one of these parameters is increased, the others must suffer.

DISPLAYING AND RECORDING A 2-D IMAGE

As described above, a 2-D sector image comprises a number of radial B-mode scans, which can be displayed on an oscilloscope and the image photographed directly as in Figure 4. However, in order to record moving images it is necessary to employ a video tape recorder, and to facilitate this it is very desirable to convert the image into a standard television format of a raster of horizontal lines. The exact configuration varies from country to country, the most common being NTSC (575 lines/frame: 30 frames/s) used in the U.S.A. and PAL (625 lines/frame: 25 frames/s) used in Europe, except France.

The conversion process is done with the aid of a digital frame store. This comprises a matrix of memory cells, containing typically 256 × 256 or more elements, each called a 'pixel'. The image intensity at each point on the 2-D scan is expressed in digital form on a scale of $0 - 32$ (sometimes $0 - 64$) grey levels and the value stored in the appropriate memory cell. When fully loaded, the memory matrix can be 'read' in any desired sequence, for example as a series of horizontal lines to form a T.V. image for a video recorder, or as a series of vertical lines to enable it to be printed by a fibre-optic strip-chart recorder.

DERIVED M-MODE RECORDINGS

A facility offered by most instruments is the ability to display and record echoes in M-mode format using a beam direction selected from a 2-D image. An electronic cursor is positioned manually on the sector image, for example to intersect the pulmonary valve leaflet, and the corresponding M-mode is then recorded. This technique is useful both as a means to expedite the M-mode examination, since location of structures like the pulmonary valve is easier on a 2-D image, and also it enables the position of the M-mode beam to be optimised, for example to determine left ventricular cavity dimensions.

With a mechanical scanner, the cursor line is positioned on the 2-D display, and when M-mode is selected the transducer is halted in the appropriate position. Small adjustments can be made by manipulating the scanning head, but it is not possible to relate these to the sector image without switching back to the 2-D mode. Although it is possible to obtain truly simultaneous M-mode and 2-D images from a mechanical transducer, the quality is so poor as to render them virtually useless. This is because only one ultrasound beam can be used to construct the M-mode image per 2-D scan. For a typical scan rate, this means that the M-mode recording has only 25 lines per second, compared with the 1000 or more normally used.

One of the advantages of the electronic beam steering is that the ultrasound beam direction can be varied at will, simply by controlling the electrical pulsing sequence. Thus it is possible, for example, to use alternate pulses from a 2-D image to form an M-mode image. By this means sufficient pulses can be made available to give one, or even two good quality M-mode recordings at the same time as 2-D images are being displayed. However, it must be remembered that by diverting pulses for M-mode recordings, the total left for the 2-D image is reduced, and its quality must suffer to some extent.

IMAGE PROCESSING

Once the sector image has been converted into digital form and stored in a memory matrix, it can be manipulated in a number of ways designed to improve the visual impression of 'quality'. Some of the techniques now being employed are described briefly below.

Gamma control

The difficulty of registering the full dynamic range of the echo signals will be discussed later. The grey level of each pixel in the store can be adjusted to alter the overall transfer characteristic, for example to eliminate low level noise, or to reduce or increase the slope of the gamma curve, thus changing the contrast.

Spatial interpolation

The structured noise introduced by the scan lines degrades the image considerably, particularly at extreme ranges and with wide scan angles. Those pixels lying in the gaps between B-mode lines can be filled with an average value of the signal intensities of the nearest points through which the scan lines pass. This has to be done carefully so as to avoid generating even more unsightly scan interference patterns akin to Moiré fringes.

Temporal averaging: variable persistence

Various techniques can be employed to improve image quality by mixing the information from two or more scans prior to displaying the image. For example, if there are four successive scans: A, B, C and D, the first displayed image could be (B + A), the second (C + B), the third (D + C), and so on. This would improve the signal: noise ratio because random noise would tend to cancel out, but rapidly moving structures would smear. An improvement would be to display first (C + 1/2B + 1/4A) then (D + 1/2C + 1/4B). Each presented image thus would contain a proportion of older information, the result being similar to increasing the persistence (after-glow) of a conventional oscilloscope display.

Alpha-numeric data

Information such as patient identification, date, time and videotape storage location can easily be added to the image.

Measurements from the display

By using a light pen or joystick-controlled cursor, it is possible to make measurements and perform calculations directly from the displayed image. However, practical problems such as parallax errors with a light pen and the manipulative skill needed to control a joystick tend to make it preferable to perform measurements from recorded hard-copy images.

PARAMETERS WHICH DETERMINE IMAGE QUALITY

To measure the 'quality' of an image is not easy, since different observers perceive 'quality' as meaning different things. The psycho-perceptual aspects of image quality are exceedingly complex, and space does not permit any discussion of them here. However, before any consideration of the eye/brain aspects of image analysis, it is necessary first to be able to measure the purely physical parameters which determine the characteristics of an image. They are:

Resolution

Grey Scale

Noise

We will consider each of these.

Resolution

The resolution of an imaging system measures its ability to distinguish objects which are close together. In 2-D echocardiography, it is necessary to consider separately *axial* resolution, along the direction in which the pulses travel, and *lateral* resolution, at right angles to the beam. For 2-D scanners, lateral resolution must further be divided into *azimuthal* resolution, at right angles to the beam axis, and in the plane of the sector scan; and *elevation* resolution, at right angles to the beam axis and at right angles to the plane of the scan. Axial resolution is limited primarily by the duration of the ultrasound pulses. If a pulse encounters two tissue interfaces in rapid succession, the front of the pulse may reach the second interface before the back of it has finished crossing the first interface. In this case the two echoes from the two interfaces merge together and only one structure is shown on the display. If the total pulse duration can be reduced, the minimum separation of interfaces needed to prevent this effect is reduced and axial resolution is thereby improved. This can be achieved, for example, by increasing wave frequency, reducing transmitter power or damping the crystal. Axial resolution of a commercial machine is typically 1 – 2 mm.

Lateral resolution is limited by beam width and side-lobe characteristics. If there are two separate targets, each just illuminated by the edges of the beam, but identical distances from the transducer, their echoes will return at the same instant; the echoes will be superimposed, and shown as though they represented objects on the central beam axis. Even echoes from objects illuminated by the side lobes will be shown as coming from axial targets. Since the main beam 10 cm from the transducer is typically 10 – 20 mm wide, lateral resolution will be of this order (i.e. 10 times worse than axial resolution) unless steps can be taken to improve beam characteristics. Poor lateral resolution is the major limitation to image quality in most commercial machines.

Grey Scale

There is a basic difficulty in recording any ultrasound image, caused by the great disparity between the dynamic range of the echo signals and that available in the recording system. The difference in amplitude between the strongest echoes (e.g. the pericardium) and the weakest that can be distinguished from the noise is typically about 1 000 000:1 (120db). Echo amplitude is represented by the intensity of the light spot on the cathode-ray tube, or by blackness of the recorded image. However, the range of intensities that can be distinguished on photographic film is only about 10:1 (20db). This can be increased somewhat by using a colour display, but is still far lower than the range of the echo signals. The tendency is thus for all strong echoes to be shown as having equal intensity, and for weak echoes not to be registered at all. This difficulty can partly be overcome by use of a non-linear video-transfer characteristic, commonly called a 'gamma' control. This is a signal amplifier which, instead of having a linear relationship between input and output amplitudes, (for which a graph showing input versus output amplitude would be a straight line) has an S-shaped input/output relationship. Over a central region, the curve is approximately linear, but at high and low levels it becomes nearly flat. Thus fairly good amplitude differentiation is provided in the middle of the range while still retaining some, though not much, at the extremes. Each stage of the signal processing tends to affect the picture gamma, and it is important for the equipment designer to be able to adjust it on each display, so that information on the oscilloscope corresponds to that recorded on videotape and printed by the recorder.

Noise

Noise in an imaging system is defined as anything not wanted. In the context of a 2-D echocardiographic system, there are three major sources of noise.

Firstly, there is random electronic noise generated in the amplifier and arising from the transducer. Added to this is physiological noise: echoes from small tissue inclusions, and from off-axis structures generated as a result of less than perfect lateral resolution. The extent to which noise artefacts are seen is determined by the overall gain level of the amplifier, and by the level of 'reject' used to supress low level signals.

However, echoes from small targets also have low amplitude, since the smaller the target the less it acts as a specular reflector. The factor limiting the *target acquisition* ability of a system is therefore the noise level. In practice, it is very difficult to determine the smallest target which can be detected. Not only is the nature of the target itself important, but the characteristics of the surrounding tissue must also be considered (an object is much easier to detect when surrounded by echo-free blood than by echogenic tissue), and detection is greatly aided by relative motion of the target and its surroundings.

The third major noise source is 'structured' noise arising from the manner in which the display is generated. In older machines, which did not have a digital scan converter, the 'spoke' pattern of the sector lines was highly evident. Use of a scan converter with spatial interpolation has improved this a lot, but there remains the raster pattern of the T.V. scan, and in some cases the pixel structure of the image is evident. This forms a good illustration of the difficulty of defining image quality: if a very high resolution recorder is used, the line and pixel structure become obvious, and most users prefer a picture which is degraded slightly by de-focussing, to the point where its resolution is not good enough to show the structured noise.

IMPROVING LATERAL RESOLUTION

One way to improve lateral resolution is to reduce the beam width by use of a focussing lens. This comprises a disc of plastic material attached to the crystal face, which acts in the same way as an optical lens, though not so effectively. It can, however, reduce the main beam width by a factor of $2-3$ at optimal focussing range.

An electronically steered beam can also be focussed electronically (Figure 5). A lens works by delaying portions of the wavefront; equivalent delays can be introduced a part of the beam steering process, and the pulsing sequence set to focus the beam at a chosen range. However, this reduces beam width only in the azimuthal plane and does not affect elevation resolution.

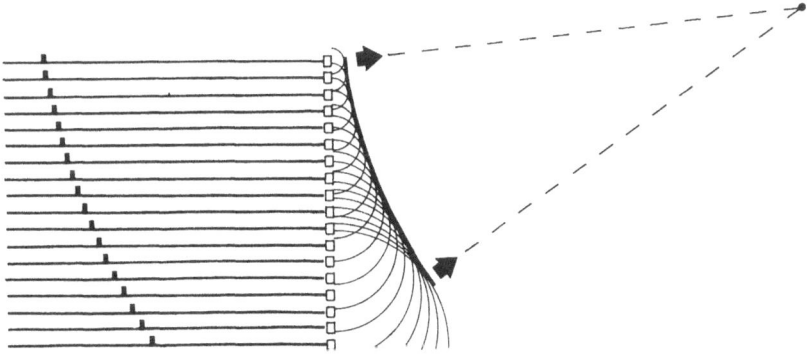

Figure 5. Pulsing sequence to provide azimuthal focussing.

14

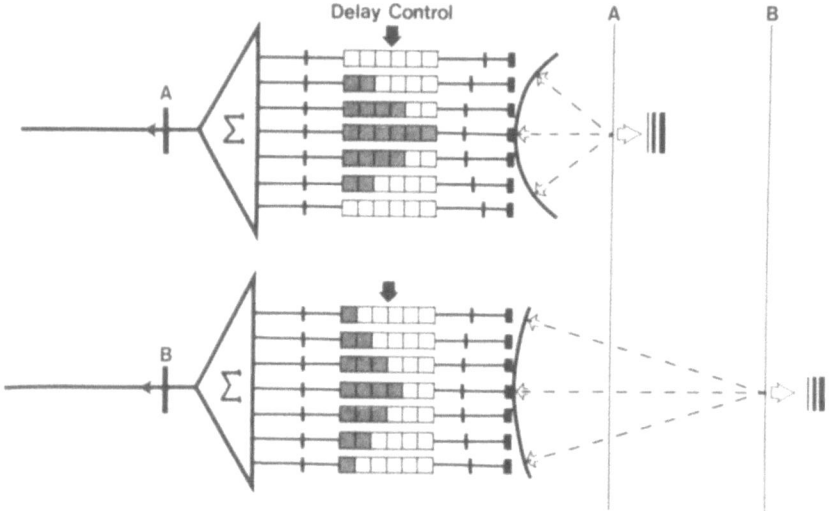

Figure 6. Principle of dynamic focussing.

Dynamic focussing

Another technique which can be used with electronically steered scanners is called 'dynamic focussing'. Referring to Figure 6, if a pulse is transmitted across two
interfaces, A and B, the first echo to return comes from A. Its wavefront is curved, so it reaches the central transducer elements before those at the edges of the
array. The electronic delay circuits are adjusted to compensate for this, and then
the signals are added together. A few microseconds later, echoes from B arrive.
The wavefront is less curved, so the delay pattern is altered. The receiver thus
changes its focal distance as echoes from more distant structures arrive, rather as
a pair of binoculars can be adjusted to keep an aeroplane in focus as it flies past.
This technique not only extends the axial range over which adequate focussing is
available but, because it acts to reject off-axis echoes, it has the effect of reducing
the number of echoes detected from objects illuminated by the side-lobes.
However, like electronic beam focussing, it acts only in the azimuthal plane and
does not improve elevation resolution.

COMPARISON OF MECHANICAL AND ELECTRONIC SCANNERS

A good deal or rivalry exists between the manufacturers of mechanically and
electronically steered scanners. Such competition is generally healthy, and will
ensure continuing product improvements which can only benefit the users and
thence the patients. However, the increasingly sophisticated technology is dif-

ficult to understand, and it is becoming hard even for a specialist to judge equipment performance critically. Thus, it is not surprising that some salesmen are making unjustified claims for the superiority of one technique over the other which are allowed to go un-challenged.

We must beware of emotional attraction to a particular technology. From the user's point of view, it is strictly irrelevant precisely how a machine functions and we should be concerned only with the end results: performance, reliability, cost and so on.

What, then are the relative merits of the two types of system? In the majority of respects, comparable technical features can be provided on both types of scanner. Thus, for example, video-tape recorders with automatic search, fast review, etc. can be fitted to any machine. The scan converter can have equally good performance, with facilities such as direct measurement and gamma control. There is also now little to chose between them in terms of size and portability.

The electronically steered transducer has no moving parts, hence should be more reliable. It is also somewhat smaller and a lot lighter than the mechanical scanner, which must house a motor. However, in some cases this advantage is negated by the cable, which has to house many individual wires, being stiff and heavy. Some mechanical scanners are an awkward shape, making it difficult to manoeuvre them into desired examination locations (e.g. suprasternal).

The superiority of the electronically steered system for obtaining a simultaneous M-mode has already been discussed; how important this is in practice will vary from user to user.

It is, however, the differences in beam characteristics of the two systems that are hardest to appreciate. For the mechanical scanner, the beam profile is straightforward: the transducer crystal is usually circular, about 12 mm in diameter, and has an acoustic focussing lens. This gives a minimum main beam diameter of $3 - 5$ mm, about $5 - 8$ cm from the transducer. Because the beam is circular, azimuthal and elevation resolution are the same. When the beam is deflected, its characteristics do not alter. The zone of optimal resolution is therefore as indicated diagrammatically in Figure 7(a).

Because its transducer area is larger, the electronically steered beam should have a slightly wider near field beam, but smaller side-lobes and less far field divergence. However, not all of the transducer area is 'active', since there must be small gaps between the crystal elements. These gaps, and the finite size of the elements, also mean that the concept of building up a beam from a large number of small wavelets cannot be realised perfectly. Undesirable interactions of the waves from the elements give rise to 'grating lobes', and in the proximal portion of the near field the beam has many discontinuities which degrade the image, an important consideration when examining neonates. Any imperfections in the crystals, or any deviations from a perfect pulsing sequence, also serve to degrade beam quality. Further degradation occurs when the beam is deflected through large angles. In part this is due to reduction in the effective transducer area (since

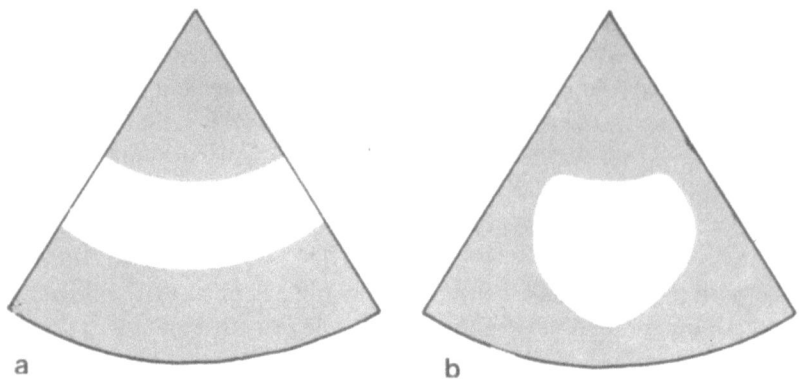

Figure 7. Optimal performance zones of (a) mechanically and (b) electronically steered systems.

it does not move, its area projected in the beam direction is reduced by the cosine of the deflection angle). Deflection also tends to unbalance the side-lobes, leaving a stronger component on the side of the beam nearest the mechanical axis of the transducer. As a result, it is generally the case that side-lobe intensity is greater with electronically steered beam systems.

To a significant extent, this disadvantage is overcome by dynamic focussing, which extends the depth of the focussing zone and even though off-axis echoes are generated by the side lobes, these are supressed. Like electronic transmit focussing, however, dynamic focussing improves the beam characteristics only in the azimuthal plane. The result is to give an optimal performance region as indicated in Figure 7(b).

It will be seen from the above considerations that mechanical beam steering is simpler, giving acceptable beam characteristics more easily, and at lower cost. The important feature that it lacks is dynamic focussing, since this can be achieved only with a multi-crystal array. We may perhaps see hybrid systems developed, which combine the advantages of mechanical beam steering with a multi-element crystal, possibly in the form of an anular array, together with an acoustic lens, for focussing.

2. COMPREHENSIVE M-MODE AND TWO-DIMENSIONAL ECHOCARDIOGRAPHIC EXAMINATION: ANATOMY, TECHNIQUE, IMAGE ORIENTATION AND SPECIFIC CLINICAL APPLICATIONS

J. ROELANDT

INTRODUCTION

Correct interpretation of echocardiograms requires technically adequate recordings and this undoubtedly represents the single most difficult aspect of echocardiography. An integrated knowledge of cardiac anatomy, pathology, normal and abnormal structure function as well as an understanding of the physical and instrumentation aspects of the ultrasound method are mandatory to perform a diagnostic examination [1, 2].

M-mode echocardiography provides a one-dimensional graphics of the heart, but an excellent resolution of structure motion because of its high sampling rate (1.000 transmit-receive cycles/sec). The disadvantage of M-mode echocardiography is the absence of spatial geometry. This lack of a spatial reference makes most information potentially available from many cardiac cross-sections meaningless. Consequently, clinical useful information is only obtained from a few cardiac cross-sections with readily recognizable structures and landmarks (mainly the long axis cross-section of the heart). In contrast, two-dimensional echocardiographic images provide more familiar images of the heart comparable to angiography and contain spatial information. A multitude of tomographic planes of the heart can be obtained from several chest wall transducer positions providing a wealth of diagnostic information. As a consequence the number of nondiagnostic examinations is significantly lower than with M-mode echocardiography. Temporal resolution (typically 50 frames/sec), however, is not as good as that available from M-mode recordings. The relative advantages of M-mode and two-dimensional echocardiography are presented in Table 1.

It is obvious that the combination of M-mode and two-dimensional methods is best for analysis of puzzling cardiac conditions and best serving the patient by virtue of its comprehensive approach. Most phased array sector scanning instruments presently available can simultaneously display the two-dimensional image while repeatedly sampling any selected area of the image for M-mode recording (Figure 1).

Roelandt, J. (ed.) The practice of M-mode and two-dimensional echocardiography
© *1983, Martinus Nijhoff Publishers. The Hague / Boston / London*
ISBN 978-94-009-6792-2.

18

Table 1. Relative advantages of echocardiographic examination techniques

M-mode Echocardiography
- Excellent time resolution
- Accurate dimensional measurements
- Timing of events against other parameters
- Easy storage and retrieval

Two-dimensional Echocardiography
- Anatomical relationships
- Shape information
- Lateral vectors of motion
- Easier to understand

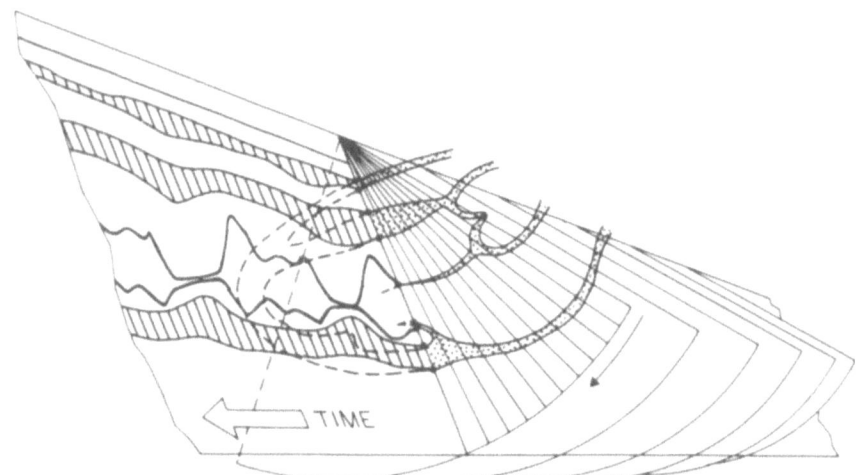

Figure 1. Diagram illustrating the relationship between the two dimensional and the M-mode echocardiogram. The motion pattern of the small part of the mitral valve hit by the sound beam is accurately tracted (1000 transmit- receive cycles/sec). However, no information on its anatomical relationships is obtained. This is available from the two-dimensional images.

TWO-DIMENSIONAL ECHOCARDIOGRAPHIC EXAMINATION

Real-time sector scanning devices have proven most useful for cardiac imaging [3 – 5]. Because of their small transducer size, problems of transduce-to-skin contact and rib shadows are minimal. They allow optimal use of the limited number of small echocardiographic windows to the heart and interrogation of most areas of the heart because of their high maneuverability [1]. Most recent instruments have a wide-angle up to 90°-field of view. Comparative advantages and limitations of each instrument are continually changing and their sophistication is increasing which makes differences between them less pronounced [6].

Recently, the American Society of Echocardiography (ASE) has published

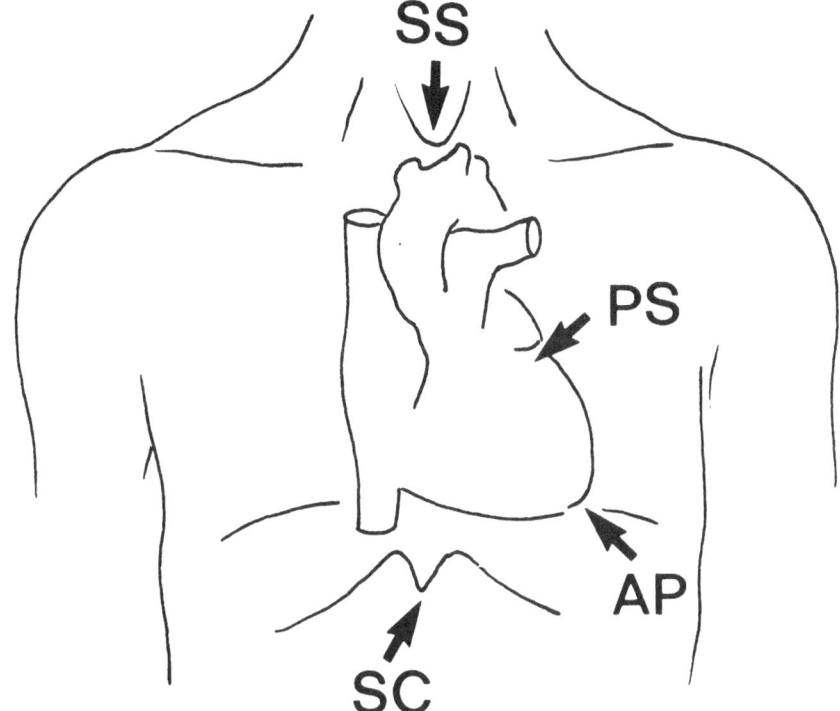

Figure 2. Schematic diagram demonstrating the four standard transducer positions on the chest wall. AP: apical; PS: parasternal; SC: subcostal; (subxiphoidal); SS: suprasternal.

recommendations for nomenclature and image orientation standards [7]. These standards will obviously make studies from different laboratories comparable and literature more understandable for the novice echocardiographer.

TRANSDUCER POSITIONS

There are four transducer positions from which the heart can be imaged using two-dimensional echocardiography (Figures 2 and 3).

In the *parasternal position*, the transducer is placed along the left sternal border in the third, fourth or exceptionally the fifth intercostal space over the anterior precordium. In the *apical position*, the transducer is placed on the lower left side of the chest over the palpable apical impulse. It is important to realize that this is not the anatomical apex of the heart. When the transducer is placed below the xiphoid process or along the lower left costal margin near the midline, it is in the *subcostal location* (also called the subxiphoid position). The fourth standard transducer location is the *suprasternal position*, with the transducer located in the suprasternal notch and directed inferiorly.

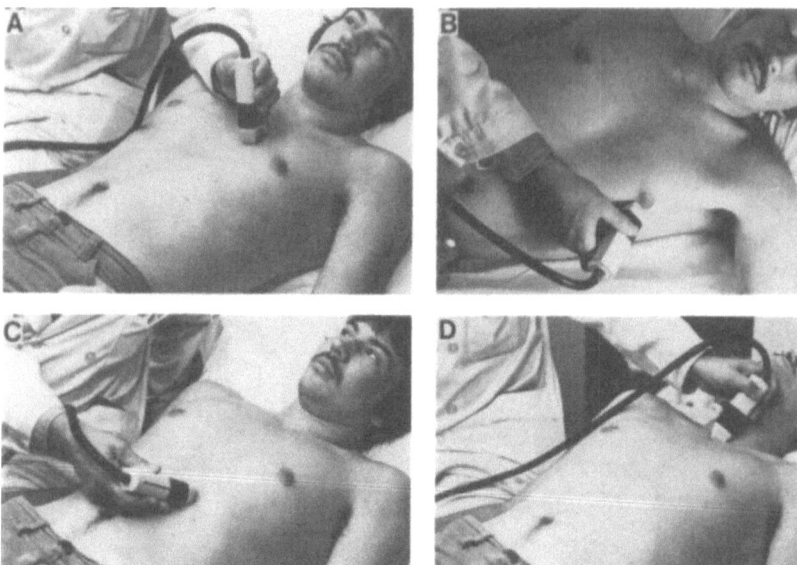

Figure 3. Technique of two-dimensional echocardiographic examination using the four standard transducer positions shown in Figure 2. A: parasternal transducer position. The transducer is along the left sternal border in the third or fourth intercostal space. B: Apical transducer position. The patient is in the left lateral decubitus position and the transducer is placed over the palpable apical impulse. C: Subcostal (subxiphoidal) transducer position. The patient is supine and the knees flexed to allow relaxation of the upper abdominal muscles. D: Suprasternal notch transducer position. The patient is supine with hyperextension of the neck.

BASIC PLANES OF IMAGING

The heart should be considered as a three-dimensional object within the thorax through which we can draw lines (axes) along which planes (cross-sections) can be obtained. An axis of the heart is a straight line about which the left ventricle may be supposed to rotate and two axes can thus be defined: (1) a *long axis* formed by the line from the base to apex, and (2) a *short axis* formed by a line at right angles to the long axis. Using this framework, three families of orthogonal planes may be defined to describe all tomographic views of the heart (Figure 4).

The *long-axis plane* is parallel to the left ventricular long axis. It is perpendicular to the anterior and inferior surfaces and parallel to the right and left lateral surfaces of the heart. Long axis views are obtained from the parasternal and apical transducer positions.

The plane perpendicular to the long axis and parallel to the short axis of the heart is referred to as the *short axis plane*. Short axis views are obtained from the parasternal and subcostal transducer positions.

The third orthogonal plane transects the heart parallel to its anterior and in-

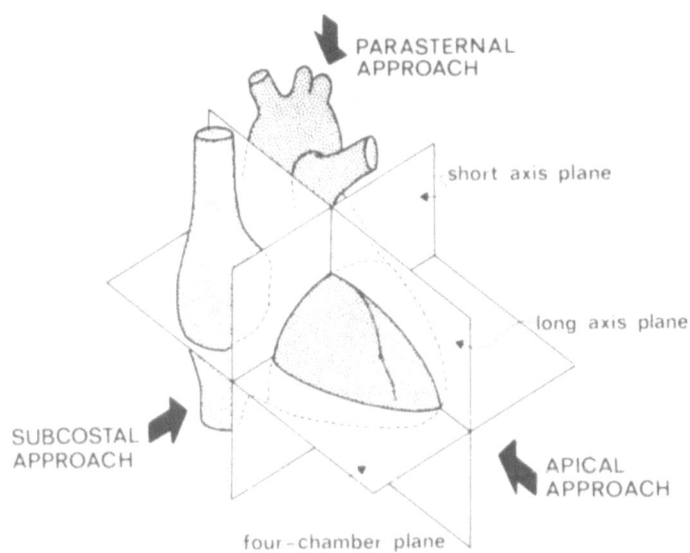

PARASTERNAL
APPROACH

short axis plane

long axis plane

SUBCOSTAL
APPROACH

APICAL
APPROACH

four-chamber plane

Figure 4. Diagram of the three orthogonal planes used to visualize the heart with two-dimensional echocardiography. The three best and most commonly echocardiographic approaches (transducer positions) to the heart correspond approximately to the points where the three standard planes intersect. From each of these, two standard planes can be examined.

ferior surfaces along its long axis and is called the *four-chamber plane* because all four cardiac chambers are included. Four chamber planes are obtained from the apical and subcostal transducer positions. Thus, from each of the three basic transducer locations, two orthogonal planes can be imaged by rotating the transducer approximately 90°. Similarly a long axis and short axis plane of imaging of the left aortic arch can be obtained from the suprasternal notch transducer position. Note that each of these planes should not be considered as a single plane but rather as a family of planes, so that from a given transducer position several cardiac planes can be imaged: e.g. tilting the transducer when interrogating the parasternal short axis view allows to image left ventricular cross-sections at the apical, papillary muscle, mitral valve and the level of the great arteries.

We shall now describe the technique of routine two-dimensional echocardiographic examination and discuss the anatomy and diagnostic utility of each of these standard cardiac views in more detail.

PARASTERNAL TRANSDUCER POSITION

The examination begins by placing the transducer in the left parasternal location, with the patient in a slight left lateral decubitus position, the head and thorax

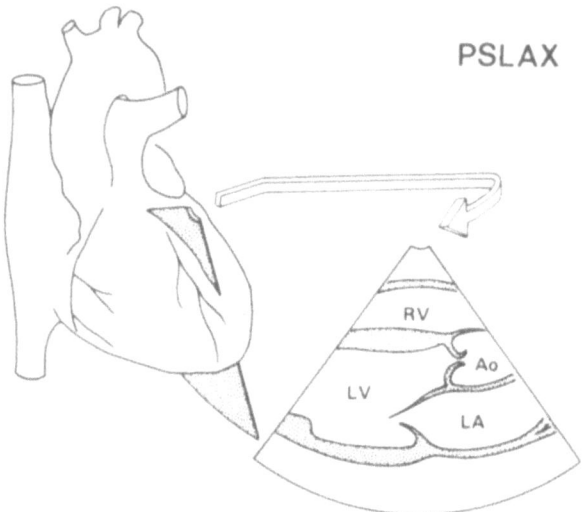

Figure 5. Diagram of plane of imaging of the parasternal long axis view (PSLAX) and orientation of the image displayed. Ao: aorta; LA: left atrium; LV: left ventricle; RV: right ventricle.

slightly elevated (Figure 3A). Recordability of parasternal views is highly influenced by body build and age. From this position, a sector image of the heart along its long and short axes can be obtained.

Long axis view (PSLAX) (Figures 5 and 6)

The standard long axis view of the left ventricle is obtained in a plane extending from the right shoulder towards the cardiac apex. The transducer is located parasternally in the second to fifth intercostal space depending on body build. This is an important diagnostic view, and represents the scan plane through which the single sound beam is swept in M-mode echocardiography. The first cardiac structure seen beneath the chest wall is the right ventricular (RV) free wall. The right ventricular outflow tract (RVOT) occupies the superior portion of the RV and is anterior to the aortic root. It must be realized that the right ventricular outflow tract curves obliquely around the cylindrical left ventricular (LV) and aorta (Ao). The anterior wall of the aorta is in anatomic continuity with the interventricular septum (IVS) (aortic-septal continuity).

The upper part of the IVS visualized in this view is the outflow septum which separates the outflow tracts of both ventricles. The posterior wall of the aorta is in anatomic continuity with the anterior mitral valve leaflet (aML) (aortic-mitral continuity), which divides the basilar portion of the left ventricular (LV) in an anterior outflow tract and a posterior inflow tract.

The left ventricular outflow is thus bounded by the IVS anteriority and the

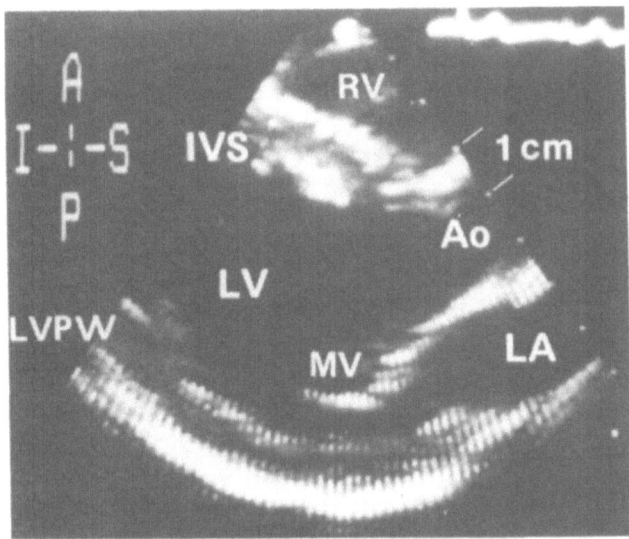

Figure 6. Parasternal long-axis view of the left ventricle of a normal subject. Aorta (Ao) is to the right and the apex of the left ventricle (LV) to the left of the image. The right ventricle (RV) is anterior and the left atrium posterior to the aorta. IVS: interventricular septum; MV: mitral valve; LVPW: left ventricular posterior wall; A: anterior; P: posterior; I: inferior; S: superior.

aML posteriorly and is normally widely patent during systole. Behind the inflow tract is the posterior mitral valve leaflet (pML). The mitral leaflets are connected by the chordae tendinae to the papillary muscles of the left ventricle.

The left atrium (LA) lies behind the posterior wall of the aorta. The left atrial and left ventricular posterior walls (LVPW) are in anatomic continuity. Immediately posterior to the lower part of the left atrium, the descending aorta can sometimes be seen. The coronary sinus, appearing as a small, circular echo-free structure, can usually be recorded in the region of the posterior atrioventricular groove. By convention, the PSLAX is displayed on the output screen as though the observer were viewing from the left side of the patient lying on his back.

In adults, the cardiac apex is not seen in this view, even with a 90° degree sector image. The PSLAX view allows a good examination of the aortic root, the aortic valve cusps, the mitral valve leaflets with their chordal and papillary muscle attachments and most of the left ventricular cavity.

The PSLAX is particularly useful in the following clinical situations.
- aortic valve disease: mobility, thickening, and calcification of valve cusps, vegegations [8, 9].
- aortic root disease: enlargement, dissection [10], sinus of Valsalva aneurysm [11].
- left ventricular outflow disease: fixed subaortic [12, 13] or valvular aortic stenosis [14], hypertrophic obstructive cardiomyopathy [15 – 17].

24

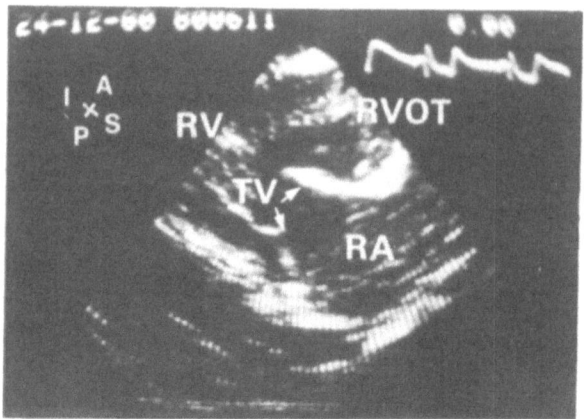

Figure 7. Parasternal long-axis view of the right ventricle. The right ventricle (RV), right ventricular inflow tract and right atrium (RA) are visualized. The tricuspid valve (TV) is well seen in this view. RVOT: right ventricular outflow tract. A: anterior; I: inferior; P: posterior; S: superior.

- ventricular septal and posterior wall thickness and motion abnormalities.
- evaluation of LV chamber dimensions.
- aortic-septal discontinuity: tetralogy of Fallot [18], truncus arteriosus [19].
- mitral-aortic fibrous discontinuity: double outlet right ventricle [20].
- mitral valve: rheumatic mitral valve disease [21], mitral valve prolapse [22, 23], flail mitral leaflet [24], vegetations [8, 9], calcified mitral annulus [25].
- left atrium: dilatation, intra-atrial thrombus, myxoma [26], and cor triatriatum.
- enlargement of the coronary sinus [27, 28].

The PSLAX view is not useful for the estimation of ventricular volumes, because of the difficulty in recording the cardiac apex. Large amplitude apical motion suggests an oblique imaging plane with foreshortening of the apex.

From the parasternal transducer position, the imaging plane can be angulated more medially and caudally with slight clockwise rotation to image the long axis view of the right ventricle and right atrium. The tricuspid valve and right ventricular inflow are usually well demonstrated in this view (Figure 7).

Short axis views (PSSAX)

Short axis views of the left ventricle can be obtained from the parasternal and subcostal transducer positions. With the transducer placed in the parasternal position, the PSSAX views are obtained by rotating it clockwise, approximately 90° so that the plane of scanning is almost perpendicular to the plane of the PSLAX (Figure 8).

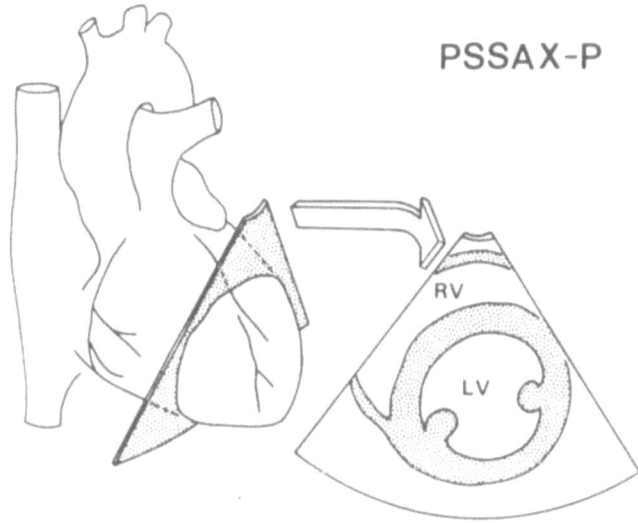

PSSAX-P

Figure 8. Diagram of plane of imaging of the parasternal short-axis view at papillary muscle level (PSSAX-P) and orientation of the image displayed. LV: left ventricle; RV: right ventricle.

PSSAX-VIEWS

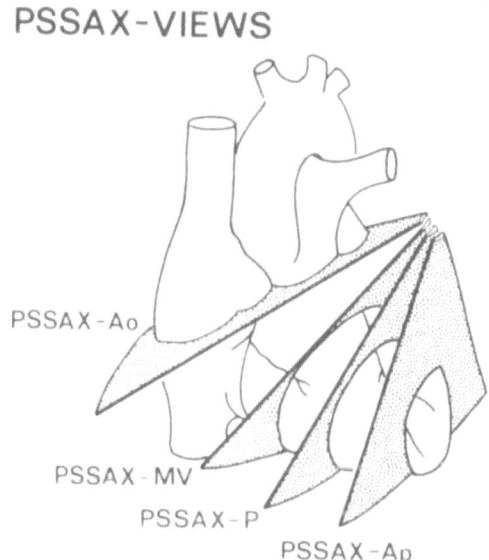

Figure 9. Parasternal short axis (PSSAX) views. A family of multiple short axis views results from sweeping the imaging plane from the base (Ao: aortic level) through the mitral valve (MV) and papillary muscle level (P), to the apical level (Ap).

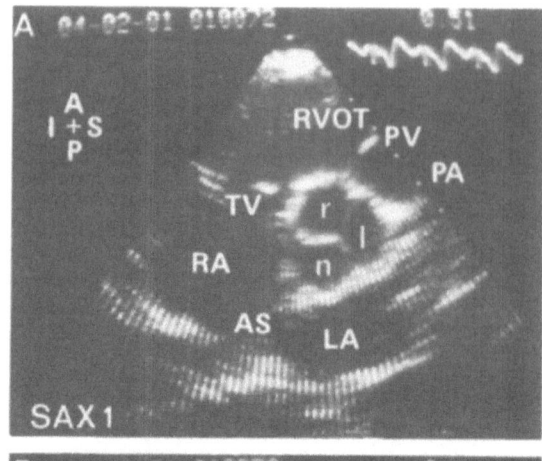

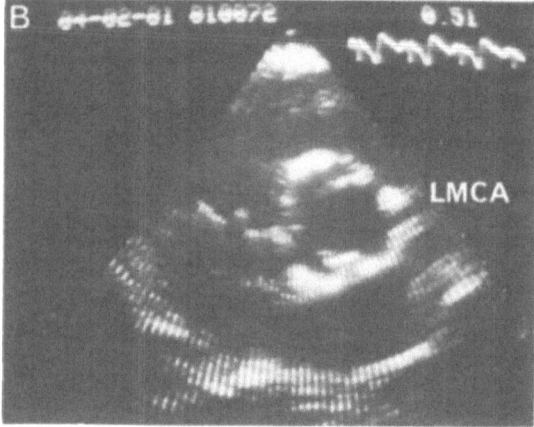

Figure 10. Stop-frame images in diastole (A) and systole (B) of the short axis view at the level of the great arteries. The aorta appears as a circular structure and the cusps are in a closed position (1: left; n: noncoronary; r: right cusp). Left atrial (LA) cavity is posterior to the aorta. Right atrium (RA) and tricuspid valve (TV) are to the left and the right ventricular outflow tract (RVOT) curves around the aorta anteriorly. The pulmonary valve (PV) and pulmonary artery (PA) are to the right. The interatrial septum (AS) is visualized. During systole, the aortic valve cusps are in an open position and the left mean coronary artery (LMCA) is well recorded. A: anterior; L: left; P: posterior; R: right.

The interrogation plane can be swept from the base of the heart to the apex to allow examination at the levels of (1) the great arteries, (2) the mitral valve office, (3) the papillary muscles, and (4) the apex (Figure 9). It is oten necessary to use two different transducer locations: a cephalad one to visualize the two first levels and a more caudal one for the two others [29]. The subcostal transducer positions often give little or no image in normal subjects and in those in whom the diaphragm is rather high in the thorax. In patients with emphysema and low diaphragms in whom the parasternal position usually gives poor results, the subcostal transducer location may yield superior short axis views at the four levels

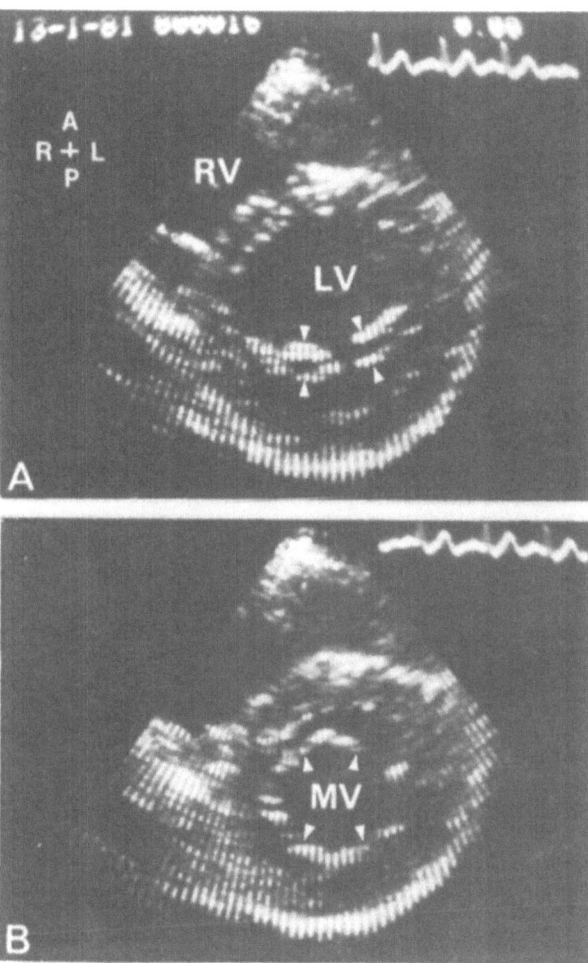

Figure 11. Parasternal short axis view at mitral valve level (PSSAX-MV). The closed mitral valve (MV) is seen in panel A and has a fish-mouth appearance when open in diastole (panel B). The right ventricle (RV) is anterior and to the left, the left ventricle (LV) appears circular and is located posteriorly. A: anterior; L: left; R: right; P: posterior.

discussed. By "scanning" the interrogating plane from base to apex, the examiner can integrate the different short axis views to obtain a three-dimensional impression of cardiac anatomy. It should be realized that short axis views of the heart are unique to two-dimensional echocardiography and are impossible to obtain with other techniques including angiography.

The images are displayed as if being viewed from the apex of the heart up towards the base. The LV is posterior and to the right and the RV anterior and to the left. The short axis image at the level of the great arteries displays the circular aortic root in the center. During diastole the three aortic leaflets appear as a letter "Y" (Figure 10). The left atrium is posterior to the aorta. The interatrial septum

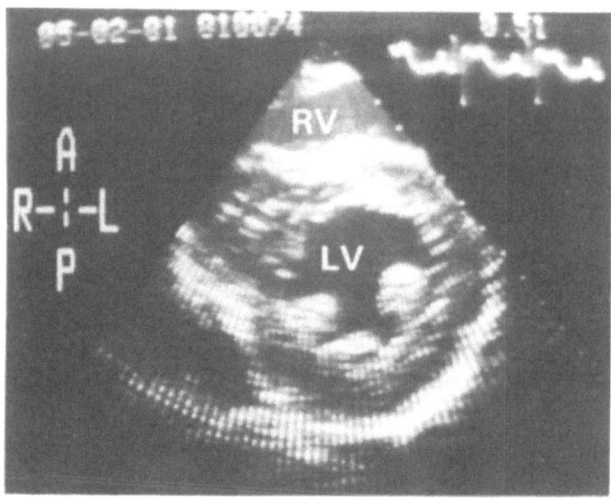

Figure 12. Parasternal short axis view of the left ventricle at papillary muscle level (PSSAX-P). The anterolateral papillary muscle projects into the left ventricular (LV) cavity at 3 and the postero-medial papillary muscle at 8 o'clock positions. The LV appears circular. RV: right ventricle; A: anterior; L: Left; P: posterior; R: right.

is seen at about 7 o'clock to the aorta and the anterior tricuspid valve leaflet is recorded at 10 o'clock to the aorta. The left atrium is posterior to the aorta and minor transducer adjustments will allow visualization of the left atrial appendage to the right on the image. The right ventricular outflow tract curves anteriorly around the aorta and the pulmonary valve is often seen about 2 o'clock. Fine changes in the plane of this view often allow visualization of the left main coronary artery in its long axis at 3 o'clock with its lumen in continuity with that of the aorta [30]. With superior tilt of the scanning plane beyond the pulmonary valve, the main pulmonary artery and its bifurcation into the right and left pulmonary arteries can be identified.

Inferior tilting of the scanning plane allows a short axis cut of the left ventricular outflow tract in the center of the image, bounded anteriorly by the upper part of the interventricular septum and posteriorly by the anterior mitral valve leaflet. Behind the latter lies at this level the left atrium. On the left of the image are, from posterior to anterior, the right atrium, the anterior tricuspid leaflet and the right ventricular outflow tract (Figure 8). In a lower section, the mitral valve is recorded with its characteristic diastolic "fishmouth" pattern. Normally the left ventricle is nearly circular and is seen in a basal cross-section at this level (Figure 11).

Further inferior and lateral angulation allows visualization of the more apical portions of the left ventricle at the level of the anterolateral and posteromedial papillary muscles. They most commonly project in the left ventricular cavity at 3 and 8 o'clock respectively (Figure 12) [31].

If the scanning plane is further tilted inferiorly and laterally, it will transect the left ventricle near its apex. The normal left ventricular cavity becomes progressively smaller at this level. Care must be taken during recording of all these short axis images to angle the transducer in a plane nearly perpendicular to the major axis. Normally, correct angulation of the sector beam results in a circular appearance of the left ventricular cavity, with symmetric opening and closing motion of the medial and lateral portions of the mitral valve. If the short axis image plane is not perpendicular to the long axis, the left ventricular cavity will appear oval in shape and one side of the mitral valve will have a larger amplitude of motion than the other.

Higher amplitude of the mitral valve leaflets medially suggests "underrotation" and higher amplitude laterally suggests "overrotation" with respect to the clockwise transducer rotation needed to obtain the correct PSSAX view from the parasternal transducer position.

The PSSAX views are useful in the following situations:

1. Aortic valve level:
   - anatomic relation of the great arteries [19, 32]
   - diagnosis of bicuspid aortic valve [31, 33]
   - thickening, calcification, and vegetations of the aortic valve [8, 9]
   - left atrial masses [26]
   - right-to-left shunts with contrast studies [34, 35]
   - visualization of orifice and main stem of left coronary artery and orifice of the right coronary artery [30]
2. Mitral valve and papillary muscle levels:
   - evaluation of regional wall motion in coronary artery disease [36, 37]
   - quantification of mitral valve orifice area [38, 39]
   - infective vegetations on mitral valve [8, 9]
   - mitral annulus calcification [25]
   - rupture of chordae tendinae [40]
   - evaluation of the papillary muscles size, location, anatomic anomalies, fibrosis, calcification, and rupture [31]
   - determination of ventricular situs

APICAL TRANSDUCER POSITION

The transducer is placed directly upon or just medial to the palpable apical impulse with the patient turned in a left lateral decubitus position (Figures 2 and 38). Optimal images are usually recorded during held expiration.

Patients who lack a palpable cardiac impulse or who suffer from lung disease have poor quality images. On the other hand, there is a high success rate of good quality images in patients who have dilated hearts or apical aneurysms.

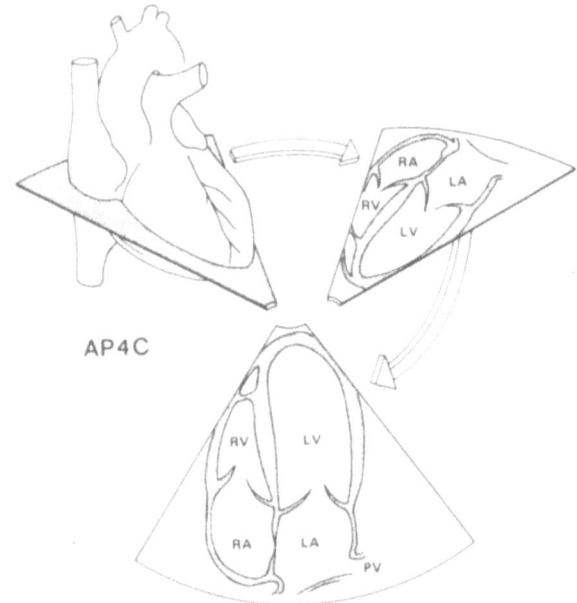

Figure 13. Diagram of plane of imaging of the apical four-chamber view (AP4C) and orientation of the image displayed. LA: left atrium; LV: left ventricle; PV: pulmonary veins; RA: right atrium; RV: right ventricle.

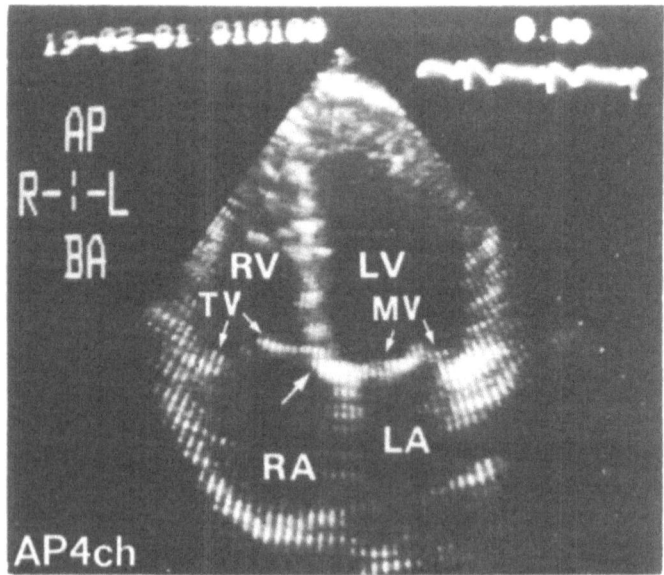

Figure 14. Stop-frame photo- graph of the apical four-chamber view (AP4ch) and obtained from a normal subject. Note lower insertion of septal leaflet of tricuspid valve on the interventricular septum as compared to anterior mitral valve leaflet. LA and RA: left and right atrium; LV and RV: left and right ventricle; MV and TV: mitral and tricuspid valve; AP: apical; BA: basal; R and L: right and left.

APICAL FOUR-CHAMBER VIEW

DISPLAY OPTIONS

OPTION 1   OPTION 2

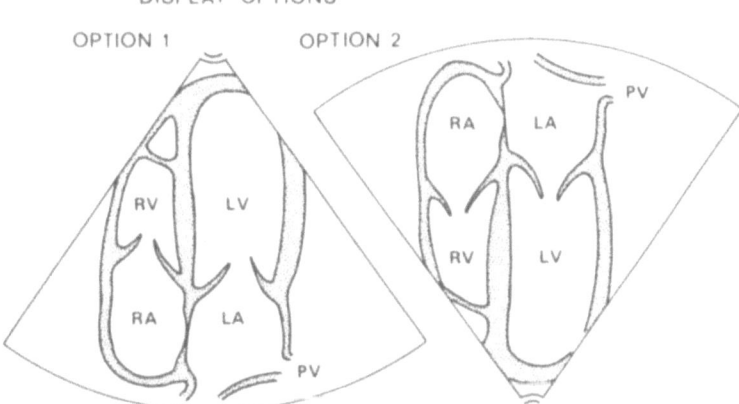

Figure 15. Diagram of apical four-chamber views and two display options. Option 2 is obtained by activation of an image inversion switch which results in the near signals of the display option 1 being inverted from the top of the bottom of the output screen.

Apical four-chamber view (AP4C)

The apical examination is begun with the scanning plane directed superiorly and medially toward the right scapula in an orthogonal plane parallel to the dorsal and ventral surfaces of heart. This plane transects and is perpendicular to the mitral and tricuspid valve orifices, and both the ventricular and atrial septa. It is called the four-chamber view, because it displays simultaneously the four chambers of the heart, and the interrelationships of the septa and both atrioventricular valves (crux cordis) (Figures 13 and 14). The transducer must be slightly tilted in order to maximize atrioventricular valve motion and ventricular area.

There has been considerable variation in orientation of this image on the output screen. The ASE has recommended two options for display. Most commonly, the apex is displayed at the top of the output screen and the atria at the bottom, while the right chambers are on the left and the left chambers on the right.

This option results in the heart being viewed from behind the patient. The other option can be obtained when an image inversion switch is available for up-down reversal: the apex is at the bottom of the display screen, the atria at the top, with the same left-right orientation (Figure 15).

The right ventricle can be identified from the presence of the moderator band. However, it is more easy to identify the two ventricular chambers by the observation of the atrioventricular valves [32]. The insertion of the tricuspid valve leaflet on the interventricular septum is 5 to 10 mm inferior (more apical) to the insertion of the anterior mitral leaflet (which is in the anatomic left ventricle). The in-

AP4C-VIEWS

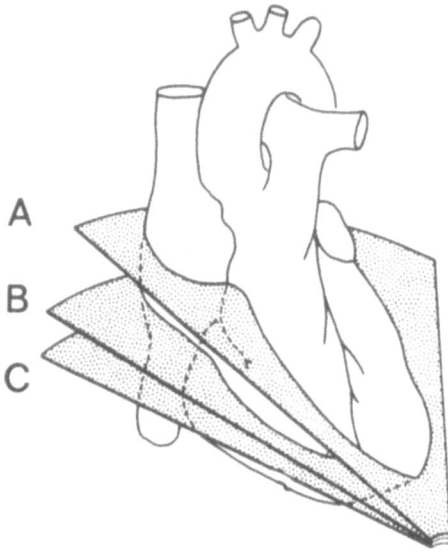

Figure 16. Diagram showing three planes of views which can be obtained with the transducer in the apical position. A: anterior tilting of the interrogating plane allows recording of the aorta, B: apical four-chamber plane, C: posterior tilting allows recording of the coronary sinus.

terventricular septum interposed between the two atrioventricular valves is the inflow septum and the remaining septum towards the apex is the trabecular septum.

From the same transducer position, the interrogating plane can be swept anteriorly to record the left ventricular outflow tract and the aortic valve and posteriorly with mild clockwise rotation to record the coronary sinus in its long axis with its ostium opening in the right atrium (Figure 16).

The AP4C view is useful for the evaluation of:

- complex congenital heart disease [41]: diagnosis of endocardial cushion defects [42], tricuspid atresia [43], Ebstein's anomaly [44]
- atrial and ventricular septal defects (with contrast studies) [34, 35]
- coronary heart disease: evaluation of regional wall motion abnormalities [37, 45, 46]
- diagnosis of ischemic aneurysm [47] and pseudoaneurysm [48, 49]
- demonstration of right and left-sided (atrial or ventricular) cardiac masses (tumors or thrombi), analysis of their movements [50 – 53]
- size of the cardiac chambers [54]
- calculation of left ventricular surface and long axis length for quantitation of volumes [55 – 60]
- evaluation of the coronary sinus

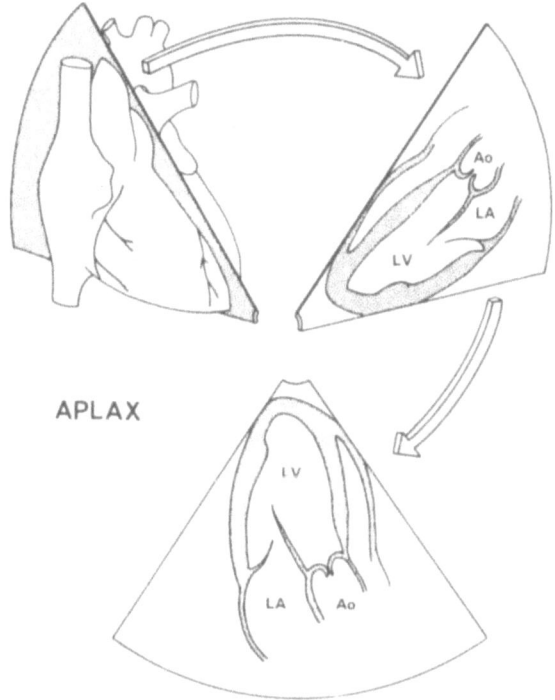

APLAX

Figure 17. Diagram of plane of imaging of the apical long axis view (APLAX) and orientation of the image on the output screen. Ao: aorta; LA: left atrium; LV: left ventricle.

— assessment of prosthetic valve function [61]
— connection of pulmonary veins to the left atrium [31]

Apical long axis view (APLAX)

When the transducer remains in the apical location and is rotated nearly 90° counter-clockwise, the scanning plane returns to a long axis plane (Figure 4). Two different views are described in the literature and confusion between these two must be avoided, because they do not represent the same perimeter of the left ventricle, but they are both perpendicular to the PSSAX:

a. the first one intersects the PSSAX view approximately at 11 and 5 o'clock. The examiner must try to define motion of aortic valves and anterior mitral leaflet. The right ventricle is seen as a small area, because the beam transets the interventricular septum in its anterior portion near the junction of the right ventricle, and the anterior LV free wall. The apex and segments of posterolateral wall of the LV are also recorded (Figures 17 and 18). This view is close to the left ventricular silhouette seen on the right anterior oblique (RAO) ventriculogram.

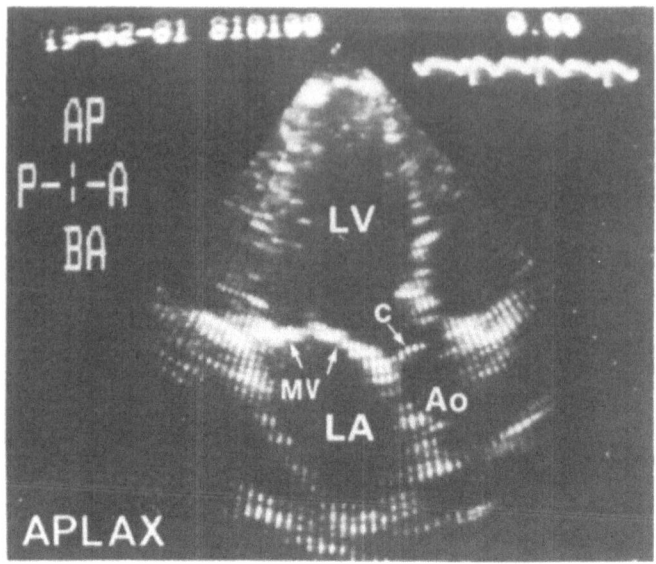

Figure 18. Stop-frame photograph of the apical long axis view (APLAX) obtained from a normal subject. Ao: aorta; C: aortic valve cusps; LA and LV: left atrium and ventricle; MV: mitral valve. AP: apical; A: anterior; BA: basal; P: posterior.

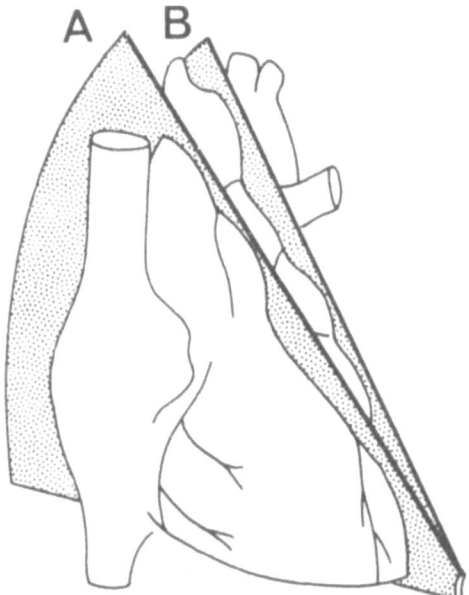

Figure 19. Diagram showing two planes of imaging from the apical transducer location. A: apical long axis view; B: apical two-chamber view.

This explains why some authors have called this view the "RAO equivalent" view. The ASE has termed this view the apical long axis view.

b. a variant of this APLAX view is obtained by rotating the transducer clockwise so that the plane intersects the short axis view at approximately 1 and 7 o'clock (Figure 19). The ultrasonic beam is then nearly parallel to the septum and includes neither the aorta not the right ventricle. Two chambers (the left atrium and left ventricle) and segments of the anterolateral apex and inferior walls are recorded. The ASE proposes that this view be called the apical two-chamber view.

The APLAX view is useful for the evaluation of:

– segmental wall motion abnormalities
– diagnosis of complications of myocardial infarction (ventricular aneurysm, pseudoaneurysm or thrombus)
– calculation of left ventricular volumes and ejection fraction (from our experience it is often difficult to record the apex in this view).

SUBCOSTAL TRANSDUCER POSITION

The transducer is positioned in the subxiphoid position in the midline or just to the right of the midline (Figures 2 and 3C). Subcostal images are best recorded with the patient supine, the head not elevated, and the knees flexed to allow relaxation of the abdominal musculature and sufficient pressure of the transducer into the abdominal wall. In normal adults, subcostal images are often of poor quality. The subcostal location provides the highest diagnostic yield in patients with lung disease and low diaphragms, because hyperinflation of the lungs usually effaces precordial and apical windows. Best images are obtained when the recording is performed during held inspiration.

From the subcostal transducer location, images can be recorded following a short-axis plane or a four-chamber plane (Figure 4).

Subcostal short axis views (SCSAX)

A family of short axis views can be recorded by sweeping the imaging plane from base to apex similar to those obtained from the parasternal transducer location (Figures 20 and 21) [29, 32, 62].

The transducer is tilted inferiorly and slightly to the right in order to obtain the inferior vena cava-right atrial junction and the drainage of the hepatic veins into the inferior vena cava (Figure 22).

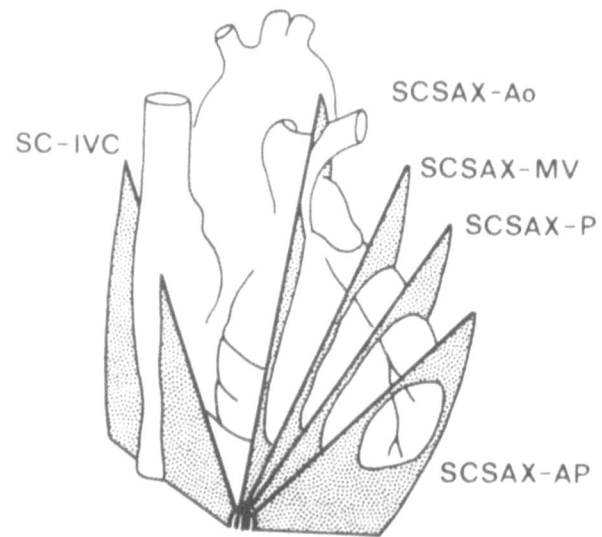

Figure 20. A family of multiple subcostal short axis (SCSAX) views results from sweeping the imaging plane from the base to the apex of the heart, analogous to those in the parasternal transducer position. For abbreviations see Figure 9. SC-IVC: subcostal view of the inferior vena cava.

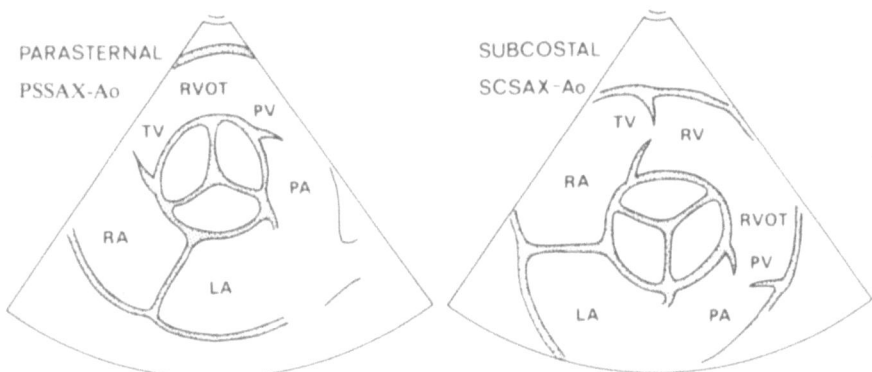

Figure 21. Diagram of the short-axis views that result when the transducer is used to visualize the parasternal short-axis view at aortic valve level (PSSAX-Ao) and the same view when the transducer is placed in the subcostal position (SCSAX-Ao). Note differences in image orientation on the display. LA: left atrium; PA: pulmonary artery; PV: pulmonary valve; RA: right atrium; RVOT: right ventricular outflow tract; TV: tricuspid valve.

Subcostal four-chamber view (SC4C)

If the image plane is rotated 90° clockwise from the SCSAX view, a foreshortened four-chamber view similar to the AP4C is obtained (Figures 4 and 23). The atrial septum is largely perpendicular to the ultrasound beams and is best evaluated in this view. In approximately 25% of patients, the hepatic parenchyma is interposed between the transducer and the right ventricle (Figure 24).

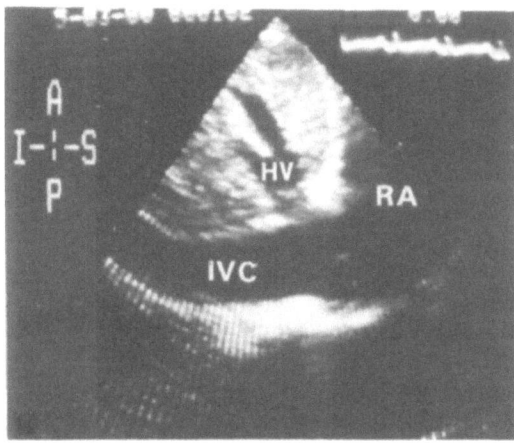

Figure 22. Stop-frame image through the base of the right atrium (RA) and inferior vena cava (IVC) following the plane indicated on Figure 20 – SC-IVC. HV: hepatic vein; A: anterior; I: inferior; P: posterior; S: superior.

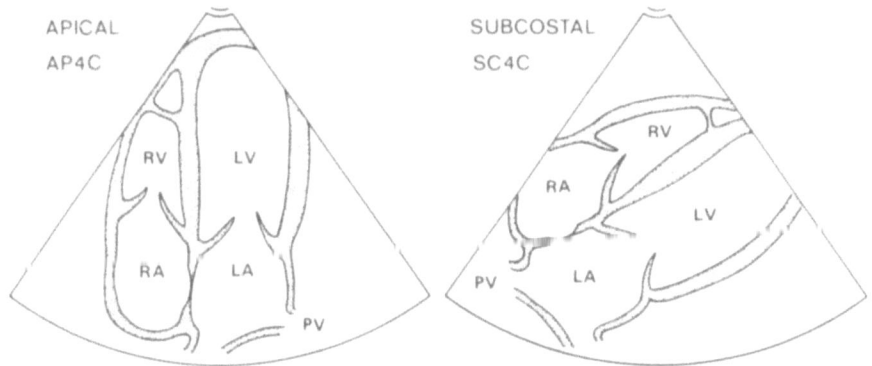

Figure 23. Diagram illustrating the differences in image orientation on the output screen of the four-chamber view when the transducer is in the apical location (AP4C) and in the subcostal location (SC4C). LA: left atrium; LV: left ventricle; PV: pulmonary veins; RA: right atrium; RV: right ventricle.

The ASE has recommended two display options for the SC4C view: a. with the sector apex above and the right ventricle at the top of the display, the apex of the left ventricle on the right and the two atria on the left, and b. with the sector apex below, the right ventricle is at the bottom of the display, the apex of the left ventricle is on the right, and the atria on the left [7].

In addition to the indications of the PSSAX and AP4C views, the subcostal views are most helpful for:

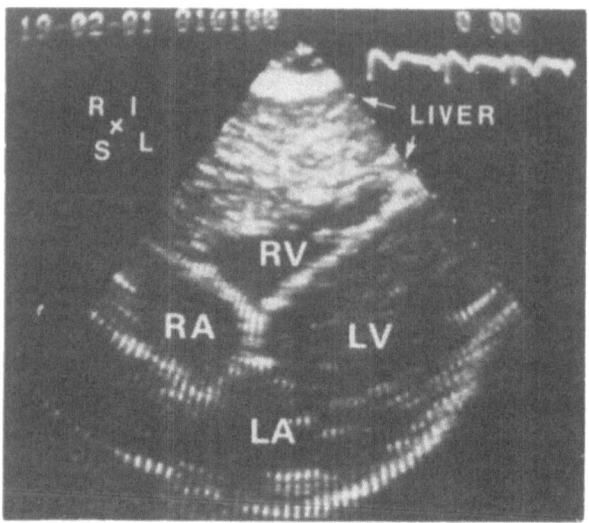

Figure 24. Subcostal four-chamber view (SC4C). Note interposed liver between transducer and the heart. LA: left atrium; LV: left ventricle; RA: right atrium; RV: right ventricle; I: inferior; L: left; R: right; S: superior.

- diagnosis of tricuspid regurgitation [63]
- diagnosis and localization of atrial and ventricular septal defects [64, 65]
- analysis of atrial septal motion.

SUPRASTERNAL TRANSDUCER POSITION

The fourth location from which clinically useful views can be recorded is the suprasternal notch (Figure 2) [66]. The examination is best performed with the patient supine and with hyperextension of the neck (Figure 3D).

Suprasternal long axis view (SSLAX)

For visualization of the aortic arch in long axis, the transducer is positioned with the scanning plane aligned with the aortic arch. This plane of imaging corresponds with the plane of aortic arch (Figure 25).

The ascending aorta, transverse aorta with the major arterial branches (innominate, left carotid and left subclavian artery origins), and descending aorta are visualized in long axis. The ascending aorta is on the left of the output screen and the descending aorta on the right. Posterior to the ascending aorta and inferior to aortic arch, the right pulmonary artery is seen in its short axis as a circular structure. The left atrium is recorded below the right pulmonary artery

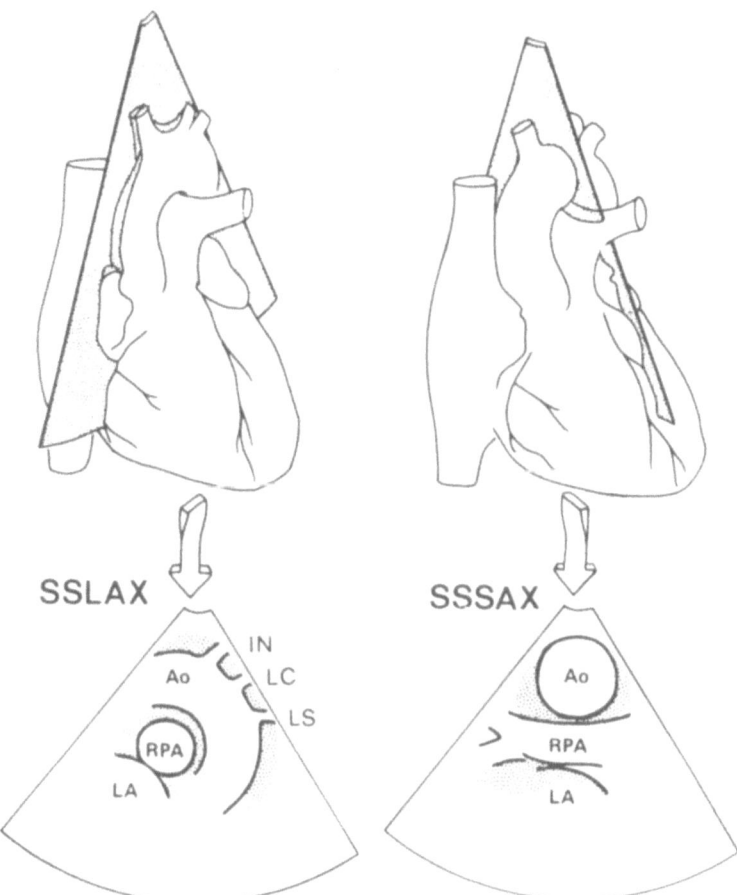

Figure 25. Diagram of planes of imaging with the transducer in the suprasternal transducer position. On the left, the long axis plane (SSLAX) is shown with the image displayed. The short-axis plane (SSSAX) and resulting image are shown on the right. Ao: aorta; IN: inominate artery; LA: left atrium; LC: left carotid artery; LS: left subclavian artery; RPA: right pulmonary artery.

(Figure 26A). Sometimes the inominate vein is recorded anterior to the aorta. Slight degrees of transducer rotation are necessary to inspect the different segments of the aorta, because the ascending and descending aorta are not in the same plane.

Suprasternal short axis view (SSSAX)

By rotating the transducer 90°, the ascending aorta is seen in its short axis as a circular, pulsating structure and the right pulmonary artery is imaged inferiorly in its long axis with the left atrial cavity inferior to it (Figure 25).

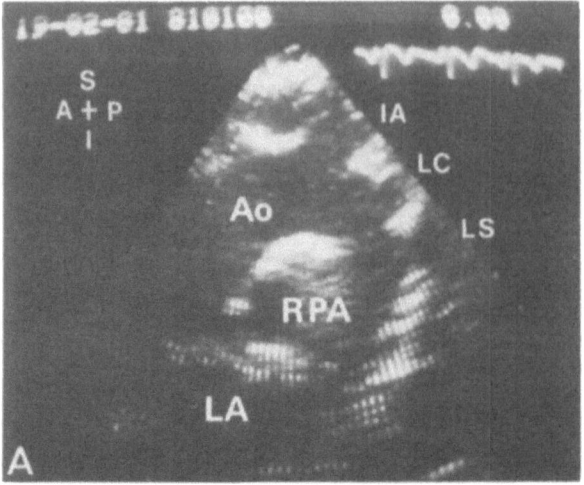

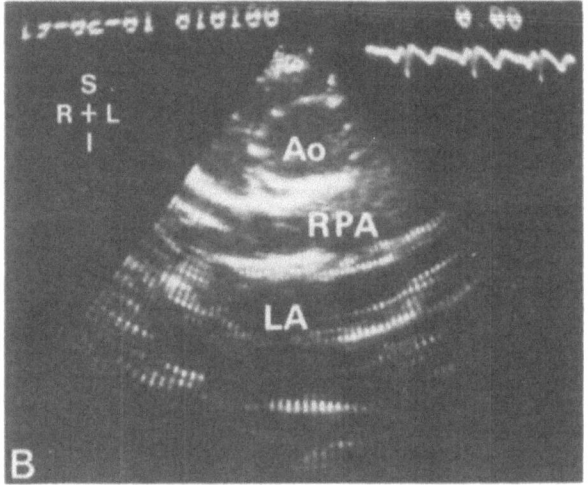

Figure 26. Suprasternal long axis (panel A) and short axis views (panel B) of a normal subject. For abbreviations see Figure 25. A: anterior; I: inferior; P: posterior; S: superior.

Occasionally, the first bifurcation of the right pulmonary artery can be visualized to the left (Figure 26B). The superior vena cava can be seen on the left of image in some patients.

Suprasternal views are useful for:

- detection of dilatation or dissection of the ascending aorta
- diagnosis of supravalvular aortic stenosis [67] and coarctation of the aorta [68].
- identification of the great vessels using peripheral contrast injections
- evaluation of the size of the pulmonary artery
- imaging of the ductus arteriosus [69]

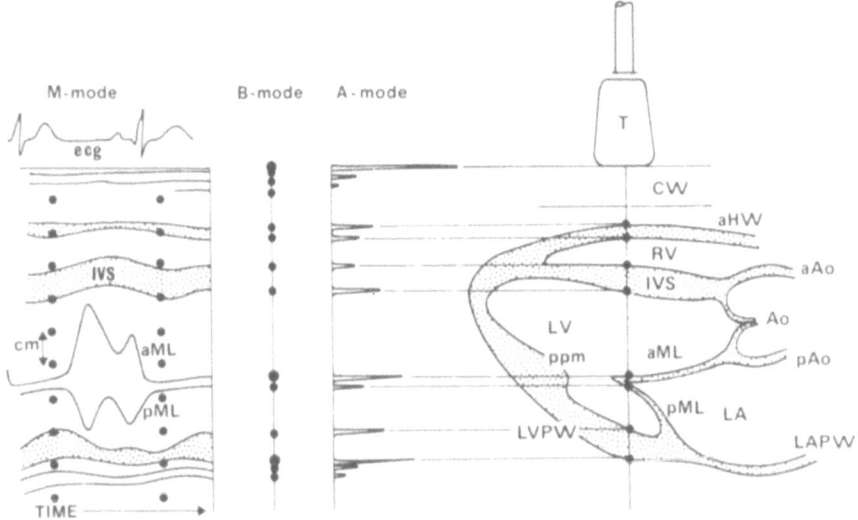

Figure 27. Schematic cross-section of the heart from the base towards the apex with cardiac structures included. The single element transducer (T) in front is aimed so that the sound beam traverses from anterior to posterior; the anterior heart wall (aHW), right ventricle (RV), interventricular septum (IVS), left ventricular cavity (LV), the tips of the mitral valve leaflets and the left ventricular posterior wal (LVPW). The echoes which originate from these boundaries are classically represented in three types of oscilloscope display and are referred to as the "A", "B" and "M-mode". Ao: aorta; c: valve cusps; aML and pML: anterior and posterior mitral valve leaflets; LA: left atrium; LAPW: left atrial posterior wall; aAoW and pAoW: anterior and posterior aortic walls; ppm: posteromedial papillary muscle.

M-MODE EXAMINATION TECHNIQUES

Ultrasonic examination of the heart with a single element can be made with the transducer located at the same four positions as for two-dimensional imaging but useful diagnostic information is mainly recorded from the parasternal location scanning the PSLAX. Figure 27 shows the transducer in its appropriate position on the chest wall to study the mitral valve.

The beam traverses from anterior to posterior: the anterior heart wall, the RV cavity, the IVS, the LV cavity, the free edges of both anterior and posterior mitral leaflets and the LV posterior wall. The echoes which originate from these structure boundaries are converted into dots of which the brightness indicates their relative intensities (Brightness or B-mode).

The M-mode is produced by adding the dimension of time to the B-mode. When recorded with a strip chart recorder, the change in range of any echo source is displayed as a function of time. A detailed analysis of the motion pattern of cardiac structures is thus obtained. By sweeping the sound beam through the PSLAX from the aorta to the apex, the interrelationship of cardiac structures

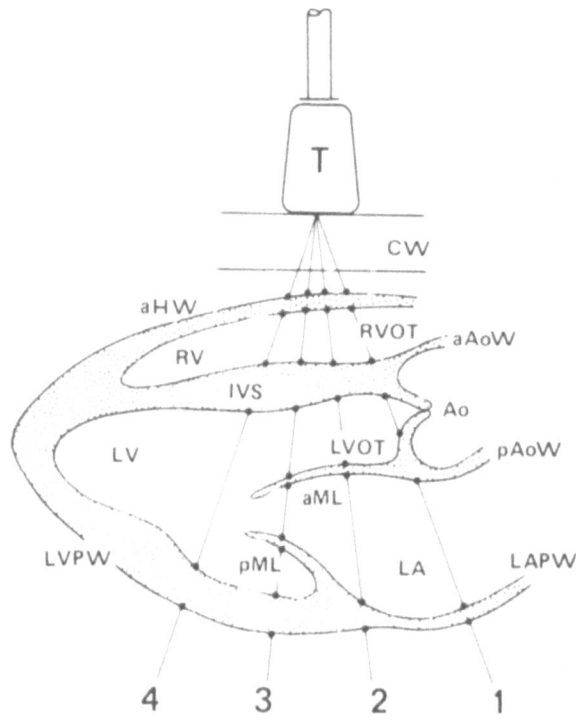

Figure 28. Schematic cross section of the heart. A sector scan or M-scan is performed when the transducer is swept from the aorta (direction 1) towards the apex (direction 4). For abbreviations see Figure 27).

and their anatomic continuity can be evaluated. This is called the M-mode scan of the heart [70, 71].

M-MODE SCAN OR M-SCAN

The examination is performed from the parasternal transducer position with the patient in the supine or a slight left lateral decubitus position with the head and thorax elevated approximately 30°.

Since the mitral valve is a central structure, it should be used as a landmark and all other cardiac structures should be related to it [71]. Therefore, the transducer is placed on the chest wall in the intercostal space where the motion amplitude of the anterior mitral leaflet is maximally recorded while the transducer is perpendicular to the chest wall and as close as possible to the left sternal border. From this "standard" position, the sound beam is scanned through the PSLAX from aorta to apex. Four anatomic areas with specific cardiac structures and motion patterns, corresponding to four sound beam directions can be distinguished.

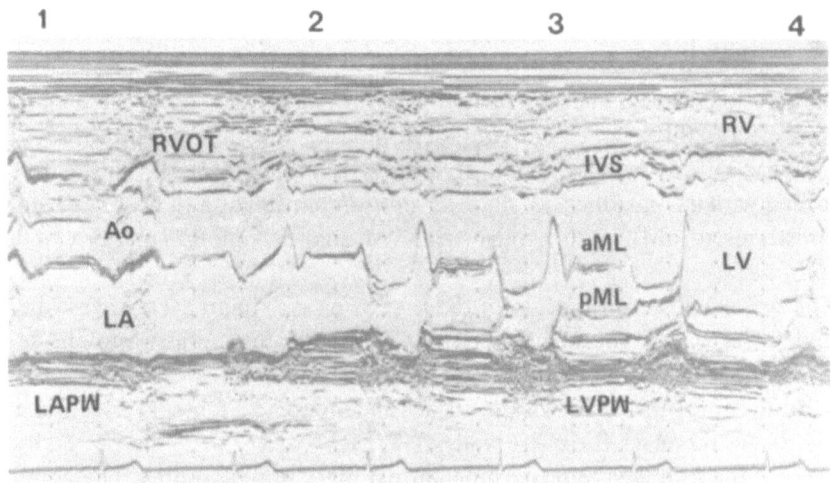

Figure 29. M-mode scan of the heart following the sagittal plane through the outflow tract or long axis of the left ventricle. The directions of the sound beam labelled 1 to 4 on the diagram of Figure 28 correspond to the areas labelled 1 to 4 on this record. For abbreviations see Figure 27.

Figures 28 and 29 show these basic sound beam directions and resulting M-mode patterns.

1. the first beam direction is obtained by superior and medial tilting of the transducer from the mitral valve position. The sound beam traverses successively the chest wall, aHW, RVOT, anterior aortic wall, the aortic valve cusps, posterior aortic wall, left atrial cavity and left atrial posterior wall. In systole, the aorta moves anteriorly and is recorded towards the transducer and a nearly parallel systolic anterior motion of the two aortic walls is recorded on the tracing. The aortic valve cusps are seen during diastole in their closed position in the middle of the aortic root; at the onset of left ventricular ejection, they open abrupty towards the aortic walls and close at the end of ejection. Both the anterior (right-coronary) and the non-coronary cusps can be recorded. The left coronary cusp is rarely seen. The left atrial posterior wall does not move at this level because it is attached to the mediastinum.

2. the second beam direction is obtained by tilting the transducer slightly laterally and inferiorly from the first direction (Figures 28 and 29, direction 2). At this level, the sound beam traverses the chest wall, aHW, RV cavity, IVS, LV cavity, aML, LA cavity and the LAPW. The scan from direction 1 to direction 2 demonstrates the anatomic continuity of aAoW with the IVS and of the pAoW with the aML. The motion pattern of the aML is characteristic. During systole, slight anterior motion of the aML is recorded due to the anterior displacement of the mitral valve apparatus. During diastole, it has a typical "M-shaped" motion pattern related to the diastolic hemodynamics. At this level, the LAPW

demonstrates motion concommitant with the "a" and "v" waves of the left atrial pressure tracing.

3. direction 3 is obtained by further inferior and lateral transducer angulation with respect to direction 2. The sound beam passes through the chest wall, aHW, RV cavity, IVS, LV cavity with aML and pML and the LVPW. The aML is still recorded with its diastolic "M-shaped" motion pattern and the pML is recognized posterior to aML with a reciprocal "W-shaped" motion pattern of lesser amplitude.

The systolic posterior motion of the LAPW as seen in area 2 changes when the sound beam passes the atrioventricular junction and merges into the typical systolic anterior motion of the LVPW.

4. In the fourth M-mode beam, direction (Figures 28 and 29, direction 4) the sound beam traverses the chest wall, aHW, RV cavity, IVS, the LV cavity and LVPW at the level of the posteromedial papillary muscle (ppm). The amplitude of the "M-shaped" motion pattern of aML decreases progressively as the sound beam passes from the free edge of the leaflet to the chordae tendinae which float over the endocardium of LVPW and merge with a thick posterior band of echoes representing the ppm.

In the area between beam direction 3 and 4 (called the "standard LV area"), RV and LV cavity dimensions, wall thickness and motion patterns of IVS and LVPW can be analysed. In order optimize the sound beam direction and record the largest cavity diameter and smallest LV wall thickness in this cross-section, a transverse scan ("T-scan") can be performed in the plane perpendicular to the long axis in the LV area between sound beam directions 3 and 4. In fact, only subtle changes of sound beam direction have to be performed to optimally display the endocardium.

From the same standard position of the transducer on the chest wall, the pulmonary and tricuspid valves can be studied using the mitral valve as a landmark.

Examination of the pulmonary valve

From the mitral valve position the transducer must be angled in a superior and slightly lateral direction to examine the pulmonary valve (Figure 30). In this position, the beam passes obliquely through the chest wall, aHW, RVOT, the left pulmonary valve cusp, the pulmonary artery or atriopulmonic sulcus and eventually posteriorly to it the LA cavity. Because of the oblique beam direction, only the left pulmonary cusp (posteriorly located) is recorded. The success rate in its detection varies with the patient population (75% in adults, 90% in children) and especially with the skill and experience of the examiner.

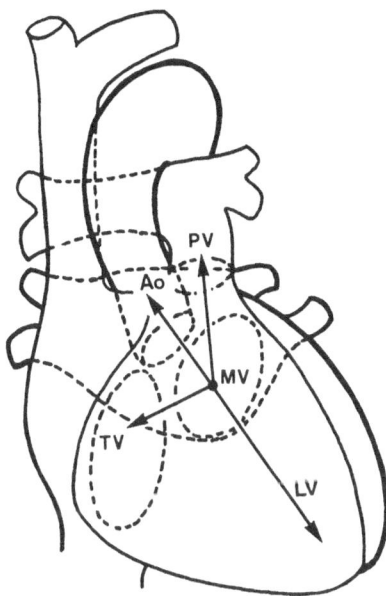

Figure 30. Sequential directions of the sound beam to examine the four cardiac valves from the standard position on the chest wall. Ao: aorta; LV: left ventricle; MV: mitral valve; PV: pulmonary valve; TV: tricuspid valve (From Roelandt J: Practical Echocardiology. Research Studies Press, 1977).

Examination of the tricuspid valve

From the standard mitral valve position, the transducer is tilted in a medial and slightly inferior direction (Figure 30). The anterior tricuspid leaflet (aTL) is usually the one recorded and is recognized by its "snapping" motion in early diastole.

When the RV cavity is enlarged, the septal tricuspid leaflet may be recorded with the same motion pattern as the posterior mitral leaflet. Figure 31 shows a M-mode scan including the four cardiac valves.

Other transducer locations

The three other transducer locations used for two-dimensional echocardiography can also be used with a single element. The apical location can be useful for the study of a valve prosthesis in the mitral valve position. In order to optimally record motion of a prosthetic valve the ultrasound beam must be directed along the longitudinal axis of the prosthetic valve. The transducer must be placed at the cardiac apex and directed medially and superiorly. Unfortunately, adequate recordings are not always obtained from this position. The transducer can also be

NORMAL HEART

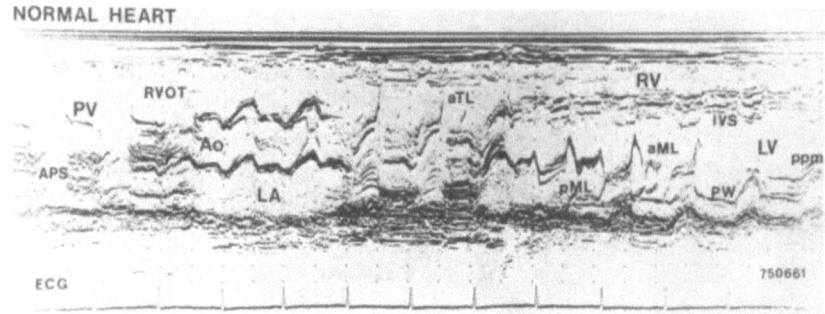

Figure 31. M-mode scan obtained from a normal subject including the four cardiac valves. Ao: aorta: aML: anterior mitral valve leaflet; APS: atriopulmonic sulcus; aTL: anterior tricuspid valve leaflet; IVS; interventricular septum; LA: left atrium; LV: left ventricle; pML: posterior mitral valve leaflet; ppm: posteromedial papillary muscle; PV: pulmonary valve; PW: left ventricular posterior wall; RV: right ventricle; RVOT: right ventricular outflow tract (From Roelandt J: Practical Echocardiology. Research Studies Press, 1977).

placed in the suprasternal notch. The beam then traverses the aortic arch, right pulmonary artery and left atrium and their respective diameters can be determined. This approach is more successful in infants and children than in adults [72].

The subxiphoid approach is especially useful in patients with barrel chest or emphysema, when the parasternal window is obliterated [73]. The diaphragm must be low to obtain optimal records. This approach is useful in patients with coronary artery disease, because it allows study of the inferior part of the IVS and the lateral wall of the LV, areas of the LV different from those seen with the parasternal transducer location.

Sliding the transducer across the ribs over the chest – called linear scanning – has been proposed for evaluation of the LV in patients with coronary artery disease. However, significant dropout limits this method and two-dimensional echocardiography is the superior method for LV study in these patients.

ACKNOWLEDGEMENT

I am very thankfull to Mr D.M. Simons of the Audiovisual Department for his excellent art-work. We are also greatfull to Mr W.B. Vletter for his technical assistance and Miss Machtelt Brussé for her secretarial help.

REFERENCES

1. Roelandt J: Ultrasonic two-dimensional imaging of the heart with multiscan. Thesis. Erasmus University, Rotterdam, the Netherlands, 1980, ch 14, 141 – 52.
2. Roelandt J. Van Dorp WG, Bom N, Laird JD, Hugenholtz PG: Resolution problems in echocardiology: a source of interpretation errors. Am J Cardiol 37:356 – 62, 1976.

3. Griffith JM, Henry WL: A sector scanner for real-time two-dimensional echocardiography. Circulation 49:1147 – 52, 1974.

4. Von Ramm OT, Thurstone FL: Cardiac imaging using a phased array ultrasound system: I System design. Circulation 53:258 – 62, 1976.

5. Kisslo L, Von Ramm OT, Thurstone FL: Cardiac imaging using a phased array ultrasound system: II CLinical techniques and application. Circulation 53:262 – 7, 1976.

6. Helak JW, Plappert T, Muhammed A, Reichek N: Two-dimensional echographic imaging of the left ventricle: comparison of mechanical and phased array systems in vitro. Am J Cardiol 48:728 – 35, 1981.

7. Henry WH, DeMaria AN, Gramiak R, et al: Report of the American Society of Echocardiography Committee on Nomenclature and Standards in two-dimensional echocardiography. Circulation 62:212 – 7, 1980.

8. Martin RP, Meltzer RS, Chia BL, Stinson EB, Rakowski H, Popp RL: Clinical utility of two-dimensional echocardiography in infective endocarditis. Am J Cardiol 46:379 – 92, 1980.

9. Stewart JA, Silimperi D, Harris P, Wise NK, Fraker TD jr, Kisslo JA: Echocardiographic documentation of vegetative lesions in infective endocarditis: clinical implications. Circulation 61:374 – 80, 1980.

10. Victor MF, Mintz GS, Kotler MN, Wilson AR, Segal BL: Two-dimensional echocardiographic diagnosis of aortic dissection. Circulation 48:1155 – 59, 1981.

11. DeMaria AN, Bommer W, Neumann A, Weinert L, Bogren H, Mason DT: Identification and localization of aneurysms of the ascending aorta by cross-sectional echocardiography. Circulation 59:755 – 61, 1979.

12. Weyman AE, Feigenbaum H, Hurwitz RA, Girod DA, Dillon JC, Chang S: Cross-sectional echocardiography in the evaluation of patients with discrete subaortic stenosis. Am J Cardiol 37:358 – 61, 1976.

13. Krueger SK, French JW, Forker AD, Caudill CC, Popp RL: Echocardiography in discrete subaortic stenosis. Circulation 59:506 – 13, 1979.

14. Weyman AE, Feigenbaum H, Dillon JC, Chang S: Cross-sectional echocardiogdraphy in assessing the severity of valvular aortic stenosis. Circulation 52:828 – 34, 1975.

15. Martin RP, Rakowski H, French JW, Popp RL: Idiopathic hypertrophic subaortic stenosis viewed by wide-angle phased array echocardiography. Circulation 59:1206 – 17, 1979.

16. Tajik AJ, Seward JB, Hagler DJ: Detailed analysis of hypertrophic obstructive cardiomyopathy by wide-angle two-dimensional sector echocardiography. Am J Cardiol 43:348, 1979.

17. DeMaria AN, Bommer W, Lee G, Mason DT: Value and limitations of two-dimensional echocardiography in assessment of cardiomyopathy. Am J Cardiol 46:1124 – 31, 1980.

18. Caldwell RL, Weyman AE, Hurwitz RA, Girod DA, Feigenbaum H: Right ventricular assessment by cross-sectional echocardiography in tetralogy of Fallot. Circulation 59:395 – 402, 1979.

19. Henry WL, Maron BJ, Griffith JM: Cross-sectional echocardiography in the diagnosis of congenital heart disease: identification of the relation of the ventricles and great arteries. Circulation 56:267 – 72, 1977.

20. Diessa TG, Hagan AD, Pope C, Santow L, Friedman WF: Two-dimensional echocardiographic characteristics of double outlet right ventricle. Am J Cardiol 44:1146 – 54, 1979.

21. Nichol PM, Gilbert BW, Kisslo JA: Two-dimensional echocardiographic assessment of mitral stenosis. Circulation 55:120 – 8, 1977.

22. Gilbert BW, Schatz RA, Von Ramm OT, Behar VS, Kisslo JA: Mitral valve prolapse: two-dimensional echocardiographic and angiographic correlation. Circulation 54:716 – 23, 1976.

23. Morganroth J, Jones RH, Chen CC, Naito N: Two-dimensional echocardiography in mitral, aortic and tricuspid valve prolapse. The clinical problem, cardiac nuclear imaging considerations and a proposed standard for diagnosis. Am J Cardiol 46:1164 – 77, 1980.

24. Mintz GS, Kotler MN, Parry W, Segal BL: A statistical comparison of the M-mode and two-dimensional echocardiographic diagnosis of flail mitral leaflets. Am J Cardiol 45:253 – 9, 1980.

25. D'Cruz I, Penetia E, Cohen H, Glick G: Submittal calcification or sclerosis in elderly patients: M-mode and two-dimensional echocardiography in mitral annulus calcification. Am J Cardiol 44:31 – 8, 1979.

26. Lappe DL, Bulkley BH, Weiss JL: Two-dimensional echocardiographic diagnosis of left atrial myxoma. Chest 74:55 – 8, 1978.

27. Slosky DA, Fraker TD jr, Steward JA, Kisslo JA: Identification of persistent left superior vena cava by two-dimensional echocardiography, Am J Cardiol 43:385, 1979.

28. Cohen BE, Winer HE, Kronzon I: Echocardiographic findings in patients with left superior vena cava and dilated coronary sinus. Am J Cardiol 44:158 – 61, 1979.

29. Popp RL, Fowles R, Coltart J, Martin RP: Cardiac anatomy viewed systematically with two-dimensional echocardiography. Chest 75:579 – 85, 1979.

30. Weyman AE, Feigenbaum H, Dillon JC, Johnston KW, Eggleton RC: Non-invasive visualization of the left main coronary artery by cross-sectional echocardiography. Circulation 54:169 – 74, 1976.

31. Bansal RC, Tajik AJ, Seward JB, Offord KP: Feasibility of detailed two-dimensional echocardiographic examination in adults. Prospective study of 200 patients. Mayo Clin Proc 55: 291 – 308, 1980.

32. Tajik AJ, Seward JB, Hagler DJ, Mair DD, Lie JT: Two-dimensional real-time ultrasonic imaging of the heart and great vessels: technique, image orientation, structure identification and validation. Mayo Clin Proc 53:271 – 303, 1978.

33. Fowles RE, Martin RP, Abrams JM, Schapira JN, French JW, Popp RL: Two-dimensional echocardiographic features of biscuspid aortic valve. Chest 75:434 – 40, 1979.

34. Fraker TD jr, Harris PJ, Behar VS, Kisslo JA: Detection and exclusion of interatrial shunts by two-dimensional echocardiography and peripheral venous injection. Circulation 59:379 – 84, 1979.

35. Weyman AE, Wann LS, Caldwell RL, Hurwitz RA, Dillon JC, Feigenbaum H: Negative contrast echocardiography: a new method for detecting left-to-right shunts. Circulation 59:498 – 505, 1979.

36. Heger JJ, Weyman AE, Wann LS, Dillon JC, Feigenbaum H: Cross-sectional echocardiography in acute myocardial infarction: detection and localization of regional left ventricular asynergy. Circulation 60:531 – 8, 1979.

37. Morganroth J, Chen CC, David C, Naito M, Mardelli TJ: Echocardiographic detection of coronary artery disease. Detection of effects of ischemia on regional myocardial wall motion and visualization of left main coronary artery disease. Am J Cardiol 46:1178 – 87, 1980.

38. Wann LS, Weyman AE, Feigenbaum H, Dillen JC, Johnston KW, Eggleton RC: Determination of mitral valve area by cross-sectional echocardiography. Ann Inter Med 88:337 – 41, 1978.

39. Martin RP, Rakowski H, Kleiman JH, Beaver W, London E, Popp RL: Reliability and reproducibility of two-dimensional echocardiographic measurement of the stenotic mitral valve orifice area. Am J Cardiol 43:560 – 8, 1979.

40. Mintz GS, Kotler MN, Segal BL, Parry W: Two-dimensional echocardiographic recognition of ruptured chordae tendinae. Circulation 57:244 – 50, 1978.

41. Silverman NH, Schiller NB: Apex echocardiography: a two-dimensional technique for evaluating congenital heart disease. Circulation 57:503 – 11, 1978.

42. Hagler DJ, Tajik AJ, Seward JB, Mair DD, Ritter DG: Real-time wide-angle sector echocardiography. Atrioventricular canal defects. Circulation 59:140 – 50, 1979.

43. Beppu S, Nimura Y, Tamal N, et al: Two-dimensional echocardiography in diagnosing tricuspid atresia. Br Heart J 40:1174 – 83, 1978.

44. Ports TA, Silverman NH, Schiller NB: Two-dimensional echocardiographic assessment of Ebstein's anomaly. Circulation 58:336 – 43, 1978.

45. Kisslo JA, Robertson D, Gilbert BW, Von Ramm O, Behar VS: A comparison of real-time, two-dimensional echocardiography and cineangiography in detecting left ventricular asynergy. Circulation 55: 134 – 41, 1977.

46. Edwards WD, Tajik AJ, Seward JB: Standardized nomenclature and anatomic basis for regional tomographic analysis of the heart. Mayo Clin Proc 56:479 – 97, 1981.

47. Weyman AE, Peskoe SM, Williams ES, Dillon JC, Feigenbaum H: Detection of left ventricular aneurysms by cross-sectional echocardiography. Circulation 54:936 – 43, 1976.

48. Roelandt J, Van den Brand M, Vletter WB, Nauta J, Hugenholtz PG: Echocardiographic diagnosis of pseudoaneurysm of the left ventricle. Circulation 52:466 – 72, 1975.

49. Gatewood RP, Nanda NC; Differentiation of left ventricular pseudoaneurysm from true aneurysm with two-dimensional echocardiography. Am J Cardiol 46:869 – 78, 1980.

50. Ports TA, Schiller NB, Strunk BL: Echocardiography of right ventricular tumors. Circulation 56:439 – 47, 1977.

51. Ports TA, Cogan J, Schiller NB, Rapaport E: Echocardiography of left ventricular masses. Circulation 58:528 – 36, 1978.

52. Meltzer RS, Guthaner D, Rakowski H, Popp RL, Martin RP: Diagnosis of left ventricular thrombi by two-dimensional echocardiography. Br Heart J 42:261 – 5, 1979.

53. Asinger AW, Mikell FL, Sharma B, Hodges M: Observations on detecting left ventricular thrombus with two-dimensional echocardiography: emphasis on avoidance of false positive diagnosis. Am J Cardiol 47:145 – 56, 1981.

54. Schiller NB, Ports TA, Silverman NH: Quantitative analysis of the adult left heart by echocardiography. In: Echocardiology, Rijsterborgh H (ed), Martinus Nijhoff, The Hague, 1981, p. 145 – 161.

55. Eaton LW, Maughan WL, Shoukas AA, Weiss JL: Accurate volume determination in the isolated ejecting canine left ventricle by two-dimensional echocardiography. Circulation 60:320 – 6, 1979.

56. Schiller NB, Acquatella H, Ports TA, Drew D, Goerke J, Ringertz H, et al: Left ventricular volume from paired biplane two-dimensional echocardiography. Circulation 60:547, 1979.

57. Folland ED, Parisi AF, Moynihan PF, Jones DR, Feldman CL, Tow DE: Assessment of left ventricular ejection fraction and volumes by real-time, two-dimensional echocardiography. Circulation 60:760, 1979.

58. Silverman NH, Ports TA, Snider AR, Schiller NB, Carlsson E, Heilbron DC: Determination of left ventricular volume in children: echocardiographic and angiographic comparisons. Circulation 62:548, 1980.

59. Erbl R, Schweizer P, Meijer J, Grenner H, Krebs W, Effert S: Left ventricular volume and ejection fraction determination by cross-sectional echocardiography in patients with coronary artery disease: a prospective study. Clin Cardiol 3: 377, 1980.

60. Starling MR, Crawford MH, Sorenson SG, Levi B, Richards KL, O'Rourke RA: Comparative accuracy of apical biplane cross-sectional echocardiography and gated equilibrium radionuclide angiography for estimating left ventricular size and performance. Circulation 63:1075, 1981.

61. Schapira JN, Martin RP, Fowles RE, et al: Two-dimensional echocardiographic assessment of patients with bioprosthetic valves. Am J Cardiol 43:510 – 19, 1979.

62. Meltzer RS, Roelandt J, Meltzer C: Sector scanning views in echocardiography: a systematic approach. Eur Heart J 1:379 – 94, 1980.

63. Meltzer RS, Van Hoogenhuyze D, Serruys PW, Haalebos MMP, Hugenholtz PG, Roelandt J: Diagnosis of tricuspid regurgitation by contrast echocardiography. Circulation 63:1093 – 9, 1981.

64. Bierman FZ, Williams RG: Subxiphoid two dimensional imaging of the interatrial septum in infants and neonates with congenital heart disease. Circulation 60:80 – 90, 1979.

65. Lange LW, Sahn DJ, Allen HD, Goldberg SJ: Subxiphoid cross-sectional echocardiography in infants and children with congenital heart disease. Circulation 59:513 – 22, 1979.

66. Snider AR, Silverman NH: Suprasternal notch echocardiography: a two-dimensional technique for evaluating congenital heart disease. Circulation 63:165 – 73, 1981.

67. Weyman AE, Caldwell RL, Hurwitz RA, et al: Cross-sectional echocardiographic characteriza-

tion of aortic obstruction. Supravalvular aortic stenosis and aortic hypoplasia. Circulation 57:491 – 7, 1975.

68. Weyman AE, Caldwell RL, Hurwitz RA, et al: Cross-sectional echocardiographic detection of aortic obstruction. 2. Coarctation of the aorta. Circulation 57:498 – 502, 1978.

69. Sahn DJ, Allen HD: Real-time cross-sectional echocardiographic imaging and measurement of the patent ductus arteriosus in infants and children. Circulation 58:343 – 54, 1978.

70. Feigenbaum H: Echocardiography. 3rd ed. Philadelphia, Lea and Febiger, 1981.

71. Roelandt J: Practical echocardiology. Forest Grove, Oregon, Research Studies Press, 1977.

72. Goldberg BB: Suprasternal ultrasonography. Jama 215:245 – 50, 1971.

73. Chang S, Feigenbaum H: Subxiphoid echocardiogdraphy. J Clin Ultrasound 1:14, 1973.

II. PROBLEMS RELATED TO QUALITATIVE AND QUANTITATIVE ANALYSIS OF M-MODE, TWO-DIMENSIONAL AND DOPPLER ECHOCARDIOGRAPHY

Echocardiography can be used in a variety of ways. A number of echocardiographic diagnoses are based on the application of qualitative criteria. In some instances a definitive diagnosis can be made (e.g. pericardial effusion, rheumatic mitral valve stenosis). In others important independent information is obtained which confirms or rejects a diagnosis already suspected on clinical grounds (e.g. vegetative endocarditis). In the assessment of function, quantitative measurements are used which may have important implication for patient management (e.g. decision to replace a valve in minimally symptomatic patients). These applications are nowadays increasingly employed.

The quantitative use of the echocardiographic method for clinical decision making, however, is extremely complex and subject to many pitfalls. A diagnosis based on quantitative measurements requires among others "normal values" of which the meaning and application are not always well understood. With respect to the method itself, physical limitations and an incorrect examination technique are important factors. Finally, measurements from echocardiograms are limited by several potential errors affecting their accuracy and reproducibility. All these aspects are extensively discussed in chapters 3 and 4.

Doppler echocardiography is a method related to M-mode and two-dimensional echocardiography and allows to examine blood flow. Its role in clinical decision making although promising is still limited by technologic limitations and these are discussed in chapter 5.

Roelandt, J. (ed.) The practice of M-mode and two-dimensional echocardiography
© *1983, Martinus Nijhoff Publishers. The Hague / Boston / London*
ISBN 978-94-009-6792-2.

3. LIMITATIONS AND PITFALLS OF M-MODE AND TWO-DIMENSIONAL ECHOCARDIOGRAPHY

J. Roelandt and J. Lubsen

Many factors may lead to an erroneous or inaccurate diagnosis of cardiac disease when reading clinical M-mode and two-dimensional echocardiograms.

These include: failure to recognise physical limitations of the method, improper examination technique, inadequate clinical information, misinterpretation of the echocardiographic data, and inadequate consideration of specificity and sensitivity of the criteria applied. It is obvious that with the increasing role of echocardiography in the management of patients with heart disease, understanding and recognition of these problems is of major importance.

1. PHYSICAL LIMITATIONS OF M-MODE AND TWO-DIMENSIONAL ECHOCARDIOGRAPHY

To produce two-dimensional echocardiographic images, some compromises have been made in comparison with M-mode echocardiography of which the sampling rate and display format are the most important to consider. Resolution in the lateral directions constitutes a physical limitation to both M-mode and two-dimensional echocardiography. It must be realized, however, that resolution by ultrasound is superior to other noninvasive cardiac imaging techniques. Drop-outs and reverberations are other physical limitations which may lead to an incorrect diagnosis.

1.1. Sampling rate (time resolution)

M-mode echocardiography uses a sampling rate of 1.000 transmit/receive cycles/sec and is able to record continuously the most rapid intracardiac events such as valve opening, closure, fluttering and subtle abnormalities of wall motion. Two-dimensional images are build up by a number of radial lines each displaying echoes in B-mode format. Building up a tomographic plane takes time and hence results in a limited frame rate (usually 50 frames/sec) determined by the scan angle (typically 85°), pulse repetition rate, number of lines per degree and image view depth (determining the number of lines as ultrasound velocity in the body is 1560 meter/sec).

Roelandt, J. (ed.) The practice of M-mode and two-dimensional echocardiography
© *1983, Martinus Nijhoff Publishers. The Hague / Boston / London*
ISBN 978-94-009-6792-2.

The resolution of motion of two-dimensional imaging systems in thus limited by the frame rate which is too low to record rapid intracardiac events. Both M-mode and two-dimensional echocardiography are therefore complementary and mutually supportive for the analysis of cardiac conditions where anatomic and functional abnormalities overlap. Modern phased-array two-dimensional sector scanners can simultaneously display the two-dimensional image while sampling any selected area of the cardiac cross-section for M-mode recording. These integrated systems have advantages for studying the heart since they allow a combination of optimal qualitative assessment and standardized quantitative measurements.

1.2. Display format

Two-dimensional images are displayed on a cathode ray tube during the examination. They are recorded on videotape using a standard TV camera or a digital scan converter for a permanent record and subsequent analysis. This process may deteriorate image quality. When these images are reviewed in the stop-frame mode, there is an inherent loss of the visual integration by the observer of structural motion. In addition, in most systems only half of the scan lines, and thus only one-half of the information available during the real-time study, is available for off-line analysis.

Representing a sectorial image on a TV output using a digital scan converter requires writing of diagonal lines across the rectangular storage grid. This results in a "moiré pattern" on the display which may interfere with proper interpretation of cardiac structures.

Al together, video tape remains a difficult, expensive and cumbersome medium for data storage and retrieval.

1.3. Axial resolution

The axial or depth resolution is the minimum axial distance at which two reflecting structures may be recognized as separate entities. It is determined by the length of the echoes which is directly dependent upon the length of the transmitted ultrasound pulses. Long pulses do not resolve closely lying boundaries along the sound beam axis as they result in overlapping echoes. Thus, the shorter the transmitted pulses, the shorter the echoes and the better the axial resolution. Axial resolution is similar in M-mode and two-dimensional echocardiography and is good (in the range of 1 to 2 mm).

M-mode and two-dimensional transducers presently used are designed to produce a pulse of 4 or 5 cycles irrespective of their frequency of operation. Thus, increasing the ultrasound frequency (e.g. from 2.25 to 5 MHz) produces a shorter

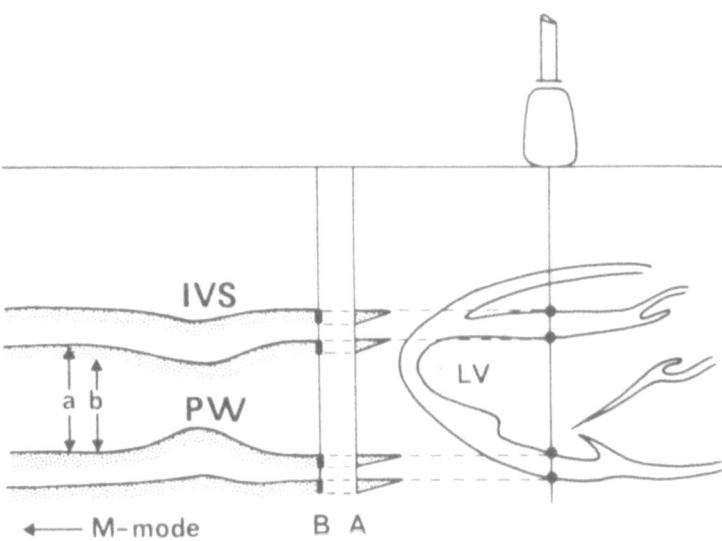

IVS

LV

a b   PW

◄———— M-mode   B A

Figure 1. Diagram illustrating how high gain settings may cause lengthening of echoes. The position of the blood-endocardial interfaces is represented by the leading edges of their echoes on the recording. Therefore the measurements of dimensions should be made from leading to leading edges (measurement a for the left ventricular cavity dimension). Increasing the gain of the receiver causes lengthening of the echoes. If the measurement is made from the trailing edge to leading edge, the left ventricular cavity dimension is underestimated by an unknown and variable quantity (measurement b). A, B and M-mode: amplitude and motion mode, brightness representation of the echo information, LV: left ventricle; PW: posterior wall.

pulse and improves axial resolution considerably. However, application of these higher ultrasound frequencies is limited by their higher absorption in tissues. Nevertheless, they are used to great advantage in examining newborns and infants. Too high gain settings of the ultrasound system may also cause lengthening of the echoes and degrading definition and axial resolution. In addition, high gain settings increase the amount of nonstructural echoes (e.g. clutter in the near field and noise). Therefore, the lowest possible gain settings of the instrument must be used during examination.

1.3.1. Clinical implications
Optimal gain settings are necessary to avoid a false-negative diagnosis in the presence of pericardial effusion since the echo-free space can be obliterated when using too high gain settings.

Errors in the measurement of left ventricular internal dimensions may result from a similar problem. It follows from acoustic theory that the location of an interface on the display is represented by the leading edge of its echo and not by the trailing edge [1]. High gain settings to visualize the interventricular septum will lengthen the trailing edge of the left sided endocardial echo into the left ventricular cavity. If the internal left ventricular dimension is then measured from the trailing edge of the septal echo to the leading edge of the posterior wall echo, the dimension

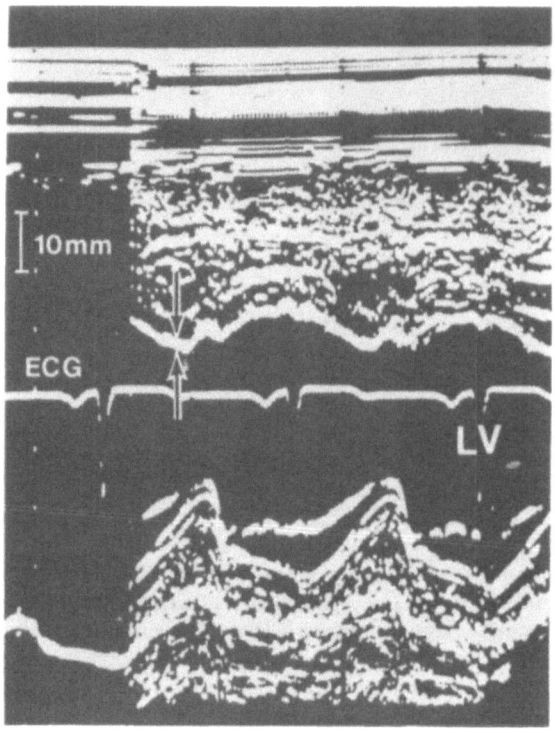

Figure 2. Polaroid representation of a left ventricular M-mode echogram. The endocardial echo of the left side of the septum has a thickness of 3 mm. Measuring the left ventricular dimension from the leading edge, which is the correct measurement, yields an internal dimension of 43 mm. If the trailing edge is taken, the cavity dimension is 40 mm. Thus, an error of 7% may be introduced. In infants and children, the error is proportionally larger because the ventricles are smaller (From Roelandt J: Practical Echocardiology. Research Studies Press, 1977).

is underestimated by the width of the septal echo (Figures 1 and 2). The implications of this type of error are discussed in the next chapter. This principle also applies to two-dimensional echocardiography but in practice, measurements are more often made from M-mode recordings. Thus, if quantitative measurements are considered, a sensitive instrument, the use of the lowest possible gain settings, a high-resolution display, and measurements between the leading edges of echoes are required to achieve accuracy and improve reproducibility (see chapter 4).

1.4. Lateral resolution (off-main axis or spurious echoes)

One of the most serious limitations of echocardiographic systems in current use is the width of the ultrasound beam, which determines lateral resolution [2, 3]. The ultrasound system regards the line of sight of the transducer as a thin line and any echo received from targets within the beam width is displayed on this line. Thus, an echo from a target on the edge of the ultrasound beam is displayed as if it were in the middle and this echo will therefore not represent the true location of the target (spurious echo). It must further be realized that the sound field generated by a transducer remains the same as the width of the active transducer surface over a short distance and then begins to diverge. Thus the lateral resolution deteriorates with increasing depth.

The ultrasound beam produced by a conventional single element ultrasonic transducer either on M-mode or mechanical sector scanning instruments has a circular shape. The lateral resolution is represented by the diameter of the circle and is the same in all directions. Electronic phased-array scanners, however, have a rectangular transducer configuration and a different resolution in the two lateral (perpendicular) directions (one parallel to the length and one parallel to the width of the active transducer surface). Thus, lateral resolution of phased array systems must be considered in two perpendicular planes. Unfortunately, little attention has thus far been given to resolution in the plane perpendicular to the imaging plane. It should be stressed, however, that many of the interpretation problems resulting from lateral resolution problems (spurious echoes) on M-mode recordings and two-dimensional stop-frame images are alleviated by real time two-dimensional echocardiography because of the unsurpassed pattern recognition capabilities of the human eye-brain system.

1.4.1. Clinical implications of limited lateral resolution

1.4.2. Spurious echoes from the mitral valve
With an ideal "pencil-like" sound beam the recorded echoes would represent the correct position of each reflecting structure in the sound beam axis. In Figure 3 this situation is schematically shown for that part of the anterior mitral valve leaflet through which the beam passess vertically. Imperfections in the beam width will result in visualization of off-axis areas of the mitral valve. The areas of the mitral valve labeled 1 and 3 are also struck in a predominantly vertical manner, and the echoes will be recorded. They will be displayed behind each other due to small differences in travel time and seen as multiple parallel moving echoes on the M-mode recording. This is demonstrated on the M-mode scan obtained from a patient with an atrial septal defect of the secundum type and a large left-to-right shunt (Figure 4). Multiple mitral valve echoes during systole suggested an abnormality but at open heart surgery the mitral valve was found to be normal. Thus, it is evident that an echo on the display does not necessarily represent a cardiac structure in that location. It is obvious that the systolic mitral valve pattern, as shown in Figure 4 cannot be interpreted as leaflet separation and therefore the diagnosis of mitral incompetence should not be made. We are aware of several instances in which misinterpretations of this pattern led to a false diagnosis of mitral incompetence was made.

Another example of superimposition of laterally spaced targets seen on routine

58

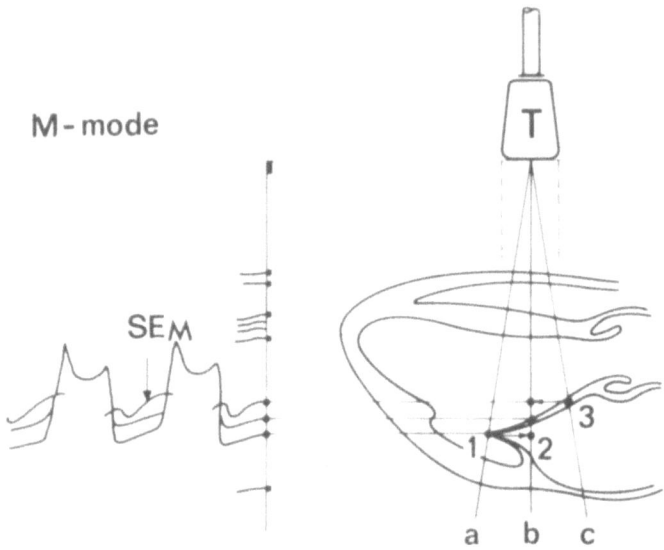

M-mode

SEM

T

1   2   3

a   b   c

Figure 3. Diagram illustrating how spurious echoes of the mitral valve (SEM) may appear on the M-mode echocardiogram of the mitral valve (see text for explanation) T: transducer.

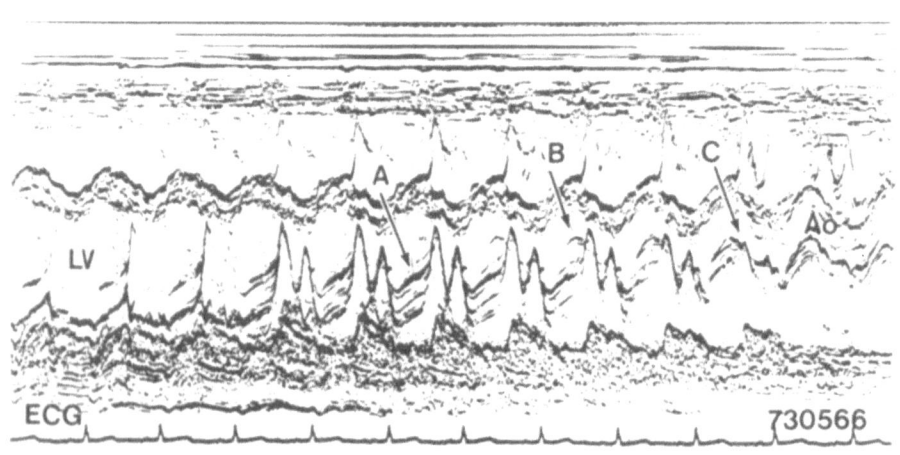

LV
A
B
C
Ao
ECG
730566

Figure 4. M-mode scan from the left ventricle (LV) toward the aorta (Ao) obtained from a patient with an atrial septal defect (type II). Patterns caused by spurious echoes are indicated by arrows: A) multiple mitral valve echoes in systole, B) overlay echo on mitral valve originating from base of aorta, and C) mixture of echo patterns from posterior aortic wall and anterior mitral valve leaflet. (From Roelandt J: Practical Echocardiology, Research Studies Press, 1977).

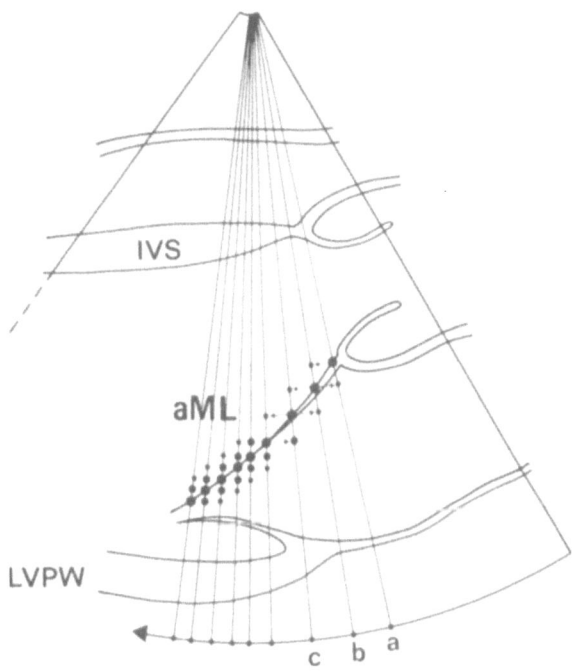

Figure 5. Multiplication of the spurious echoes of the anterior mitral valve (aML), resulting from each single sound beam as shown in Figure 3, on two-dimensional images. These spurious echoes lead to distortions altering the size and thickness of the valve. IVS: interventricular septum; LVPW: left ventricular posterior wall.

M-mode echocardiograms is that where echoes of the chordae tendinae interfere with the mitral valve echogram.

Additional linear echoes in systole are often seen draped over the mitral valve echogram in patients with dilated cardiomyopathy. This pattern too has been suggested to be indicative of leaflet separation. It probably results from the stretched mitral valve apparatus caused by both the dilatation of the left ventricle and the papillary dysfunction present in this condition [4]. The low-amplitude wave form most likely originates from the areas closer to the mitral valve ring and papillary muscles whereas the higher amplitude wave form originates from the mid-portion of the mitral valve. Multiple systolic echoes are commonly recorded in patients with mitral valve prolapse syndrome. In this condition, multiple areas on the valve leaflets reflect ultrasound because of their ruggedness and redundancy. As a consequence, differentiation between anterior and posterior leaflet prolapse from M-mode echocardiograms, as was suggested in some earlier publications, is unreliable [45, 6]. Sometimes shallow early systolic humps may be seen in addition to the midsystolic prolapse. This pattern most likely represents different motion of the valve away from the prolapsing segment, both patterns being superimposed as a result of the beam width [7].

A single sound beam with a finite width will display multiple adjacent areas on

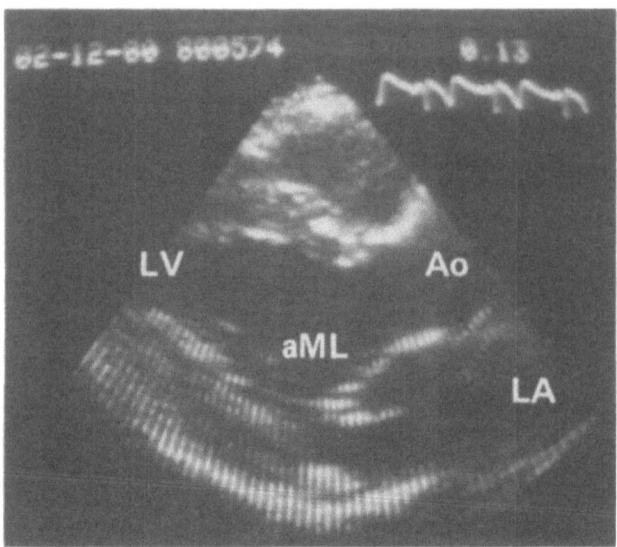

Figure 6. Distortions of the normal anterior mitral valve (aML) on a stop-frame image of the parasternal long axis view. For explanation see text and Figure 5. Ao: aorta; LA: left atrium: LV: left ventricle.

an obliquely oriented mitral valve as if they were located behind each other (Figure 3). When a two-dimensional image is build up with echoes of many such sound beams, these off-axis echoes will give a different appearance of structures on the resulting images. The mitral valve is represented by a set of "horizontal" echo complexes altering both its size of shape (Figure 5 and 6).

These distortions of the mitral valve are equally seen in two-dimensional views created with focused transducers used in mechanical scanning systems and phased-array systems.

1.4.3. Spurious echoes from the aorta

Echoes originating from the posterior wall of the aorta and/or mitral valve ring, both being strong reflectors, may be picked up when the transducer is aimed at the mitral valve and interfere with its motion pattern, especially in systole. The off-axis origin of these echoes is inferred from their motion pattern and their timing within the cardiac cycle, since they are similar to the echoes obtained when the main sound beam is aimed to the base of the aorta (Figure 4).

Spurious systolic echoes of the posterior aortic wall overlaying the mitral valve could suggest systolic anterior motion of the anterior mitral valve leaflet (false-SAM) and, hence, the false-positive diagnosis of functional outflow obstruction. These spurious echoes of the base of the aorta are often seen in patients with mitral valve prolapse syndrome [8]. This may be because the mitral valve leaflets move towards the left atrium and are thus closer to the base of the aorta facilitating mixture of motion patterns from both structures. Echoes originating from the mitral valve or ring may interfere with the posterior aortic root echoes and suggest duplication of the posterior aortic wall. In addition, the echocardiogram recorded from the base of the aorta is a mixture of echoes from both the sinus of Valsalva and the aortic root. The pattern may suggest aortic wall dissection in patients with dilated aorta.

It is difficult to assess to what extent off-axis echoes of the base of the aorta and the mitral valve ring extend into the left ventricular cavity on two-dimensional images. They may limit the accuracy of long axis measurement of the left ventricle.

1.4.4. Spurious echoes from the endocardium

Proper identification of the LV endocardial echoes is important when attempting to define cavity dimensions. Theoretically, the same principles concerning off-axis echoes apply, but because of the changing geometry of the LV during contraction certain specific problems must be considered.

The endocardium is a rough trabecularized structure which provides multiple targets for reflection. If most of these targets are in a perpendicular plane to the sound beam, the integrated information is seen as a single and relatively strong echo.

With inclination of the endocardial surface to the sound beam direction, however, echoes from parts of the endocardial surface at the edge of the sound beam will be displayed and seen as multiple echoes (the principle is similar to that shown for the mitral valve in Figure 5). The axial distance between these off-axis and true endocardial echoes in a given direction increases with the angle of inclination until, at a certain angle, no echoes return on the transducer (drop-out). Thus, the endocardium may be erroneously identified, especially in the presence of LV shape abnormalities. A standard M-mode recording of the left ventricle, obtained from a normal subject, is shown in Figure 7. When the endocardium of the posterior wall is recorded at the lowest gain, one single echo is seen (arrow A). When the gain is increased, multiple parallel moving echoes originating off the main sound beam axis are seen in diastole (arrows B and C). Thus, by carefully adjusting the gain setting controls, the true endocardium can be identified since it has the highest intensity. Note also that the echoes which move almost parallel in diastole merge during systole. This is due to a change in the angle of inclination of the endocardium to the sound beam which is becoming more "perpendicular", and causes the spurious echoes to fall closer to the endocardial echo and to merge. Spurious echoes and drop-outs of the endocardium hamper the correct identification of the endocardial contour from two-dimensional stop-frame images [3].

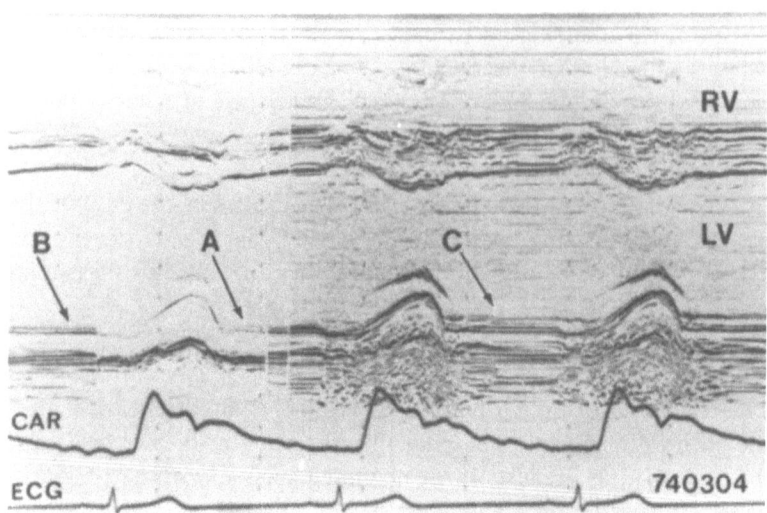

Figure 7. Spurious echoes on the M-mode echocardiogram from the endocardium of the left ventricular posterior wall, recorded at three different gains: A, B and C; for explanation see text. CAR: carotid artery tracing; LV: left ventricle; RV: right ventricle. (From Roelandt J: Practical Echocardiology, Research Studies Press, 1977).

1.5. Side-lobes

A problem of the phased-array scanners is the existence of beam "side-lobes" which occur when the main beam direction is deviated from the central axis of the transducer. These side-lobes result in the appearance of "ghost" echoes originating from strong reflectors outside the main interrogating beam. Although the exact cause is not well understood, it is believed that these side-lobes mainly are caused by gaps between the elements of the transducer array. Characteristically, side lobes produce extended echoes from prominent cardiac structures (pericardium, calcified valves, etc.) which are depicted throughout the full sectorial image.

1.6. Reverberations (phantom echoes)

The most common axial multiple reflection artifact is caused by an ultrasound pulse which travels twice the distance between the transducer and the reflecting structure when the echo bounces back from the transducer. The resulting reverberation echo will be displayed twice as far from the transducer and its amplitude will be twice as large. It does not correspond to a real interface.

These 're-echoes' or 'reverberations' can eventually produce a duplication of

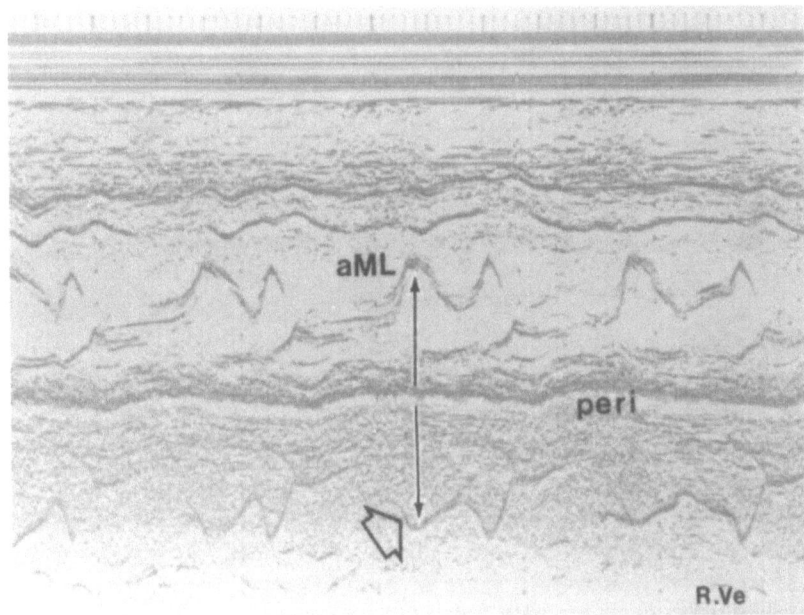

Figure 8. Reverberations between the anterior mitral valve leaflet (aML) and pericardium (peri) result in an inverted mitral valve echogram behind the heart. (From Roelandt J: Practical Echocardiology, Research Studies Press 1977).

the heart, thus giving the appearance of a 'phantom' heart behind the real heart.

The stationary echoes seen in the first few centimeters of the M-mode recordings are most likely reverberations between the transducer and skin or structures in the chest wall and may obscure proximal structures such as the anterior heart wall and occasionally the tricuspid valve.

The reverberation phenomenon may also occur between structures within the heart. This results in apparent deepening of the position of a structure and inverts the phase of its motion pattern. This is illustrated by the example shown in Figure 8, where an inverted image of the mitral valve is seen behind the posterior wall. Here, the phantom image of the mitral valve resulted from a reverberation between the pericardium and the mitral valve. In normal-sized hearts these reverberations rarely cause difficulties in interpretation. Difficulties may arise in dilated hearts where, e.g., a phantom of the aorta may be seen within the dilated left atrial cavity and suggest a thrombus. Ultrasound may also bounce back and forth within a structure. This is demonstrated in an vitro experiment with the transducer in a water tank aimed to a glass plate (Figure 9). The ultrasound reverberates within the glass plate resulting in multiple echoes of decreasing amplitude on the display. This phenomenon is encountered within a disc valve (Björk-Shiley) prosthesis and in cardiac catheters. The resulting patterns may simulate a mass lesion.

REVERBERATIONS WITHIN A GLASS PLATE

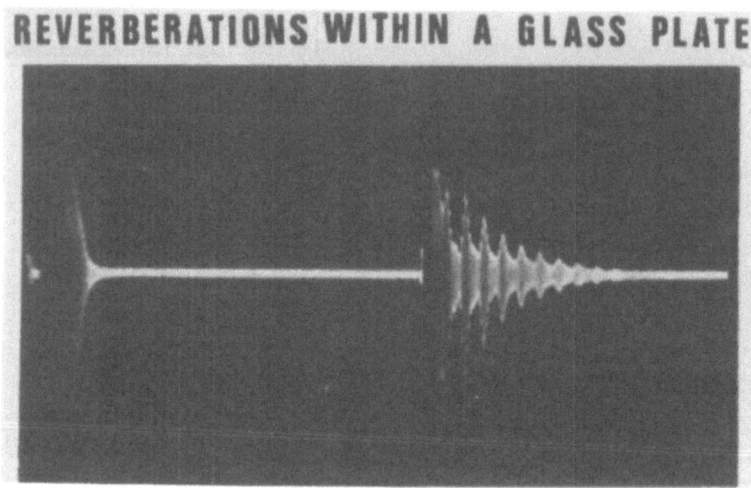

Figure 9. In vitro experiment in a water tank illustrating the effect of multiple reflections within a glass plate. (From Roelandt J: Practical Echocardiology. Research Studies Press, 1977).

Likewise, reverberations may occur within a fibrotic or calcified valve such as in mitral stenosis, and this partially explains its multi-layered appearance in this condition and invalidate thickness measurements. The pattern of an atrial myxoma may be mimicked. A peculiar artifact can be observed in images obtained with the rotating mechanical sector scanners. These appear as linear rapidly oscillating echoes in the near field. They are most probably due to reverberations between the transducer and its plastic housing which is in contact with the patient.

It is not clear to what extent multiple non-axial reflections may affect the display. Here the ultrasound pulse is reflected away from the main beam direction, strikes another interface and is reflected back to the transducer. Non-axial reverberations could theoretically occur within the heart but are difficult to prove [2].

1.7. Drop-outs of structures

The intensity of echoes from reflecting structures may vary widely since they depend on several physical factors. These are the attenuation of the energy with distance travelled due to tissue absorption, differences in acoustic impedance, and the angle of incidence of the sound beam. Thus, only structures that are relatively perpendicular to the ultrasonic beam will be recorded on M-mode and two-dimensional echocardiograms. Furthermore, ultrasound systems can only display echoes within a limited range of intensities. As a consequence, anatomic structures may not be seen in the display (drop-outs).

1.7.1. Clinical implications
Drop-outs of parts of the interventricular septum may result from LV shape irregularities and unfavorable angles of structures to the sound beam. Drop-outs of the interventricular septum may falsely suggest the existence of an interventricular septum defect. On the other hand, ventricular septal defects will not be detected when the size of the defect is smaller than the beam width (see section 1.4.) or when the shape of the defect is not favorable to the sound beam. Unless there is an overriding aorta (aortic-septal discontinuity) which is diagnostic, the detection of a ventricular septal defect requires considerable experience.

Drop-outs are also seen where there is a posterior displacement of the mitral valve apparatus when the left ventricle dilates. This gives a discontinuity pattern of the anterior mitral valve leaflet and aorta. Repeating the M-scan from another intercostal interspace might adjust the angle of the sound beam to the "drop-out area" so that echoes will be recorded.

Drop-outs occur on M-mode echocardiograms when the aortic-septal axis is angulated. This angulation problem is seen in patients with poststenotic aortic dilatation, an unfolded aorta, or right ventricular dilatation (see section 2.). Two-dimensional systems obviate most of these difficulties since they allow direct visualization of the aortic-septal axis [9]. Because the sound beams are parallel to the interventricular septum and lateral LV wall when apical two-dimensional views are used, significant drop-outs of the endocardium occur in most diagnostic studies. This is a major limitation for the estimation of LV volumes.

1.8. Analysis of motion patterns

It should be realized, that motion of structures occurs in a three-dimensional space. Only the motion along the sound beam axis is displayed correctly on M-mode recordings. Structures that move obliquely within the beam show only the components of their motion that are parallel to the sound beam axis. Thus, the observed amplitude of motion is diminished by the angular relationship. When the structure moves perpendicular to the sound beam axis, its echo is motionless on the resulting record.

On the other hand, structures may move in and out the sound beam during the cardiac cycle which may lead to false M-mode echo patterns (Figure 10). Two-dimensional echocardiography is most helpful in overcoming these problems as motion perpendicular to the sound beams is recorded in one plane and structures can be followed throughout the cardiac cycle in their correct spatial relationship.

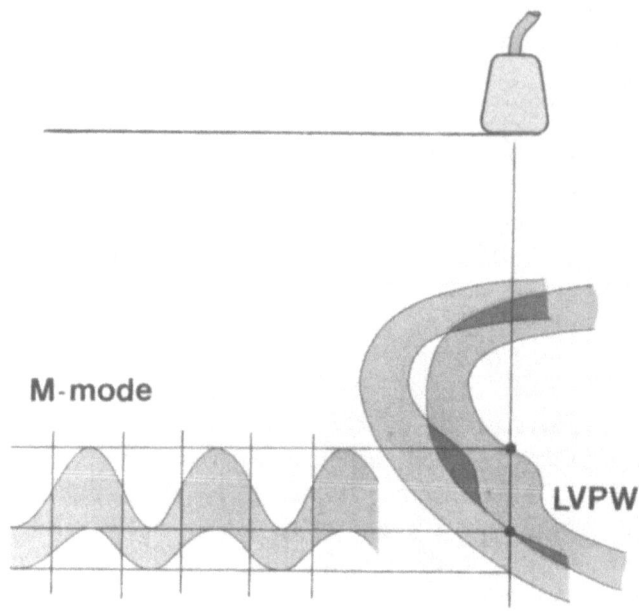

M-mode

LVPW

Figure 10. False M-mode echo pattern of systolic wall thickening which results when the infarcted segment in the papillary muscle area moves in and out the sound beam. LVPW: left ventricular posterior wall.

2. PITFALLS RELATED TO IMPROPER EXAMINATION TECHNIQUE

Transducer position on the chest wall will influences motion patterns on M-mode echocardiograms and suggest cardiac disease. The "standard" transducer position for recording M-mode echocardiograms is over the middle of the heart [10]. Unfortunately one cannot rely on the intercostal space to determine the appropriate transducer position since the relationship of the heart to the chest wall varies from one individual to another. The mitral valve is a central cardiac structure and can thus be used as an intracardiac landmark. The intercostal space from which its maximal amplitude of motion is recorded with the transducer perpendicular to the chest wall is therefore the "standard position" and is equidistant from the anterior aortic wall and interventricular septum [10, 11]. When the transducer is at a higher interspace, the anterior aortic wall is closer to the transducer than the septum and a false pattern of aortic-septal discontinuity is recorded since the improper angle of sound beam incidence may cause echoes of the outflow septum to "drop-out" (see section 1.7.). This discontinuity pattern may also result from an anteriorly displaced and/or dilated aorta and in the presence of a dilated right ventricle (Figures 11 and 12).

Similarly, an aortic-mitral valve discontinuity is not uncommon in patients

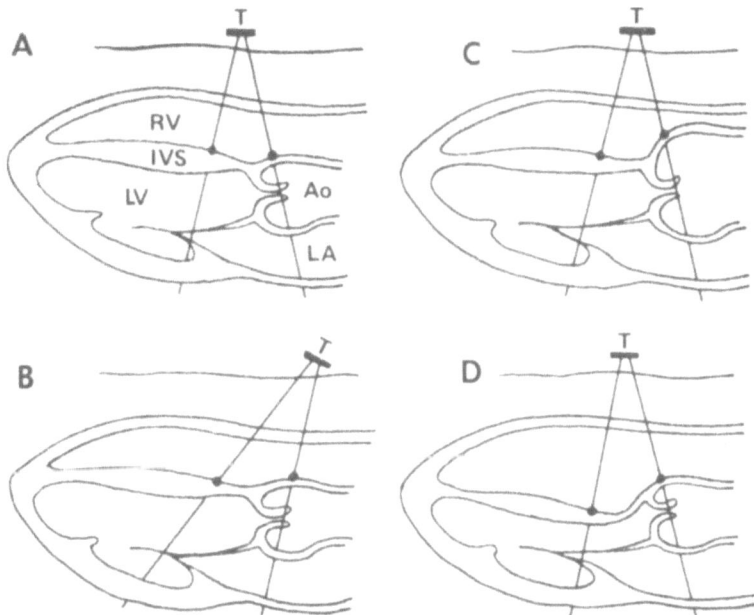

Figure 11. A: normal transducer position on the chest wall; B: too high transducer position which may lead to a false pattern for overriding aorta; C: a dilated aortic root and; D: a dilated right ventricle may also lead to false patterns of overriding aorta on M-mode recordings (For explanation see text). Ao: aorta; IVS: interventricular septum; LA: left atrium; LV: left ventricle.

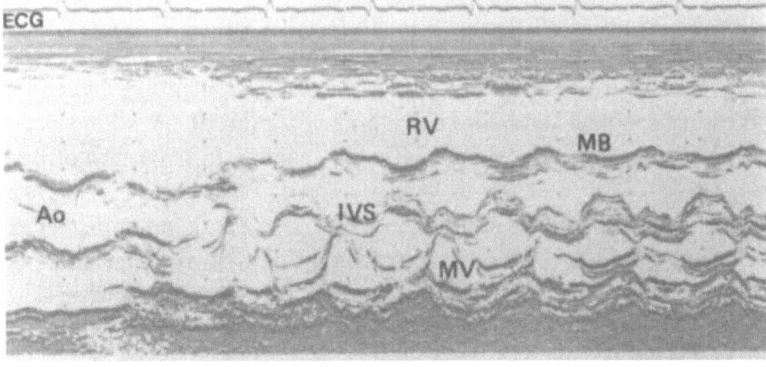

Figure 12. False pattern of overriding aorta (Ao) in patient with dilated right ventricle (RV) due to pulmonary hypertension (see also diagram D of Figure 11).

with a dilated left ventricle. Repeating the M-scan from another intercostal space might adjust the angle of incidence so that echoes from these area's will not "drop-out".

A high transducer position can give a pattern suggestive of mitral valve pro-

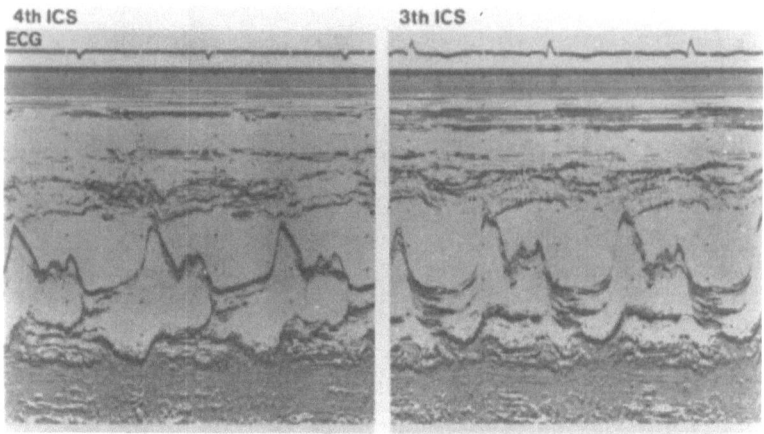

Figure 13. Recording the mitral valve from the 3rd intercostal space results in an echo pattern simulating mitral valve prolapse. The systolic prolapse is not seen when the valve is recorded from one intercostal (4th ICS) lower. The clinical findings in this normal subject were not consistent with mitral valve prolapse syndrome.

lapse in normal subjects as the mitral valve leaflets move away from the transducer during systole when the base of the LV moves towards the apex [12] (Figure 13). With a too low transducer position on the chest wall, the mitral valve leaflets will move towards the transducer in systole producing a pattern in normal subjects which mimics systolic anterior movement (false SAM).

When LV internal dimensions are recorded with the transducer placed one or more interspaces too high or too low, an oblique chord of the LV is obtained measurement of LV dimensions and LV wall thickness are likely to be inaccurate.

Oblique chords of the aorta and left atrium are also measured when the aortic cusps are not used as a landmark for standardization of the sound beam direction. Aiming the transducer too medially may cause a false pattern of pericardial effusion [10].

It appears that most of the limitations which result from an improper examination technique relate to M-mode echocardiography. Two-dimensional echocardiography is therefore the superior technique for studying structural relationships.

3. LIMITATIONS TO QUANTITATION OF LEFT VENTRICULAR FUNCTION

M-mode echocardiography, initially a qualitative technique rapidly became a quantitative method for measurement of LV dimensions and its wall thickness. There are several limitations, however, in measurement accuracy related to the physics of echocardiography and the examination technique. These were discussed in previous sections. M-mode echocardiography only provides information of a limited LV area which is not representative for the entire ventricle in many cardiac disorders. Improper measurement techniques further compromise the accuracy and precision of these measurements (see chapter 4 by Lubsen). Despite these limitations, several simple measurements of the LV from M-mode echocardiogdrams have proven to be of value. For example, the LV internal dimensions at end-diastole and end-systole (preferably end-ejection) can be measured directly from the M-mode echocardiogram with a caliper after the LV endocardial echoes of the septum and posterior wall and the timing of the events in the cardiac cycle have been identified. Other quantities which can be measured directly from the tracing involve time and further allow the determination of the change of LV dimension per unit of time. Finally, some directly measurable quantities relate various measurements to each other and express them to a single parameter. An example is the fractional shortening defined as the change in dimension devided by the enddiastolic dimension and expressed in percent. Furthermore, from two-dimensional echocardiographic stop-frames we can directly measure LV surface areas and the dimensions.

Apart from such directly measurable quantities, parameters are often used which cannot be measured directly. An obvious example is left ventricular volume. LV volume is not measured as such but derived by the application of a formula to a measured quantity. Thus, LV volume is obtained from an M-mode echocardiogram by cubing the LV dimensions times a constant ($1.047 D^3$) [10]. These are important distinctions between directly measured and derived quantities. It should be obvious that cubing an internal, dimension a directly measured quantity, and multiplying it by a constant, amounts to only a rescaling of the original units of measurement to a different one, i.e. from mm to mm^3. No independent information is generated and such quantities have limited usefullness. Two-dimensional echocardiography overcomes some of the limitations of M-mode echocardiography when both methods are used in combination. Animal studies where angiographically determined LV volumes were used as a standard for comparison have shown good agreement. In humans, the correlation has been less good and LV volume was consistently underestimated by echo. Several reasons for these conflicting results have been discussed in previous sections. They include: incomplete visualization of the endocardium due to dropouts (section 1.7.), poor visualization of the apical zone as a result of non structural echoes in the near field (section 1.3.), blurring of LV contour on stop frame images (section 1.2.), spurious echoes from the endocardium limiting correct identification of the LV perimeter (section 1.4.4.), and problems with correct echocardiographic plane selection, since total cardiac displacement during the cardiac beat may yield different views for end-diastole and end-systole.

Another factor which has to be taken in account is that angiocardiography does not measure LV volume directly. Infact no ''absolute'' standard reference is available at present.

Several groups are now working to develop geometric models of the LV most suitable for determining LV volume, while refining instrument design and display techniques. The most distressing limitation to solve, however, remains the quality of the echocardiographic image itself.

It appears that until better echocardiographic systems are available, analysis of two-dimensional images will, unfortunately, have to rely upon subjective and qualitative visual impressions.

Patient management and follow-up are preferably based on directly measurable quantities. Derived quantities are only useful to rescale measurements to more familiar indices with existing frame of reference (e.g. fractional shortening vs ejection fraction).

4. MISDIAGNOSIS OF ECHOCARDIOGRAMS

Incorrect identification and inaccurate assessment of motion of the recorded structures lead to an erroneous diagnosis. Identification of the right side of the interventricular septum is often difficult because of the many echoes interfering with the endocardial echoes. These echoes originate from trabeculae, the tricuspid valve or are often of a nonstructural nature.

In normal sized and hypertrophic ventricles, difficulties arise to differentiate the endocardium of the posterior wall from chordal echoes since both structures are in close contact. In general, the endocardium is the weakest echo and its systolic anterior motion is faster than that of the chordal echoes with usually show an early diastolic notch when the mitral valve opens [10].

A calcified mitral annulus can be mistaken for the LV posterior wall and the echo-free space between the annulus and pericardium interpreted as pericardial effusion [13]. It is obvious that subsequent measurements of LV dimension will be highly inaccurate as well. Correct identification of the anterior and posterior heart walls with their endocardium, epicardium and pericardium remains crucial for the diagnosis of a pericardial effusion (see section 1.3.). Swinging of the heart in large pericardial effusion causes pseudo-motion patterns such as systolic posterior and anterior movement of the mitral valve (Figure 14), paradoxical septal and high amplitude motion of the LV posterior wall. It should be stressed once again that the recorded motion of any cardiac structure is the addition sum of its intrinsic motion and total cardiac displacement. Thus, motion patterns should never be interpreted and preferably dimensions never measured in the presence of a large pericardial effusion [10].

When the recorded area of the interventricular septum is too close to its connection with the aorta (the upper third or outflow septum), a false diagnosis of paradoxical septal motion is made as it moves with the aorta towards the transducer during systole [14].

The differentiation between true and false systolic anterior movement of the

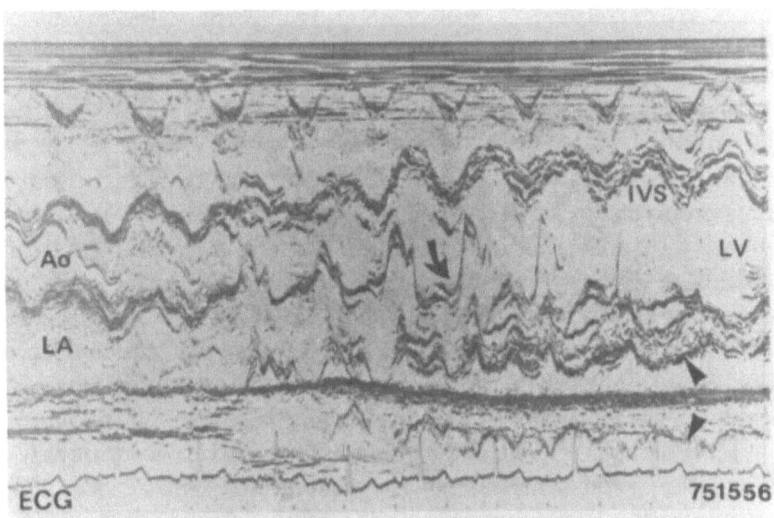

Figure 14. M-mode scan obtained from a patient with large pericardial effusion and swinging heart syndrome. Note the pseudo pattern of mid-systolic mitral valve prolapse (see arrow) and exaggeration of systolic posterior movement of the interventricular septum (IVS). Note also the reverberation between the epicardium and pericardium resulting in a mirror image of the epicardial echo behind the heart (see arrows). Ao: aorta; IVS: interventricular septum; LA: left atrium; LV: left ventricle.

anterior mitral valve leaflet, another pitfall, suggestive of functional outflow obstruction is discussed in the chapter 10 by ten Cate et al.

5. INADEQUATE CLINICAL INFORMATION

Some criteria used as a basis for diagnosis in echocardiography have a high specificity and sensitivity (e.g. those for rheumatic mitral valve stenosis, pericardial effusion) and a correct diagnosis can always be made without clinical information. For most cardiac diseases, however, current criteria are less specific and sensitive and clinical information is then highly valuable for making final conclusion. As an example: paradoxical septal motion is not a specific abnormality and seen in many conditions. Knowledge of a previous septal infarction, prior open heart surgery or the ECG findings in that situation is important for an accurate diagnosis of the echocardiographic findings. Another example is knowledge of the presence of a pacing catheter which may produce echoes mimicking vegetations on the tricuspid valve or a right sided heart tumor.

On the other hand, clinical information may bias the examiner. E.g. a pattern consistent with mitral valve prolapse is readily obtained by manipulating the transducer in long thin patients. There is always a danger searching the abnormality which fits the clinical picture.

6. INADEQUATE CONSIDERATION OF NORMAL VALUES, SENSITIVITY AND SPECIFICITY OF CRITERIA

There are many examples of misdiagnosis of heart disease which result from inadequate criteria.

In practice, a difficult diagnosis to make or to exclude is that of an hypertrophic cardiomyopathy. The criteria have limited sensitivity and specificity. Furthermore the application of these criteria require accurate measurement of septal thickness. This quantity is extremely difficult to measure and there is a large spread or range of normal values. The ratio of diastolic septal thickness to LV posterior wall thickness greater than 1.3 at one time was felt to be specific for hypertrophic cardiomyopathy. It was subsequently realized that asymmetric hypertrophy of the septum was not specific and may occur in newborns, normals, hypertension, aortic stenosis, pulmonary hypertension, coronary artery disease and congenital heart disease (see chapter 10). The echocardiographer must be aware of the accuracy and reproducibility of these measurements and in problems of the use of normal values. These problems are dealt with in chapter 4 by Lubsen et al.

There are many more examples of abnormalities initially thought to be specific for a condition, e.g. systolic anterior movement of the anterior mitral valve (see chapter 10), reduced early diastolic closure rate of the mitral valve (chapter 13), early systolic reclosure of aortic valve, etc. It must also be realized that the specificity of some criteria may change with increasing age. Early diastolic aortic valve eccentricity of more than 30% within the aorta and/or multiple cusp echoes are indicative of bicuspid aortic valve. These criteria are highly specific in young patients but loose their specificity in older patients.

Recognition of these problems is of importance to make a correct diagnosis or avoid a diagnosis of cardiac disease when none is present.

REFERENCES

1. Wells PNT: Principles of Ultrasonic Diagnosis. Academic Press, London and New York, 1969, p. 85 – 90.
2. Kossoff G, Robinson DE, Garrett WJ: Ultrasonic two-dimensional visualization for medical diagnosis. J Acoust Soc Am 44:1310 – 18, 1968.
3. Roelandt J, van Dorp WG, Bom N, Laird JD, Hugenholtz PG: Resolution problems in echocardiology: a source of interpretation errors. Am J Cardiol 37:256 – 62, 1976.
4. Millward DK, McLaurin LP, Craige E: Echocardiographic studies of the mitral valve in patients with congestive cardiomyopathy and mitral regurgitation. Am Heart J 85:413 – 21, 1973.
5. Dillon JC, Hain CL, Chang S, Feigenbaum H: Use of echocardiography in patients with prolapsed mitral valve. Circulation 43:503 – 7, 1971.
6. Kerber RE, Isaff DM, Hancock EW: Echocardiographic patterns in patients with the syndrom of systolic click and late systolic murmur. N Engl J Med 284:691 – 3, 1971.
7. Gramiak R, Wagg RC: Cardiac Ultrasound. C.V. Mosby Co, St. Louis, Mo., 1975, p. 47 – 73.

8. Sahn DJ, Allen HD, Goldberg SJ, Friedman WF: Mitral valve prolapse in children. A problem defined by real-time cross-sectional echocardiography. Circulation 53:651 – 7, 1976.

9. Welch JW, Popp RL: Variability of echocardiographic discontinuity in double outlet right ventricle and truncus arteriosus. Circulation 51:848 – 54, 1975.

10. Roelandt J: Practical Echocardiology, chapt. 2. Research Studies Press, Forest Grove, Oregon, 1977.

11. Popp RL: Effect of transducer placement on echocardiographic measurement of left ventricular dimension. Am J Cardiol 35:537, 1975.

12. Markiewicz W, Stoner J, London E, Hunt SA, Popp RL: Mitral valve prolapse in one hundred presumably healthy young females. Circulation 53:464 – 73, 1976.

13. Hirschfeld DS, Emilson BB: Echocardiogram in calcified mitral annulus. Am J Cardiol 36:354, 1975.

14. Hagan AD: Ultrasound evaluation of systolic anterior septal motion in patients with and without right ventricular volume overload. Circulation 50:248, 1974.

4. QUANTITATIVE ASPECTS OF MEASUREMENT ERROR IN ECHOCARDIOGRAPHY

J. Lubsen, J. Roelandt, H. Rijsterborgh, and R.T. van Domburg

1. QUANTITATIVE MEASUREMENTS: COMPONENTS OF ERROR

Any discussion of measurement error and its consequences in clinical practice should be based on an unequivocal definition of terms. We shall define the terms and concepts on which the following sections are based as follows:

$$M = T + B + e \qquad (1)$$

In this equation, M represents the actually observed measurement value and T the true value of the quantity being measured. B and e make up the difference between M and T, i.e. the total measurement error. B and e each represent a distinct component of that error.

B reflects the bias or systematic error in the measurement. It represents the amount by which the measurement method tends to either overestimate or underestimate the true value. We will think of it as a fixed quantity at a given level of T. On the other hand, e will reflect the random error component in the total measurement error. We will think of it as a random variable with a mean of zero (denoted by $\bar{e} = 0$) and with a certain variance, denoted by var(e).

To clarify what we exactly mean by 'bias' and 'random error', let us suppose that we have repeated the same measurement a large number of times in the same patient. We further assume T to be constant. Such repeated measurements will be denoted by M_r. The results can be represented as shown in Figure 1. Note that the respective values of M_r vary around their mean value, denoted by $\overline{M}_r$. To quantify the amount of variability of M_r around $\overline{M}_r$, we may calculate the variance of M_r, denoted by var(M_r). The variance is a standard measure of variability in statistics and its calculation may be found in any textbook. Its square root is the familiar standard deviation (sd). Note also that the figure reflects the fact that we need not necessary find that $\overline{M}_r = T$ (which we assumed to be known in the imaginary example of Figure 1 although this will rarely be the case in clinical practice).

It follows from equation (1) and the associated definitions of B (constant at a given level of T) and e (random variable with mean zero and a certain variance) that the behaviour of repeated measurements may be described as follows:

Roelandt, J. (ed.) The practice of M-mode and two-dimensional echocardiography
© *1983, Martinus Nijhoff Publishers. The Hague / Boston / London*
ISBN 978-94-009-6792-2.

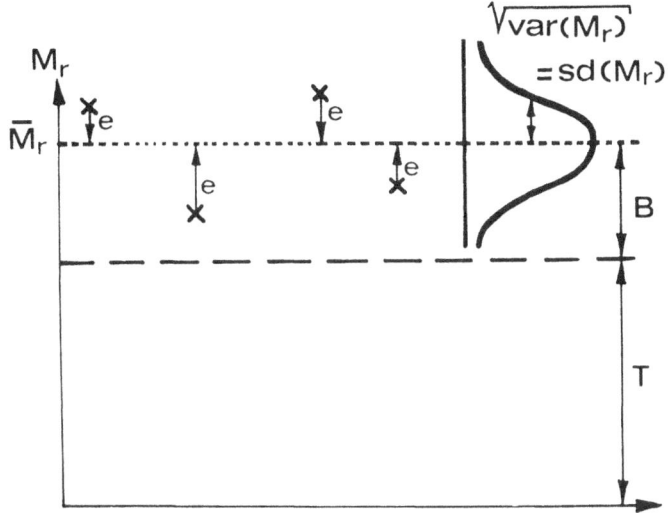

Figure 1. Diagrammatic representation of four values of repeated measurements at the same level of T (i.e. of the same quantity) and the components of error. The true value of the quantity measured (T) and the bias (B) are constant. The random error (e) varies from measurement to measurement but is zero on the avarage. The variability of M_r, represented by var(M_r) is due to the variability of e. The bell-shaped curve represents the distribution of M_r (see also text).

$$\overline{M}_r = T + B \qquad (2)$$

$$\text{var}(M_r) = \text{var}(e) \qquad (3)$$

Equation (2) follows from equation (1) because we have defined the mean of the random error, i.e. $\bar{e}$, as zero. Equation (2) demonstrates the fact that, on the average, the measurement value differs from the true value due to a bias inherent in the particular method of measurement used. Equation (3) holds, because in the case of repeated measurements, both T and B are constant and therefore do not contribute to the variability of M_r. Equation (3) demonstrates that there is a random error in the measurement method which is responsible for the fact that no two values obtained in a series of repeated measurements of the same quantity are exactly equal. It is this random error which produced the scatter of the values shown in Figure 1. It follows also from Figure 1 that bias and random error are difficult to separate. If we had had only a single measurement result M of the known quantity T, we only could have said that in this particular instance, there was a total measurement error of M − T. How much of this was due to bias and how much to random error would have been indistinguishable had we not repeated the measurement a number of times. Nevertheless, bias on the one hand and random error on the other have very different consequences, as will appear below.

In the context of definitions, a note on terminology is appropriate. In the limited amount of literature available on this topic in a medical context (see for instance [1] and [2]), one often finds the terms 'accuracy' and 'precision'. 'Accuracy' has the same connotation as 'bias'. An 'accurate' measurement method is one which produces, on the average, the true value, i.e. is without bias. 'Precision' on the other hand is used in the context of what we have called 'random error' here. A 'precise' measurement method is one which, if repeated, produces little variability in its results, i.e. has little random error. Another term often used is 'reproducibility', which has the same connotation as 'precision'. We believe that the terminology used here is more sententious and therefore more easily remembered, notwithstanding the fact that they have not found universal acceptance.

2. IMPLICATIONS OF BIAS AND RANDOM ERROR FOR THE TECHNIQUE

From the definition of bias in the previous section, it is clear that the absolute value of the bias in any particular method of measurement can only be determined if it is possible to determine the true value of the quantity being measured. In clinical practice this will rarely, if ever, be the case and it is therefore impossible to determine the bias in most methods of measurement, echocardiography being no exception. However, this must not bother us too much. Indeed, echocardiographic measurements are made in a particular patient to compare them to those made in other patients or in healthy subjects. Often, we may do repeat measurements in the same patient to follow his or her clinical condition. Random error is a prime concern in all these situations. Bias on the other hand can never be a concern as long as it is constant from measurement to measurement. The reason is that bias causes only a shift in the actual measurement values obtained but does not affect the variability of the measurements in health or disease. It cannot be overemphasized that this holds only if the bias is indeed kept constant. In echocardiography, this entails rigorous attention to detail in calibration of the equipment and in standardization of all aspects of the application of the technique. These include transducer positioning, identification of structures, timing of events in the cardiac cycle, etc., aspects which were extensively discussed in the previous chapter. Although standardization is necessary to assure constancy of bias, it should be stressed that standardization may also decrease the amount of random error. For instance, measuring at the trailing instead of the leading edge of an echo not only changes the bias but also introduces extra random error since the position of the trailing edge will depend on the gain setting. It should be stressed also that what has been said above about the lack of interest in the actual value of bias holds only for measurements obtained by the same measurement method. As soon as measurements of the same quantity made by different methods, e.g. echo- and angiocardiography, are used and compared, bias plays a very important role. This problem will be taken up again in section 3.

One general remark on the random error component e of the total measurement error and the amount of variability it produces in repeated measurements will be made here. Even in the most rigorously designed clinical study to determine the magnitude of var(e) by repeated measurements, we can almost never guarantee that the true value T is truly constant. For instance, if we repeat an echocardiogram in the same subject for a number of consecutive days, T will certainly not be the same due to within-subject biological variability. The degree to which this is the case will depend on certain aspects of the design of the study, such as e.g. the time elapsed between repeat examinations. If these are not done by the same investigator, we will further add between-investigator variability to the measurement variability and thereby to the assessment of var(e). The same is the case when the repeats are done with different machines. There are always several separate sources of random error and each will contribute to the total variability of repeated measurements. In terms of the total var(e), separate random errors certainly do not 'cancel out', notwithstanding the fact that the mean of all the random errors added together will still be zero (see note 1 of the appendix). One may conclude from this that strictly speaking, the true var(e) inherent to any clinical method of measurement can not be determined. This is not the case. What we need to know in clinical practice, and what in principle can be determined, is the var(e) of repeated measurements in stable (healthy or ill) individuals in which a certain method of measurement is applied. To what extent the var(e) of echocardiographic measurements determined in such a setting reflects random error unavoidable in ultrasound technology and/or a certain amount of clinically unavoidable within-subject biological variability, etc. is irrelevant.

3. COMPARISONS BETWEEN TWO MEASUREMENT METHODS

Echocardiography is a fairly recent technique in cardiology. Naturally, attempts have been made at various stages of its development to compare echocardiographic results with those of an established 'old' measurement technique, most commonly cineangiography. Comparisons between these two methods and consequently reports on this subject reappear every time new echocardiographic techniques are introduced.

To discuss the problems encountered when two methods of measurement are compared we shall use the framework and definitions introduced in the section 1. Let

$$M_1 = T_1 + B_1 + e_1 \tag{4}$$

represent measurements obtained with the first method, and

$$M_2 = T_2 + B_2 + e_2 \tag{5}$$

represent measurements obtained with the second. B_1 and B_2 represent the bias in each of the measurement methods and are both assumed to be constant at a certain value of T_1 and T_2 respectively. Furthermore, e_1 and e_2 represent the random errors in each of the methods. By definition they both have a mean of zero and the amount of variability they produce in repeated measurements is determined by $\text{var}(e_1)$ and $\text{var}(e_2)$ respectively.

From equations (4) and (5), it is immediately apparent what we want to know when comparing two measurement methods. First of all, we want to know the relative magnitude of B_1 and B_2. It is not really relevant (as discussed in the previous section) to determine the absolute values of both B_1 and B_2. More important is the difference between the respective biases, i.e. $B_1 - B_2$ since it is this quantity which will tell us how much larger, or smaller, measurements made with the first method will on the average be than the ones we obtain with the second method. If $B_1 - B_2 = 0$, we conclude that the biases of both methods are the same and that both methods will on the average produce the same results. On the other hand, if $B_1 - B_2 > 0$, we conclude that the first method tended on the average to produce larger results than the second one, etc. Second, we will want to know how $\text{var}(e_1)$ compares to $\text{var}(e_2)$, since the random error determines, among others, clinical usefulness. If $\text{var}(e_2)$ is smaller than $\text{var}(e_1)$, we shall certainly want to use the second instead of the first method unless its cost and/or its risk to the patient are a limitation. On the other hand, if $\text{var}(e_2) = \text{var}(e_1)$, there is not much to choose in terms of the quality of the measurements and we will prefer the method which is the simplest and/or the safest.

The important question is now how to obtain the necessary estimates of $B_1 - B_2$, $\text{var}(e_1)$ and $\text{var}(e_2)$. Obviously, a series of measurements in stable subjects repeated at least once for each of the two methods would give the answer. In practice however, such a study is often infeasible. With a non-invasive technique like echocardiography there would not be much of problem, but one can hardly repeat cineangiography to study the random error of its measurements. At best, repeated injections during one catheterization are possible. However, from measurements repeated in such a way one would obviously tend to underestimate the random error associated with repeats of the complete procedure in the same subject. In practice, we shall often have to limit ourselves to just one measurement in the same subject for each of the two methods. Comparisons between echo and angio reported in the literature are unvariably based on measurement pairs of this kind.

A pair of measurements made in a single stable subject with two different methods may be viewed as follows (see Figure 2). We have two measurement results, M_1 and M_2. Each has the structure of equations (4) and (5), i.e. is subject to its own bias and random error. Although we generally do not know T, it is reasonable to assume in a stable subject that the two measurements have been

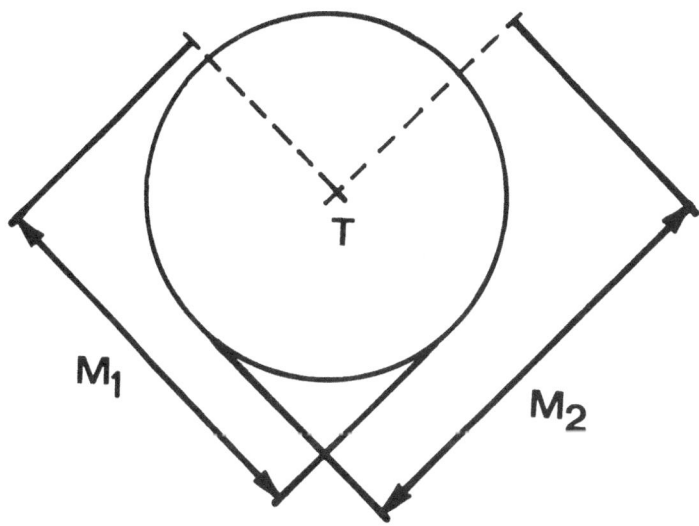

Figure 2. Structure of paired measurements. With different methods, two measurements are made of a single quantity T in a stable subject. The assumption that T is equal in both instances is reflected by drawing T as a circle (see also text).

made at the same value of T. Therefore, in paired measurements, we assume that $T_1 = T_2$. In what follows we shall omit the subscript and write T for the common true value in each pair. Now, if we have a series of pairs M_1, M_2 each made in a single stable subject, what can be said about $B_1 - B_2$, $var(e_1)$ and $var(e_2)$? Obviously, T will vary from subject to subject (between-subject variability). Therefore, although we assume T to be the same within each pair, T will vary between the pairs. We will denote the average of the T values (different for each subject!) by $\overline{T}$. Under these assumptions about the structure of paired measurements, equations (4) and (5) imply that

$$\overline{M}_1 = \overline{T} + B_1 \tag{6}$$

$$\overline{M}_2 = \overline{T} + B_2 \tag{7}$$

if we also assume that B_1 and B_2 each do not depend on T, which is a reasonable assumption if we limit the range of measurement values in the series. It follows by substraction of equation (7) from equation (6) that $\overline{M}_1 - \overline{M}_2 = B_1 - B_2$. This result implies that if we accept the assumptions mentioned above, $\overline{M}_1 - \overline{M}_2$ is, in the language of the statistician, an estimator of $B_1 - B_2$, which was one of the quantities we wanted to know when making a comparison between the two methods. In passing, we note that the familiar paired t-test is in this case a test of the null-hypothesis $B_1 - B_2 = 0$, i.e. of equality of the two biases.

Now, what about $var(e_1)$ and $var(e_2)$? Apart from the assumptions already mentioned, we shall have to introduce a few more. These are that the random errors e_1 and e_2 are independent of each other, again a perfectly reasonable assumption, and also that e_1 and e_2 are independent of the true value, which is equally reasonable if the range of measurement values in the series is not too big. Under these assumptions, we may apply to equations (4) and (5) the well known theorem from statistics, which states that the variance of the sum of two independent random variables equals the sum of the variances of each of the two variables. We then obtain:

$$var(M_1) = var(T) + var(e_1) \tag{8}$$

$$var(M_2) = var(T) + var(e_2) \tag{9}$$

These equations indicate that the total variability of each of the paired measurements is the sum of the between-subject variability (expressed by var(T)) and the variability due to its random error (expressed by var(e)). In paired measurements, the first source of variability is common to both measurements, the second on the other hand is method specific. $Var(M_1)$ and $var(M_2)$ can be calculated from the data. If we knew var(T), we could then calculate $var(e_1)$ and $var(e_2)$ from equations (8) and (9). Here, we come to a remarkable theorem, the proof of which is given in note 2 of the appendix. It says that, under the assumptions mentioned, var(T) may be estimated by the covariance of M_1 and M_2, denoted by $cov(M_1,M_2)$. The covariance is a standard measure in statistics of the covariability of two random variables; its calculation will be found in any textbook. Although it appears at first sight unlikely that we can determine from paired measurements the variance of a quantity we do not really know, i.e. T, it is not difficult to see that $cov(M_1,M_2)$ and var(T) are related. Suppose that the series of paired measurements were made in a series of subjects who were all the same (i.e. no between-subject variability). In that case var(T) = 0 and $var(M_1)$ = $var(e_1)$ while $var(M_2)$ = $var(e_2)$. The respective random errors would thus be the only sources of variability in each of the two measurements. Since e_1 and e_2 are independent random errors (i.e. $cov(e_1,e_2)$ = 0) we would expect $cov(M_1,M_2)$ to be zero also if var(T) = 0. On the other hand, as soon as there is between-subject variability (i.e. var(T) > 0) we expect a certain amount of covariability between M_1 and M_2 since for a big value of T, M_1 and M_2 will both tend to be large and for a small value of T, M_1 and M_2 will both tend to be small.

It follows from the theorem above and from equations (8) and (9) that $var(e_1)$ may be estimated by $var(M_1)$ − $cov(M_1,M_2)$ and $var(e_2)$ by $var(M_2)$ − $cov(M_1,M_2)$. A test of the null hypothesis $var(e_1)$ = $var(e_2)$ against the alternative $var(e_1) \neq var(e_2)$ is available. The test statistic may be found together with its reference in note 3 of the appendix. Thus it appears that we can obtain estimates of all quantities of interest to interpret the results of comparisons of two methods from a series of paired measurements. It is important to realize that we do not even have to know the true values of the quantity being measured although certain assumptions had to be made in the derivation of the estimators of $B_1 - B_2$, var(e_1) and var(e_2) respectively. These assumptions seem quite tenable however in many practical situations. The estimators described here were first derived in 1948 by Grubbs[3] and they are therefore known by some as the 'Grubbs estimators'.

With this background in mind, we shall now turn to a discussion of comparisons of echocardiography and cineangiocardiography based on paired measurements as they have appeared in the literature. In the vast majority of these comparisons, the following methodology is used. A scattergram is reproduced in which the paired measurements for each of the subjects studied are represented as dots. In many such diagrams, the 'line of identity' is drawn. Also we often find one or two regression lines, with or without confidence intervals and 'standard errors of the estimate' indicated. In some, all these lines are shown on the scattergrams. Invariably, the correlation coefficient calculated from the pairs of values is reported. As an example we will reproduce and discuss here one of the earlier comparisons between echocardiographic and cineangiocardiographic measurements as reported by Troy et al [4]. From this report, we will only use the data on a comparison between the left ventricular internal dimension in end-diastole, i.e. LVID(ED), as measured by M-mode echocardiography and from a cineangiocardiogram in the antero-posterior view. In their report [4], the authors have tabulated all measurement pairs on which this particular comparison is based and it was therefore possible to recreate the scattergram shown in the original report. It is reproduced here as Figure 3. Indicated also is the correlation coefficient (R) and the fact that this coefficient is statistically significant at the 1% level ($p < 0.01$). Furthermore, a so-called least squares regression line (LSRL) is drawn which represents the mean echo measurement value when the angio measurement value is known. All these were reported in the original publication also, and this way of presenting a comparison is typical for published reports dealing with similar comparisons. The question is of course whether these and related statistical methods tell us anything about the quantities of interest in a comparison of this kind, as defined before.

With respect to the correlation coefficient, the answer is: nothing. This might be fairly obvious but we shall nevertheless explain briefly why this is so. Suppose that both the echo and the angio measurement have equal bias and no random error. When we denote the echo measurement by M_2 and the angio measurement by M_1, we will have for each pair $M_2 = M_1 = T + B$. In that case the dots of Figure 3 would have fallen on the 'identity line' $M_2 = M_1$, a line which makes an angle of 45° with the horizontal (M_1) axis and goes through the origin of the scattergram. If the biases were not equal we would have, in the absence of random error, $M_2 = M_1 - (B_1 - B_2)$. The dots would fall on a line parallel to the identity line but shifted upwards or downwards, depending on the value of $(B_1 - B_2)$. In either case, it will be obvious without proof that the correlation coefficient of

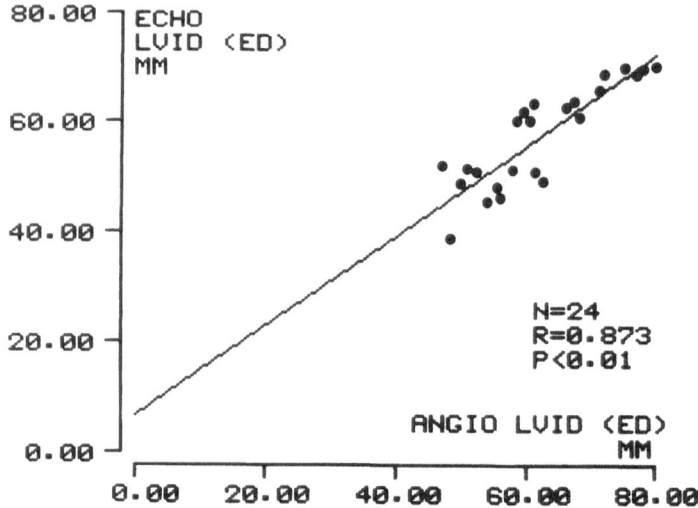

Figure 3. Paired measurements of the left ventricular internal dimension in end-diastole (LVID(ED)) derived from a cineangiocardiogram in the antero-posterior view (horizontal axis) and an M-mode echocardiogram as reported by Troy et al [4]. Explanation: see text.

M_1 and M_2, denoted by R, will be unity. However, in the real world there will be random error and any scattergram is likely to look more like Figure 3. Due to random error the dots will scatter away from the identity line. The correlation coefficient will be smaller than unity and more so the more scatter away from the identity line there is. Now the basic problem is that nor from the scattergram nor from the value of R will we be able to tell were the scatter away from the identity line comes from. It may result from a large random error in one method, even if the other method had no random error at all. Alternatively, random error in both methods may be responsible. The correlation coefficient does not distinguish between these situations. It is to a certain extent (remember that the value of the correlation coefficient depends on the range of the measurements also!) a reflection of the total random error in both methods but its value does not inform us in any way on the question how big the random error is in each of the two methods. So we have to conclude that R does not tell us anything about $(B_1 - B_2)$ and may be less than unity due to random error in any one or in both of the measurement methods compared. This fact is also apparent from the way R is calculated (see note 4 of the appendix). Troy et al [4] reported that the correlation coefficient R of the angio and echo measurements of LVID(ED) was 0.873. The fact that this figure is bigger than zero merely tells us that big ventricles appear big both to the angio- and the echocardiographer. The fact that R differs from zero at the 1%-level of statistical significance tells us only that this is unlikely to be a conclusion based on a chance finding. The fact that R is less than one is an indication that there is a less than perfect relationship between the results of angio- and echocardiography in the patients studied. This is all that can be said on the basis of the correlation coefficient reported. Next, we turn to that other often used, and abused, type of statistical analysis, the least squares regression line (LSRL). In the following we shall again denote the angio measurements of LVID(ED) by M_1 and the corresponding echo measurements by M_2. First, we have to consider the interpretation of a LSRL. The one drawn in Figure 3 gives the average value of the echo measurements (M_2) for all patients who have a certain fixed value of their angio measurement M_1. For instance, we may determine from the LSRL in Figure 3 that for all patients in whom we have measured an angio LVID(ED) of 70 mm, the average corresponding echo value is about 64 mm. Of course, this does not mean that we will always find an echo value of 64 mm in a patient in whom we have measured 70 mm on the angiocardiogram. Sometimes, the echo value will be higher, sometimes lower. Nevertheless, 64 mm is the echo LVID(ED) we expect to find when the corresponding angio measurement was 70. We will use the notation $\hat{M}_2 \mid M_1$ to denote expected values of this kind, which are determined from a LSRL. In the above example $\hat{M}_2 \mid 70 = 64$. In Figure 3, only the LSRL is drawn which describes $\hat{M}_2 \mid M_1$. The other one, which describes $\hat{M}_1 \mid M_2$ is not shown. Note however, that these two lines have very different meanings. The first gives the expected echo value $\hat{M}_2$ for a patient for whom we know the corresponding angio value M_1. The second gives the expected angio value where we know the echo value. It is always necessary to be very clear about the precise interpretation of a LSRL and to use it in the one-and-only correct way.

Now, what tell these lines us about bias and random error? The LSRL shown in Figure 3 has the following well-known general formula:

$$\hat{M}_2 \mid M_1 = a_{21}.M_1 + b_{21} \tag{10}$$

In this formula, a_{21} is called the regression coefficient. It is the tangent of the angle between the LSRL and the axis on which the so-called independent variable is plotted, i.e. the horizontal M_1-axis in Figure 3. Also, b_{21} is the so-called intercept. It is a constant and it gives the point on the axis on which the independent variable (here M_2) is plotted through which the LSRL passes. Of course, there is a second LSRL, described by:

$$\hat{M}_1 \mid M_2 = a_{12}.M_2 + b_{12} \tag{11}$$

If this line were drawn in Figure 3 also, a_{12} would be tangent of the angle between that line and the vertical (i.e. M_2-)axis and b_{12} would be the point on the horizontal (i.e. M_1-) axis through which the line passes. Now, suppose that both our paired measurements were free of random error and had equal bias. It is intuitively clear and easily shown that in that case both LSRLs would fall on the identity line. On the other hand, if there is random error, there will be scatter away from the identity line and a less perfect relationship between the paired measurements would result. This must mean that the regression coefficients become less than unity. That this is so is easily appreciated if one thinks of paired measurements with a lot of random error. The dots in the diagram will scatter all over the place and it will be impossible to say anything about, for instance, $\hat{M}_2$ if we know M_1, in which case the regression coefficient (which describes the unit change in $\hat{M}_2$ per unit change of M_1) must be zero. As is explained in note 5 of the appendix, one minus the regression coefficient is a measure of the random error in the measurement chosen as the independent variable in calculating that coefficient. Therefore, the two regression lines tell us something about the random error in each of the measurements. In that sense, they are certainly more usefull than the correlation coefficient. But they do not provide us with a direct estimate of $var(e_1)$ and $var(e_2)$. The two LSRLs also tell us something about the difference in bias. They both pass through the point $\overline{M}_1, \overline{M}_2$ a point which defines $\overline{M}_1 - \overline{M}_2$, our estimate of $B_1 - B_2$. In the figures in their publication [4], Troy et al. have drawn regression lines but their interpretation is not discussed nor are the regression coefficients and intercepts given. The LSRL in Figure 3 has the following equation:

$$\hat{M}_2 \,|\, M_1 = (0.81).M_1 + 6.88$$

From the fact that the regression coefficient is less than unity, we may draw the conclusion that the angiographic measurements are less than perfect, i.e. are subject to random error. But we would have to calculate $\hat{M}_1 \,|\, M_2$ and $\overline{M}_1 - \overline{M}_2$ to get information on the random error in the echo measurements and the difference in bias respectively.

In the context of LSRLs and comparisons of methods, a remark must be made about the standard error of the estimate (SEE). In the publication [4] from which the example discussed here was taken, SEEs are reported. It would be beyond the scope of this chapter to discuss the meaning of the SEE in detail. Suffice it to say that one interpretation of the SEE is that it provides a measure of the extent to which the LSRL fits the data points in the scattergram. An SEE of zero indicates that the points are all exactly on the LSRL. As discussed before, this means for paired measurements that both methods are free of random error. If the SEE is bigger than zero, there is a scatter around the LSRL but no direct information on random errors in each of the methods can be derived from its value.

Having thus concluded that the statistical analysis used by Troy et al [4] and similar reports does not directly address the issues in the comparison problem, we will now analyse as an example Troy et al's data on LVID(ED) by means of the Grubbs estimators. The data are tabulated in Table 1. With the help of a pocket calculator with basic statistical functions, the results given in Table 2 may be verified. From the means of the measurements we estimate $B_1 - B_2$ as 62.2 − 57.5 = 4.7 mm. This means that echocardiography tends to underestimate LVID(ED) measurements from angiograms by 4.7 mm. The paired t-test of the

Table 1. Left-ventricular internal dimension in end-diastole (LVID(ED)) in mm by angio- and echocardiography in 24 patients

LVID(ED)		LVID(ED)		LVID(ED)	
Angio	Echo	Angio	Echo	Angio	Echo
54.2	45.5	50.0	48.8	47.2	52.0
75.4	70.0	58.0	51.5	48.4	39.0
72.0	68.5	68.0	61.0	50.8	51.5
62.6	49.5	55.2	48.3	52.4	51.0
61.2	63.5	78.0	69.5	67.2	63.5
58.8	60.5	77.6	69.0	80.0	70.0
60.4	60.5	61.6	51.0	55.6	46.5
71.6	65.5	67.0	63.0	59.6	61.5

Data taken from Troy et al [4].

Table 2. Statistics calculated from Table 1

	LVID(ED) in mm			
	Angio (M_1)		Echo (M_2)	
$\overline{M}_1$, $\overline{M}_2$	62.2		57.5	t_{23} = 4.73 (p < 0.001)[a]
var(M_1), var(M_2)	97.0		84.4	
cov(M_1,M_2)		79.0		
vâr(e_1), vâr(e_2)[b]	18.0		5.4	t_{22} = 0.67 (ns)[c]
sîd(e_1), sîd(e_2)	4.2		2.3	

[a] paired t-test with 23 degrees of freedom of $\overline{M}_1 = \overline{M}_2$ versus $\overline{M} \neq \overline{M}_2$.

[b] Grubbs estimators (see text).

[c] t-test with 22 degrees of freedom of var(e_1) = var(e_2) versus var(e_1) ≠ var(e_2); see note 3 of appendix.

difference between the means is highly significant, indicating that the $B_1 - B_2$ differs indeed significantly from zero. The Grubbs estimators of the variances of the random errors in angio and echo LVID(ED) measurements are 18.0 and 5.4 mm² respectively. Although it appears that the random error in the angio is larger than in the echo measurement, the difference is not significant by the test described in note 3 of the appendix. Therefore, we conclude that we do not have strong evidence in these data that echo is indeed better than angio in terms of random measurement error.

In this context, it is worthy to note that Troy et al. had their echocardiograms measured twice by two different observers. The values used in their comparisons are the average of the two measurements, which will have removed some of the random error associated with their echo measurements. When we take the square roots of the var(e) estimates, we obtain 4.2 and 2.3 mm respectively. These represent estimates of the standard deviations of the respective random errors. In clinical practice, it is important to have such estimates, in particular when measurements are used to follow a patient's clinical condition. We derive from it the knowledge that an echocardiographic measurement of LVID(ED) in a single subject will lie between $\{ T + B - 2.(2.3) \}$ mm and $\{ T + B + 2.(2.3) \}$ mm with approximately 95% probability. Obviously, 2.(2.3) represents two times the standard deviation of the random error component in the echocardiographic measurement and the rest of the statement follows from standard statistical theory. If we have two echocardiographic measurements of LVID(ED), the difference would have to be considerably bigger than 2.(2.3) = 4.6 mm in order to conclude that there was a difference in the size of the patient's heart (in fact, the difference would have to exceed 6.6 mm to be reasonably sure, see note 6 of the appendix).

We close this discussion with a few remarks on the limitations of the Grubbs estimators. The most important one is the fact that fairly rigid assumptions had to be made in their derivation. The assumption of independence of random errors of each other is tenable by definition, i.e. in view of the behaviour of random error. On the other hand, the assumption that the bias and the random error are independent of the true value may not be reasonable in many situations unless the range of the measurements in the paired series is small. It may be necessary to do separate comparison studies in different parts of the range of values of clinical interest. Of course the assumption that the values are equal in ach pair of observations can only be met up to a certain extent. Here, however, the same remark on the impossibility and the irrelevance of keeping T truly constant in reproducibility studies made in section 2 applies. Finally, a considerable number of data pairs is required. Primarily with small sets of data, a negative estimate of var(e_1) or var(e_2) may occur. This is unacceptable. In our experience, some 75 pairs are needed to have any confidence in the results. Notwithstanding these drawbacks, one may wonder why the estimators discussed here have been so rarely applied to the study of measurement problems in clinical medicine, where their application seems self-evident. Nevertheless, as with all statistical methods, the question whether the underlying assumptions are tenable in a particular case remains a matter of careful consideration.

REFERENCES

1. Wulff HR: Rational Diagnosis and Treatment (2nd edition). Blackwell, Oxford, 1981.
2. Sokal RR, Rohlf FJ: Biometry; the principles and practice of statistics in biological research. Freeman, Chicago, 1969.
3. Grubbs FE: Errors of Measurement, Precision, Accuracy and the Statistical Comparison of Measuring Instruments. Technometrics Vol 15 – 1:53 – 65, 1973.
4. Troy BL, Pombo J, Rackley CE: Measurement of Left Ventricular Wall Thickness and Mass by Echocardiography. Circulation Vol XLV:602 – 611, 1972.
5. Maloney CJ, Rastogi SC: Significance test for Grubbs's estimators. Biometrics, vol 26 – 4:671 – 676, 1970.

APPENDIX

Note 1. On various sources of random error

If $M = T + B + e_1 + e_2 + e_3 + \ldots$, where $e_1, e_2, e_3 \ldots$ represent various sources of random error each with mean zero and a certain variance, it follows that, if we assume each of the random errors to be independent of all others:

$$\overline{M}_r = T + B \tag{1}$$

$$\text{var}(M_r) = \text{var}(e_1) + \text{var}(e_3) + \ldots \tag{2}$$

These equations illustrate the wellknown fact that various random errors 'cancel out' in terms of their mean value only but not in terms of the total scatter of repeated measurements as reflected by $\text{var}(M_r)$.

Note 2. Proof of the theorem underlying the Grubbs estimators

In what follows, $E(x)$ and $\overline{x}$ denote the expected value of the random variable x. Let $M_1 = T_1 + B_1 + e_1$ and $M_2 = T_2 + B_2 + e_2$. Assume that $T_1 = T_2 = T$ since we are dealing with paired measurements in the same subject. Assume furthermore that B_1 and B_2 are constants, $E(e_1) = E(e_2)$ 0, $E(e_1)(T - \overline{T}) = 0$, $E(e_2)(T - \overline{T}) = 0$ and $E(e_1)(e_2) = 0$. Then we have: $E(M_1 - \overline{M}_1)(M_2 - \overline{M}_2) = E(T + B_1 + e_1 - \overline{T} - B_1)(T + B_2 + e_2 - \overline{T} - B_2) = E(T - \overline{T})(T - \overline{T}) + E(e_1)(T - \overline{T}) + E(e_2)(T - \overline{T}) + E(e_1)(e_2)$. From this equality and the assumptions mentioned, it follows that the variance of T is estimated by the covariance of M_1 and M_2 since $E(M_1 - \overline{M}_1)(M_2 - \overline{M}_2)$ is $\text{cov}(M_1, M_2)$ and $E(T - \overline{T})(T - \overline{T})$ is $\text{var}(T)$ by definition.

Note 3. Significance test for Grubbs estimators

Maloney and Rastogi [5] have derived the following test for $\text{var}(e_1) = \text{var}(e_2)$ against $\text{var}(e_1) \neq \text{var}(e_2)$. Let $U = M_1 + M_2$ and $V = M_1 - M_2$. The test statistic is:

$$t = \frac{R_{uv}(n - 2)^{1/2}}{(1 - R_{uv}^2)^{1/2}}$$

R_{uv} represents the product-moment correlation coefficient of U and V, i.e.

$$\frac{\text{cov}(U,V)}{\text{sd}(U).\text{sd}(V)}, \text{ and}$$

n the number of pairs in the comparison. Under H_0: $\text{var}(e_1) = \text{var}(e_2)$, t follows student's t distribution with $(n-2)$ degrees of freedom. For the power of the test, see Maloney and Rastogi [5].

Note 4. The correlation coefficient of paired measurements

Using the notation and definitions of section 3, the correlation coefficient R of a series of paired measurements is given by the wellknown formula

$$R = \frac{\text{cov}(M_1,M_2)}{\{\text{var}(M_1). \text{var}(M_2)\}^{1/2}} \tag{3}$$

Based on the theorem proven in note 2, it is obvious that we expect R to be unity if $\text{var}(e_1) = \text{var}(e_2) = 0$. For, in that instance both the numerator and the denominator of (3) are estimators of $\text{var}(T)$. If $\text{var}(e_1)$ or $\text{var}(e_2)$ or both are greater than zero, $\text{cov}(M_1),M_2)$ will still estimate $\text{var}(T)$ (see note 2). Therefore, the numerator in (3) will be unaffected by $\text{var}(e_1)$ or $\text{var}(e_2)$. However, the denominator of (3) will increase with increasing magnitude of $\text{var}(e_1)$ or $\text{var}(e_2)$ and R will become less than unity.

Note 5. Paired measurements and regression coefficients

Let $\hat{M}_2|M_1 = a_{21}.M_1 + b_{21}$ represent the least-squares regression line (LSRL) of M_2 on M_1, M_1 and M_2 representing the two measurements respectively in a series of paired measurements. The regression coefficient a_{21} is given by the formula

$$a_{21} = \frac{\text{cov}(M_1,M_2)}{\text{var}(M_1)}$$

It is clear that we expect a_{21} to be unity when $\text{var}(e_1) = 0$ since in that case both $\text{cov}(M_1,M_2)$ and $\text{var}(M_1)$ estimate $\text{var}(T)$ (see note 2). If $\text{var}(e_1) > 0$, $\text{cov}(M_1,M_2)$ will still estimate $\text{var}(T)$ but $\text{var}(M_1)$ will estimate $\text{var}(T) + \text{var}(e_1)$. Therefore, we expect a_{21} to become smaller than one with increasing $\text{var}(e_1)$. It follows that $(1 - a_{21})$ is a measure of $\text{var}(e_1)$.

Note that in the above argument, $\text{var}(e_2)$ does not play a role. Note also that, by a symmetrical argument, $(1 - a_{12})$ is a measure of $\text{var}(e_2)$.

Note 6. Measurement error and follow-up studies

A common problem in clinical medicine occurs when two measurements made with the same method in the same patient are compared to determine whether the patient's condition has changed. Let $M_1 = T_1 + B_1 + e_1$ represent the first measurement and $M_2 = T_2 + B_2 + e_2$ the second. If we assume that the patient's condition is in fact unchanged and the method well standardized, we imply that we assume $T_1 = T_2$ and $B_1 = B_2$. In that case we expect $M_2 - M_1 = 0$. However, $M_2 - M_1$ may be non-zero due to random error. Under the assumptions mentioned we have:

$$var(M_2 - M_1) = var(e_1) + var(e_2)$$

This is so because, under the assumptions mentioned above, M_1 and M_2 are independent random variables and because the variance of the difference of two independent random variables is the sum of their respective variances. Since we have used the same measurement method, we may assume $var(e_1) = var(e_2) = var(e)$ and write $var(M_2 - M_1) = 2\ var(e)$. This means that $M_2 - M_1$ lies with approximately 95% probability between $-2.\sqrt{2\ var(e)}$ and $+2.\sqrt{2\ var(e)}$ if we assume that the patient was in fact stable. This statement is based on statistical theory indicating that, if x is a normally distributed random variable with mean $\bar{x}$ and variance var(x), 95% of its values lie within $\bar{x} \pm 1.96\ \sqrt{var(x)}$. From the data provided by Troy et al [4] we found that for echocardiographic measurements of LVID(ED), $var(e) = 5.4\ mm^2$ (see Table 2). This means that $M_2 - M_1$ would have to be either bigger than 6.6 mm (i.e. $2\ \sqrt{2.(5.4)}$) or smaller that -6.6 mm to be 95% confident that the heart had either increased or decreased in size over the period of time which passed between M_1 and M_2. This argument applies only if the decision to do M_2 was not influenced by the fact that M_1 was found to be particularly high or low. If that was the case, we would have to take the 'regression-to-the-mean' phenomenon into account with the help of a least-squares regression line which describes $\hat{M}_2|M_1$, with appropriate confidence intervals for $M_2|M_1$. A full discussion of this topic is outside the present scope.

5. DOPPLER-ECHOCARDIOGRAPHY; ITS ADVANTAGES AND LIMITATIONS IN ADULT CARDIOLOGY

R. JENNI, A. VIELI, M. ANLIKER, AND H.P. KRAYENBUEHL

Doppler-echocardiography is a new non-invasive method which ultimately may lead to quantitative measurements of blood flow in the four cavities of the heart as well as in the large vessels. The principal aim of Doppler-echocardiography is to evaluate quantitatively mitral- aortic-and tricuspid insufficiencies, and, if possible, the stenoses of the semilunar leaflets.

PREREQUISITES FOR QUANTITATIVE MEASUREMENTS OF BLOOD FLOW WITH PULSED DOPPLER ULTRASOUND

In a vessel with a circular cross-section of radius R and a velocity profile V(r), the flow Q is given by

$$Q = \frac{\pi}{\cos a} \cdot \int_{-R}^{+R} V(r) \cdot r \cdot dr \qquad (1)$$

where a : angle between the ultrasound beam and the axis of the vessel; r : Radial coordinate with $r = 0$ corresponding to the center of the vessel and $r \overset{>}{<} 0$ representing the proximal and distal half of the cross-section respectively.

If the flow is calculated according to formula (1), the following variables must be known:
1. V(r) Velocity distribution in the crosssection of the vessel.
2. a Angle between the ultrasound beam and the axis of the vessel.
3. 2R Diameter of the cross-section, which is assumed to be circular.

If instead of V(r), the average velocity within the cross-section of the vessel is known, formula (1) can be rewritten as:

$$Q = \frac{1}{\cos a} \cdot \bar{v} \cdot F \qquad (2)$$

whereby $\bar{v}$: Average velocity across the cross-section of the vessel; F : Cross-sectional area of the vessel.

Thus the prerequisite for quantitative blood flow measurements is either to:

Roelandt, J. (ed.) The practice of M-mode and two-dimensional echocardiography
© *1983, Martinus Nijhoff Publishers. The Hague / Boston / London*
ISBN 978-94-009-6792-2.

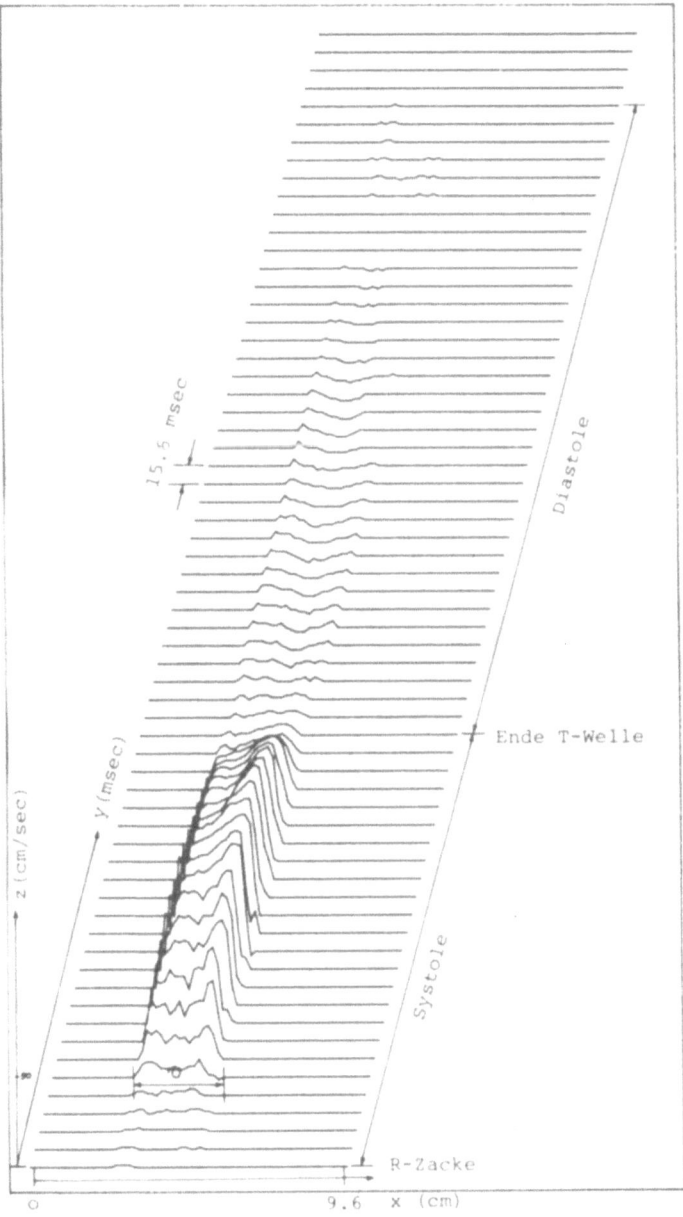

Figure 1. Velocity profiles in the ascending aorta of a healthy subject (averages of 10 heart cycles).

1. record a velocity profile along the ultrasound beam axis within the cross-section of the vessel
or
2. to determine the average velocity within the cross-section.

By means of echocardiography, the angle between the ultrasound beam and the axis of the vessel, as well as the vessel diameter can be determined.

The presently available echo-Doppler instruments are 'one channel' instruments, which only measure the velocity of the blood flow as a function of time at *one* point ("sample volume") within a vessel or a cavity of the heart.

Dynamic changes of the velocity distribution in the vessel cannot be evaluated. It is conceivable, however, that one could increase the so-called "sample volume" so that it contains the entire lumen of the vessel and accordingly provides a measure of the average velocity [1]. In this case the flow can be calculated with formula 2.

In order to record temporal variations of the velocity profiles in larger vessels or heart cavities, multi-channel Doppler instruments are necessary. With such instruments the channels are distributed along the ultrasound beam. Our Doppler instrument has a range of 9.7 cm which is divided into 128 equally spaced channels [2]. Thus it is possible to measure the blood flow velocity simultaneously at 128 different intervals Figure 1 shows the velocity profiles in the aorta ascendens of a healthy person. The profiles were recorded from the suprasternal notch.

x : Distance in (cm) divided into 128 identical distances x = 0 corresponds to the skin surface.
y : Time in msec. The profiles are separated by 16 msec, starting from the R-wave of the ECG.

Figure 2. Definition of volume-Flow.

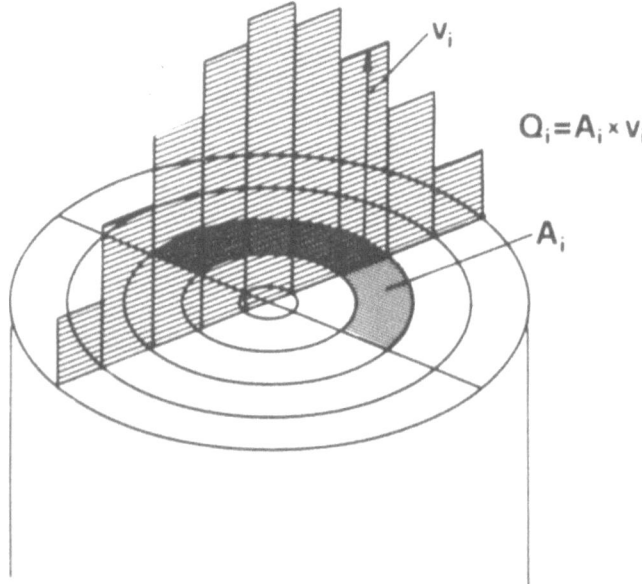

$$Q_i = A_i \times v_i$$

Figure 2. Definition of volume-Flow.

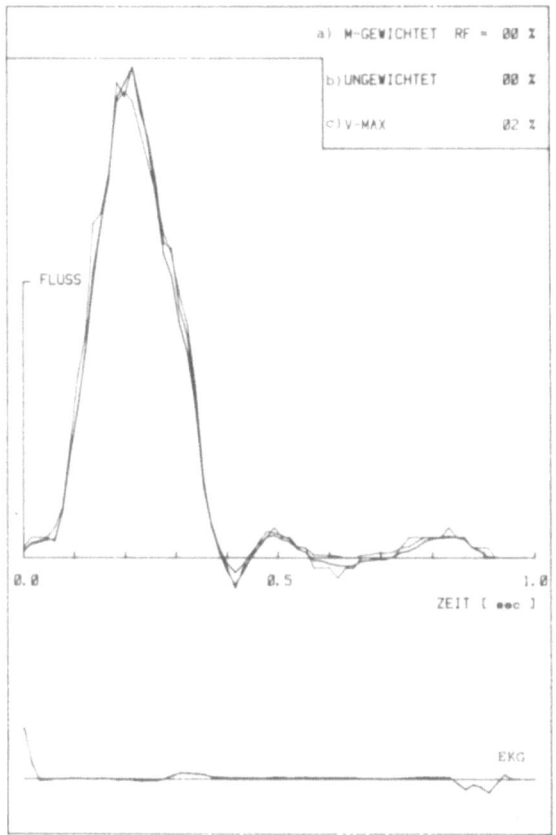

Figure 3. Volume-flow pattern calculated from the velocity profiles given in Figure 1.

z : Relative velocity in cm/sec. Positive velocities represent flow away from the heart, negative velocities flow towards the heart.

d : Diameter of the vessel in cm.

DETERMINATION OF THE VOLUME-FLOW FROM THE VELOCITY DISTRIBUTION

In Figure 1 a velocity profile is shown schematically.

v_i : Average velocity in channel i
A_i : Corresponding half-annular area
$Q_i = a_i \cdot v_i$: Flow in area A_i

The summation of the Q_i values yields the total flow [3]. As illustrated in Figure 2, the cross-section is subdivided into half-annuli whose widths correspond to the depth interval of the individual channel. The velocity determined by any one of the channels is considered to be constant over the corresponding half-annulus.

Figure 3 shows the volume-flow calculated from the velocity profiles given in Figure 1.

The three different curves represent:

a. flow pattern computed as indicated in Figure 2 (so called M-weighted-flow)
b. flow pattern based on 'unweighted' mean of velocities
c. flow pattern based on normalized instantaneous maximum velocity

The good agreement among the three flow patterns is an indication that in the case of healthy subjects the velocity field is "well behaved".

CLINICAL FUNDAMENTALS OF DOPPLER-ECHOCARDIOGRAPHY

The clinical applications of Doppler-echocardiography, as described in the literature, refers almost exclusively to the 'one-channel' Doppler device combined with a one- or a two-dimensional echography system [4].

The problems encountered in measuring flow with 'one-channel' Doppler system is illustrated by an actual situation. In Figure 4, the velocity profiles in the aorta ascendens of a patient with severe aortic insufficiency are shown. The recording was made from the suprasternal notch with a 128-channel, digital Doppler-instrument.

The lower half of Figure 4 shows the systolic profiles, the upper half the diastolic profiles. In contrast the velocity profiles indicate back flow during the entire diastolic period. The profiles were averaged synchronously with the ECG during 10 successive heart cycles.

If in the same patient, the velocity pattern would be recorded by a 'one-channel' Doppler system, the velocity as a function of time would depend very much on the position of the channel in the lumen of the aorta ascendens as illustrated in Figure 5.

The five velocity patterns were obtained from the velocity profiles given in Figure 4. The second curve (measurement near the anterior wall of the aorta) yields an aortic regurgitation fraction of about 90%, whereas in the center of the vessel the fraction is only 40%. It is thus clearly demonstrated that a 'one-channel' Doppler system does not allow for a reliable determination of the regurgitation fraction. This is not only true in the case of aortic insufficiency but also in the cases of mitral- and tricuspid insufficiencies.

DETERMINATION OF THE AORTIC REGURGITATION FRACTION

If the aortic regurgitation fraction is calculated according to Figure 2, the velocity profiles in Figure 4 yield a value of 32%. The angiographic value, however, is 80%.

If on the other hand one assumes that the instantaneous flow is proportional to

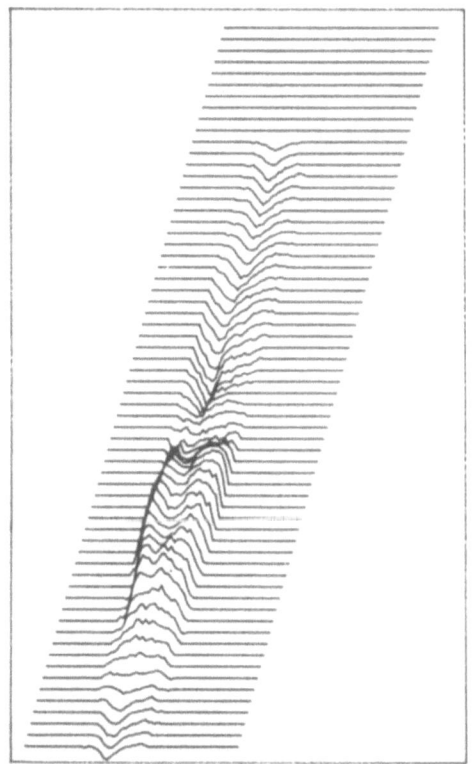

Figure 4. Velocity profiles in the aorta ascendens, of a patient with severe aortic insufficiency. The graphic parameters are aequivalent to those of Figure 1.

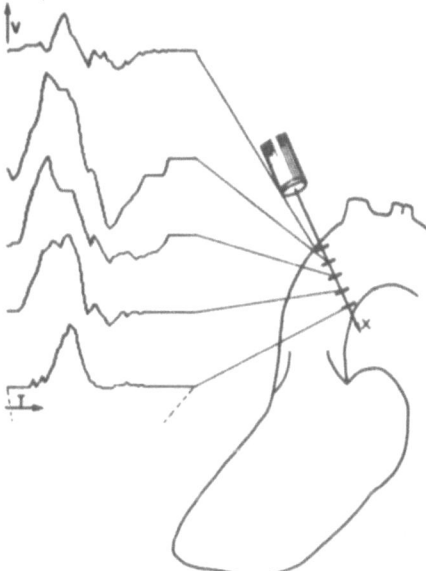

Figure 5. Blood velocity as a function of time at five different points of measurement within the aorta ascendens V = velocity, T = time, X = ultrasound beam axis.

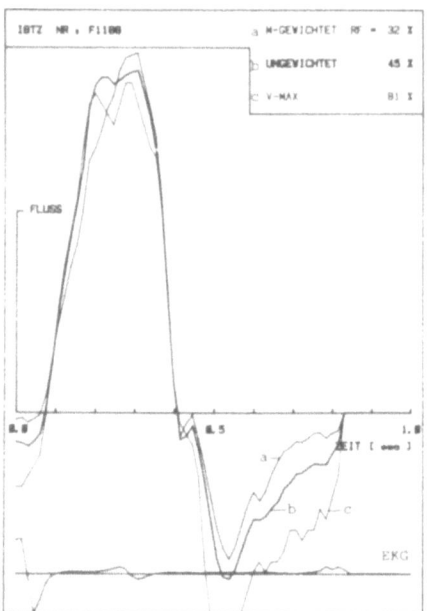

Figure 6. Flow patterns in patient with severe aortic insufficiency.

the instantaneous maximum velocity within the cross-section, the aortic regurgitation fraction is 81%. Finally, if the regurgitation fraction is calculated from the unweighted average velocity, the resulting value is 45%. Figure 6 shows the flow patterns, computed with the three methods utilized.

a. flow patterns computed according to Figure 2.
b. flow pattern based on the unweighted average velocity.
c. flow pattern based on instantaneous maximum velocities.

The large variations of the results for the regurgitation fraction based on the three methods is due to the fact that the shape of the instantaneous velocity profiles undergoes drastic changes during the cardiac cycle. In a recent study [5] it was shown that the determination of the regurgitation fraction on the basis of the instantaneous maximum velocity agrees within ± 15% with the corresponding values obtained in the catheter laboratory.

OUTLOOK

The success of quantitative Doppler-echocardiography largely depends on the realisation of a two-dimensional echograph with a multichannel Doppler system capable of measuring reliably and accurately the velocity profiles at depths up to 20 – 25 cm.

REFERENCES

1. Gill RW: Pulse Doppler with B-Mode Imaging for Quantitative Blood Flow Measurement, Ultrasound in Med and Biol 5:223 – 225, 1979.
2. Brandestini M: Signalverarbeitung in perkutanen Ultraschall Doppler Blutfluss Messgeräten, Diss. ETHZ, 1976.
3. Doriot PA: Blutflussmessung mit Hilfe eines mehrkanaligen Ultraschall-Doppler-Gerätes, Diss. ETHZ, 1976.
4. Goldberg SJ, Allen HD, Sahn DJ: Pediatric and Adolescent Echocardiography (2nd ed.); Year Book Medical Publisher, 1980.
5. Jenni R, Hübscher W, Casty M, Anliker M, HP Krayenbühl: Quantitation of Aortic Regurgitation by a Percutaneous 129-Channel Digital Ultrasound Doppler Instrument, Echocardiology, Ch. T. Lancee (ed.), Martinus Nijhoff Publishers, The Hague, 1979.

III. CLINICAL USEFULNESS OF TRANSESOPHAGEAL AND CONTRAST ECHOCARDIOGRAPHY

Transesophageal echocardiography is a recent investigational technique which offers advantages in patients in whom poor quality echocardiograms are obtained from the precordial transducer position as a result of chest deformity or obstructive lung disease.

In addition the method allows recording of M-mode and two-dimensional echocardiograms not disturbed by respiration and chest wall movements. This may be an advantage during exercise as continuous good left ventricular echocardiograms can be obtained.

Another advantage is the visualization of awkward area's of the heart which are not readily accessible from the precordial approach. The many aspects of transesophageal echocardiography are discussed in chapter 6.

Contrast echocardiography allows to image intracardiac blood flow patterns and complements standard echocardiography which only provides information on cardiac structure and function. Their combination makes it possible to obtain data which were heretofore available only from cardiac catheterization and angiocardiography. Chapters 7 and 8 in this part deal with the many modalities of cardiac investigation using contrast echocardiography in infants, children, and adults. It will become obvious to the reader that M-mode and two-dimensional echocardiography supplemented with contrast echocardiography may preclude the need for cardiac catheterization and angiocardiography in many instances.

Roelandt, J. (ed.) The practice of M-mode and two-dimensional echocardiography
© 1983, Martinus Nijhoff Publishers. The Hague / Boston / London
ISBN 978-94-009-6792-2.

6. TRANSESOPHAGEAL (M-MODE AND TWO-DIMENSIONAL) ECHOCARDIOGRAPHY

P. Hanrath, M. Schlüter, B.A. Langenstein, J. Souquet, J. Polster, and P. Kremer

Compromised image quality due to abnormal chest wall configuration, small intercostal space, obesity, emphysema, chronic obstructive pulmonary disease is the main limitation of conventional M-mode and two-dimensional echocardiography. Even in patients with a normal "echo window" it is sometime difficult to visualize certain anatomical structures (e.g. interatrial septum or LV-apex) due to anatomical or physical reasons. Another limitation of transthoracic echocardiography is its application during dynamic exercise. Transducer instability due to heavy chest wall movement and lung tissue interference with the ultrasound beam during heavy inspiration are the main reasons why exercise echocardiography is only of limited importance in clinical cardiology compared with radionucleid techniques.

In order to overcome these limitations we recently used transesophageal M-mode and two-dimensional echocardiography in clinical practice. For this purpose a special single-element transducer (3.5 or 5 MHz) (Figure 1) or a multi-element phased array transducer (3.5 MHz) (Figure 2) was incorporated into the tip of a commercially available gastroscope [1 – 9]. This allowed easy introduction of the transducer and an external control of transducer position by angulation of the tip of the gastroscope in 2 orthogonal planes, as well as up – and downward movement or rotation of the shaft of the gastroscope by the examiner.

EXAMINATION TECHNIQUE

Due to the fact that in the presently used prototypes the fibre optics system of the gastroscope has been removed, a barium X-ray examination of the esophagus must be performed prior to the ultrasound examination in order to exclude a diverticulum. The patient has to be fasted for about eight hours and receives 0.5 mg atropinsulfate s.c. one hour prior to the examination in order to avoid bradycardia or hypersalivation. The transesophageal study is done while the patient is lying in a supine position. The patient usually swallows the ultrasound gastroscope as easily as he would a normal endoscopic fiberscope. Complications were not observed in over 150 transesophageal M-mode and two-dimensional studies which were done in the last 18 months.

Roelandt, J. (ed.) The practice of M-mode and two-dimensional echocardiography
© *1983, Martinus Nijhoff Publishers. The Hague / Boston / London*
ISBN 978-94-009-6792-2.

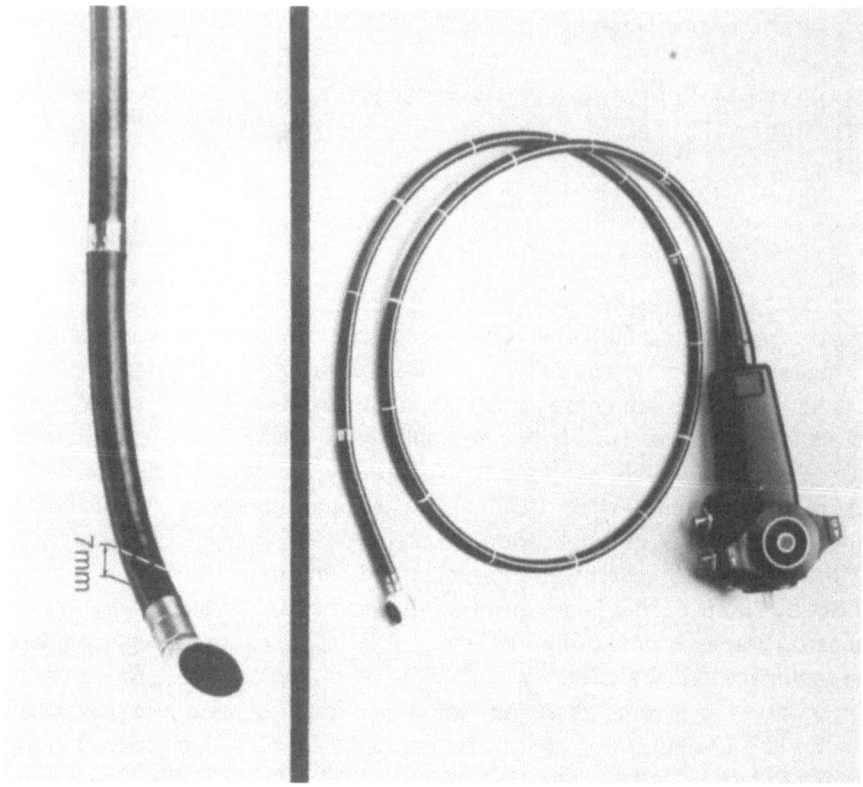

Figure 1. Gastroscope with a single element ultrasound transducer with an outer diameter of the gastroscope of 7 mm.

TRANSESOPHAGEAL M-MODE ECHOCARDIOGRAPHY

After insertion of the gastroscope to a depth of about 40 cm, the first cardiac structure that is easily identified is the aortic root with its leaflets. By further insertion and slight counter-clockwise rotation of the gastroscope the anterior and posterior mitral leaflets are visualized. The transesophageal image of the left ventricle at the level of the free edges of the mitral leaflets is an upside-down version of the normal transthoracic image. That means the left ventricular posterior wall is near to the transducer, the anterior wall of the left ventricle is far from the transducer. Due to the fact that there is no limitation of transducer orientation by ribs and lung tissue, the septal as well as the anterior region of the left ventricle can be visualized easily by rotation of the gastroscope.

Transesophageal imaging is not disturbed by respiration and chest wall excursion. So even during a severe bicycle exercise test in a supine position a continuous, good image of the left ventricle can be obtained. The recording allows a

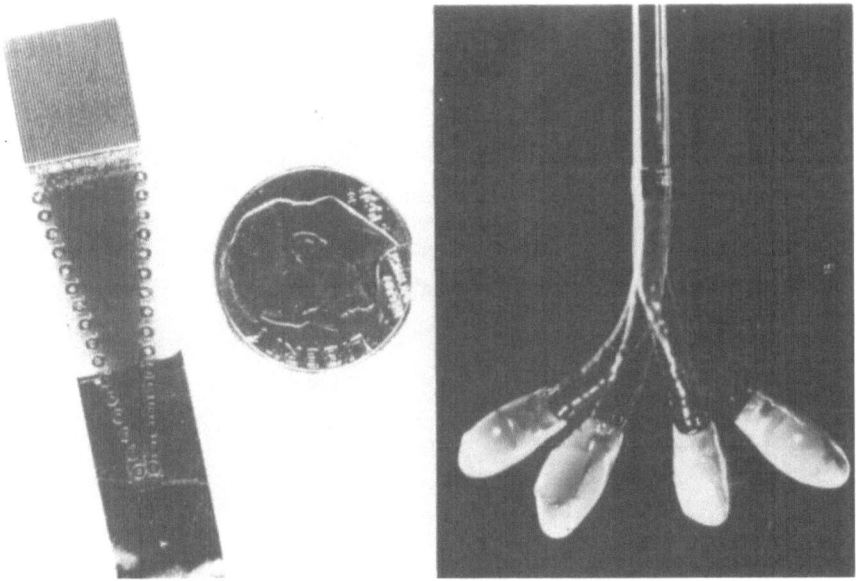

Figure 2. Gastroscope (9 mm diameter) with an array of 32 ultrasound elements for phased array imaging. The tip of the gastroscope with the transducer can be angulated in every direction by an external knob in order to guarantee a close contact between the surface of the transducer and the esophageal wall.

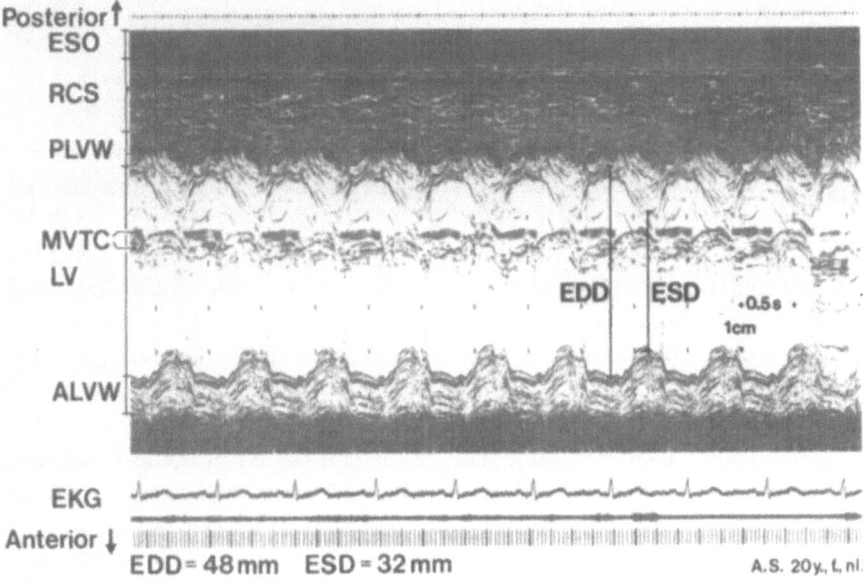

Figure 3. Transesophageal M-mode recording in a normal subject at rest. ALVW : antero-lateral left ventricular wall, MVTC : mitral valve chordae tendineae, LV : left ventricle, PLVW : posterior left ventricular wall, RCS : retrocardial space, ESO : esophageal wall.

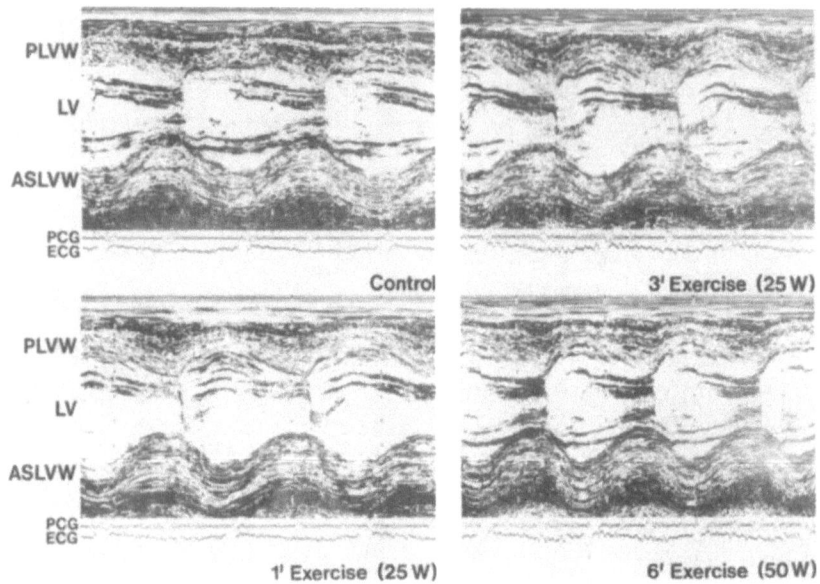

Figure 4. Transesophageal M-mode recording in a patient with hypertrophic cardiomyopathy at rest and during supine bicycle ergometry. ASLVW : antero-septal left ventricular wall, PLVW : posterior left ventricular wall, LV : left ventricle.

beat-to-beat analysis as it is exemplarily shown in a normal subject (Figure 3) and in a patient with hypertrophic cardiomyopathy (Figure 4).

TRANSESOPHAGEAL CROSS-SECTIONAL ECHOCARDIOGRAPHY

For two-dimensional cardiac imaging a special 3.5 MHz transducer array of 32 elements is fitted to the distal end of an endoscope with an outer diameter of 9 mm.

Figure 5 represents a cross-sectional view of the aortic root. All 3 cusps are visible and parts of the left atrium as well as the right and left ventricular outflow tract are clearly outlined. In some patients the origin of the right or more often of the left coronary artery can be visualized (Figure 6). By further insertion of the gastroscope and slight counter-clockwise rotation the left atrium and both mitral leaflets can be seen in a tangential plane (Figure 7a). The visualization of the left ventricle in several cross-sectional views at different levels of the left ventricular long axis can be achieved by further insertion of the gastroscope (Figure 7b – d). Depending on the anatomical relationship between the heart and the esophagus in the individual patient, both ventricles can be imaged within a 90° sector image if the heart is not dilated (Figure 8). By clockwise rotation of the gastroscope at the atrio-ventricular junction the right atrium, the interatrial septum and the right ventricle can be identified (Figure 9).

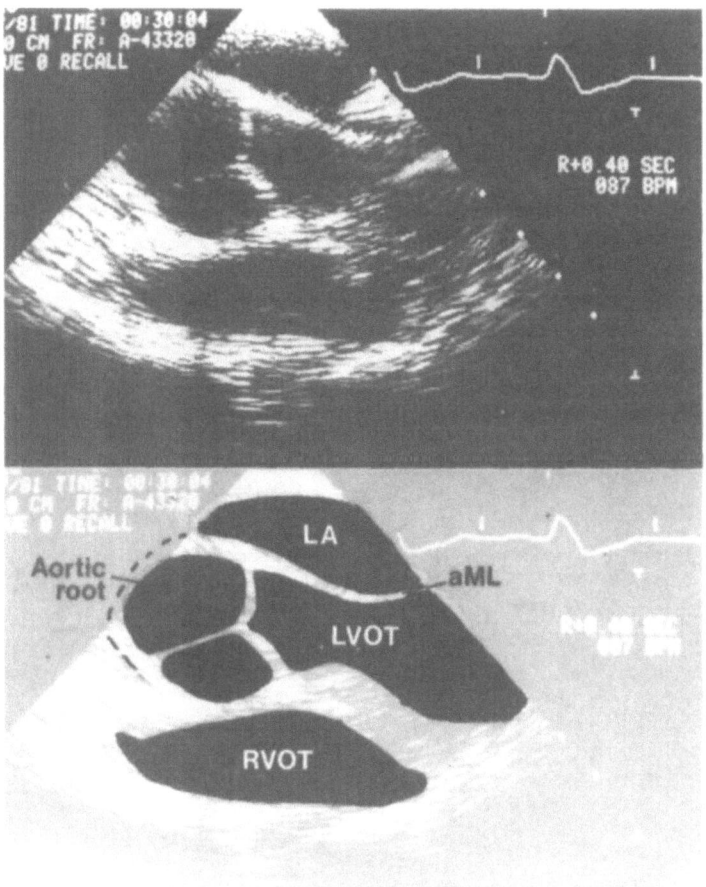

Figure 5. Cross section image of the aortic root with the aortic cusps in a closed position (Mercedes Benz-like configuration).

DISCUSSION

Since the first clinical application of transesophageal echocardiography by Frazin et al. in 1976 [10] only a few studies concerning the evaluation of left ventricular function at rest by the transesophageal approach were published [11 – 14]. This was in part due to the unique technique and partly due to the difficulty of transducer control. In order to further apply this technique as a routine method for the evaluation of left ventricular function during surgery [8] or during exercise [1 – 4] the transducer system had to be improved for a better external control. The incorporation of the ultrasound transducer into the tip of a gastroscope or bronchoscope-like instrument – as it was recently reported by

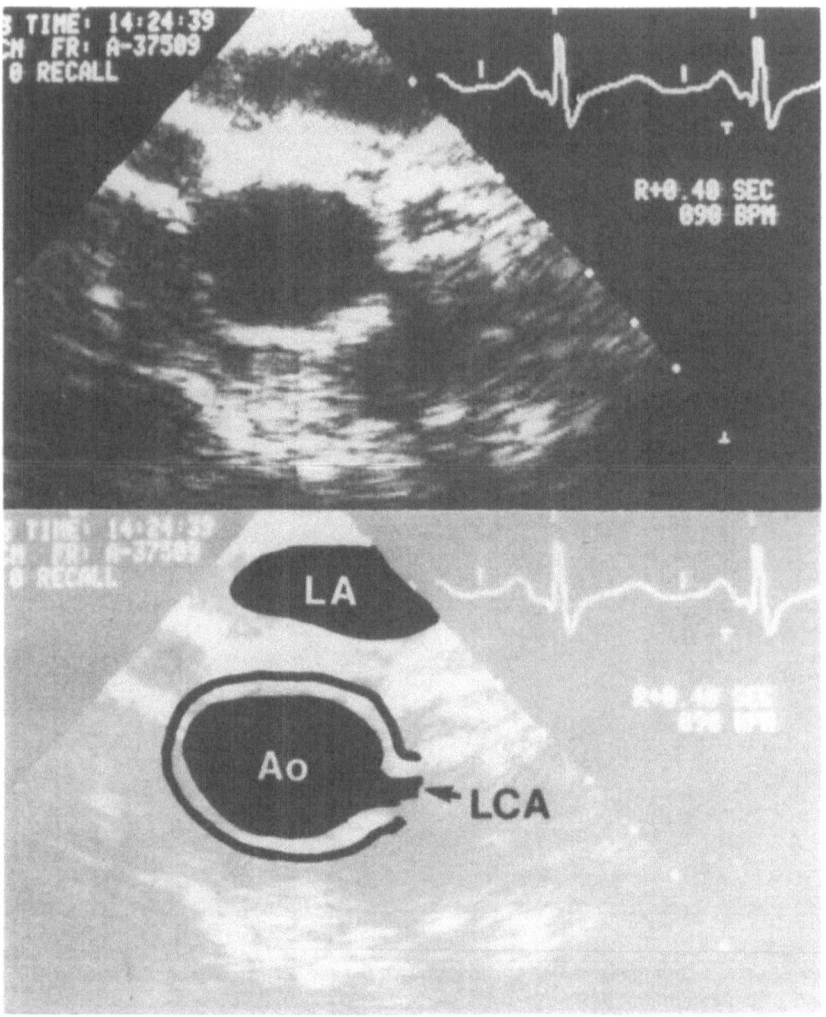

Figure 6. Cross section image of the aortic root with the origin of the left coronary artery. Ao : aorta, LCA : left coronary artery, LA : left atrium.

several authors [1 – 4, 12, 15, 16] – facilitated the recording of the cardiac structures by up- and downward movement of the ultrasonic gastroscope or rotation.
The external angulation of the transducer in 2 orthogonal planes, however,
which is only possible with the present system seems to be the major advantage.
Transesophageal exercise echocardiography is superior to transthoracic exercise
echocardiography due to the facts that there is no interposition of lung tissue between the transducer and the heart during exercise-induced hyperventilation, and
that chest wall movement does not compromise left ventricular imaging due to

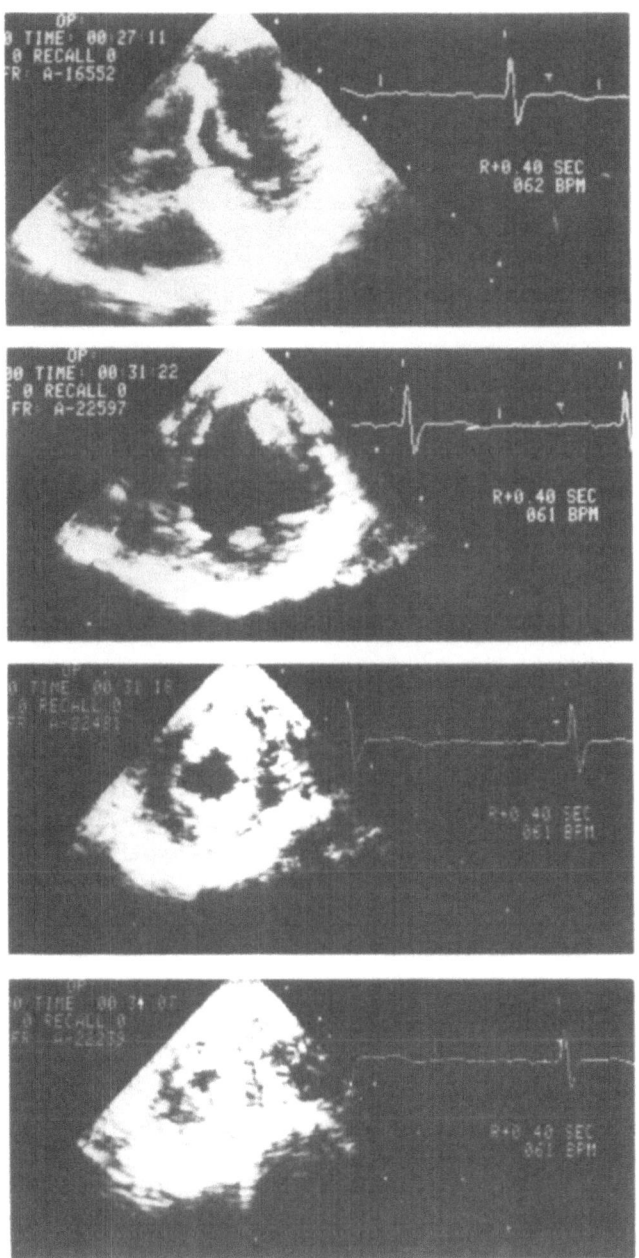

Figure 7. Cross section view of the left ventricle at different levels along the long axis of the left ventricle.

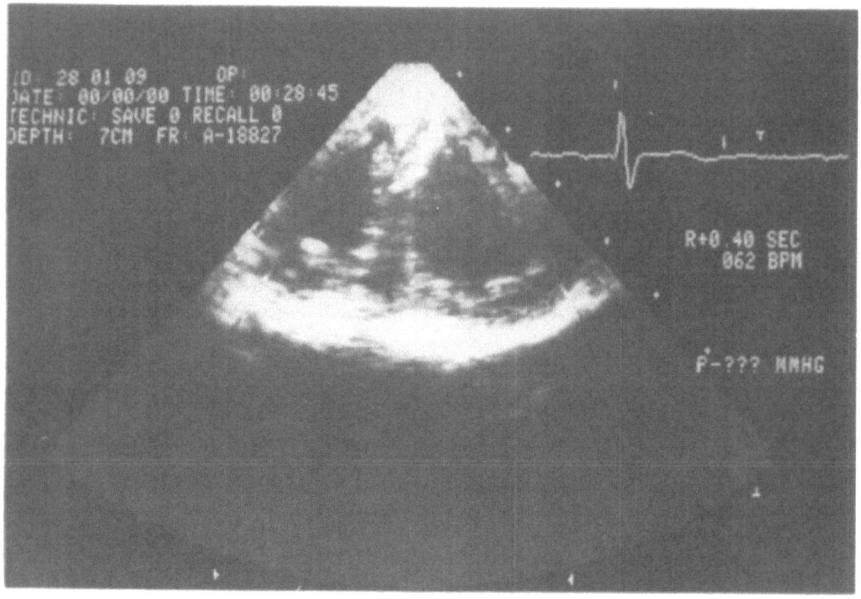

Figure 8. Cross section view of both (right/left) ventricles.

the close anatomical relationship of the esophagus and the heart.

In 1980 Hisanaga and coworkers [11] introduced transesophageal cross-sectional imaging using an ultrasonic high speed rotating scanner. In comparison with conventional cross-sectional echocardiography two-dimensional cardiac imaging from the esophagus is not limited by the configuration of the chest wall, obesity, emphysema, or hindrance from the ribs. The advantage of Hisanaga's mechanical scanner in comparison with the present 90° phased array transesophageal probe is the wide sector angle of 180° or 260° allowing the visualization of all structures of the heart in a single plane. The phased array probe with a sector image of 90° does not visualize all structures of the heart in a single plane. This can however be achieved by scanning the heart successively due to rotation of the gastroscope. The visualization of all structures of the heart in a single plane is however of minor clinical importance in adult cardiology. It may only be important in certain congenital malformations of the heart. With the present 90° phased array transesophageal transducer we are able, even in patients with dilated left ventricle, to identify the left chamber at different levels along the long axis of the heart. In most cases with nondilated heart chambers both the right and the left ventricle can be identified within one sector image.

The major advantages of the present phased array transesophageal imaging device are threefold: 1. There is no discomfort for the patient by a mechanical vibration of a rotating transducer system. 2. There is no need for an oil bag as a sound-coupling system. The external control of the transducer mounted at the tip

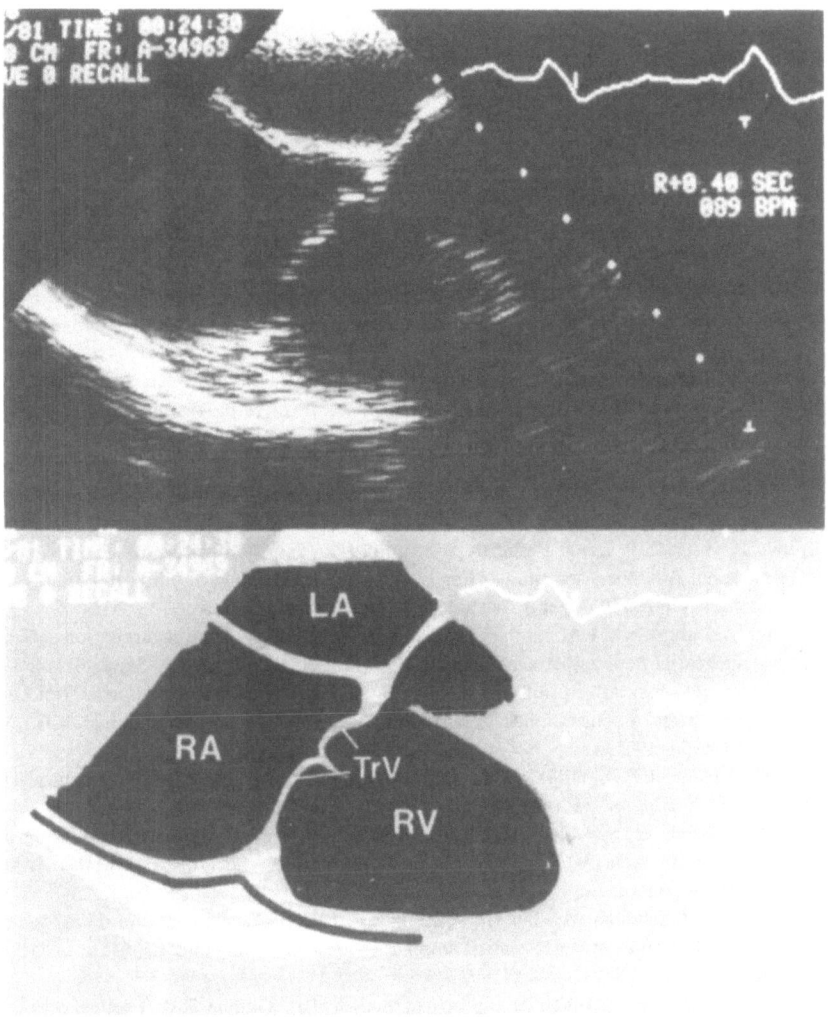

Figure 9. Cross section image at the level of both atria with the interatrial septum and the tricuspid valve apparatus. TRV : tricuspid valve, LA : left atrium, RA : right atrium, RV : right ventricle.

of the gastroscope always allows a close contact of the esophageal wall and the transducer surface. 3. The present phased array device has a higher line density within the sector image.

Although the transesophageal technique implies some discomfort to the patient and some skill is required to introduce the gastroscope into the esophagus, the high image quality due to the close anatomical relationship between the esophagus and the heart even under severe exercise, and the visualization of the heart in planes which cannot be obtained from the external approach leading to higher diagnostic accuracy, compensate for the disadvantages. Furthermore this technique enables to evaluate left ventricular function during cardiac surgery or to monitor left ventricular performance in high-risk patients undergoing anaesthesia.

REFERENCES

1. Hanrath P, Kremer P, Langenstein BA, Matsumoto M, Bleifeld W: Transösophageale Echokardiographie. Ein neues Verfahren zur dynamischen Ventrikelfunktionsanalyse. Dtsch Med Wschr 156:523, 1981.
2. Hanrath P, Kremer P, Langenstein BA: Determination of quantitative left ventricular function by M-mode echocardiography together with other noninvasive parameters, in Echocardiology ed. by H. Rijsterborgh p. 189, Martinus Nijhoff Publishers, The Hague, Boston, London, 1981.
3. Hanrath P, Matsumoto M: Transesophageal echocardiography: A new method for the evaluation of left ventricular performance during dynamic exercise. Ed. by A. Kurjak in: Recent Advances in Ultrasound Diagnosis 3:393, 1981.
4. Kremer P, Hanrath P, Langenstein BA, Matsumoto M, Tams C, Bleifeld W: The evaluation of left ventricular function at rest and during exercise by transesophageal echocardiography in aortic insufficiency (abstr.). Amer J Cardiol 47:412, 1981.
5. Schlüter M, Langenstein BA, Hanrath P, Kremer P, Bleifeld W: Mitral regurgitation detected by transesophageal pulse Doppler echocardiography (abstr.). Eur Heart J 2, Suppl A:114, 1981.
6. Langenstein BA, Hanrath P, Polster J, Schlüter M, Kremer P, Engel St, Souquet J: Detection of atrial septal defect by transesophageal cross-sectional contrast echocardiography (abstr.). Amer J Cardiol 49:956, 1982.
7. Souquet J, Hanrath P, Zitelli L, Kremer P, Langenstein BA, Schlüter M: Transesophageal phased array for imaging the heart. IEEE Trans Biomed Eng, in press, 1982.
8. Kremer P, Schwartz L, Cahalan MK, Gutman J, Schiller N: Intraoperative monitoring of left ventricular performance by transesophageal M-mode and 2-D echocardiography (abstr.). Amer J Cardiol 49:956, 1982.
9. Langenstein BA, Schlüter M, Hanrath P, Kremer P, Bleifeld W: Detection of mitral and aortic regurgitation by transesophageal pulsed Doppler echocardiography (abstr.). Amer J Cardiol 49: 959, 1982.
10. Frazin L, Talano JV, Stephanides L, Loeb HS, Kopel L, Gunnar RM: Esophageal echocardiography. Circul 54:102, 1976.
11. Hisanaga K, Hisanaga A, Hibi N, Nishimura K, Kambe T: High speed rotating scanner for transesophageal cross-sectional echocardiography. Amer J Cardiol 46:837, 1980.
12. Olson RM, Shelton DK: A nondestructive technique to measure wall displacement in the thoracic aorta. J Appl Physiol 32:147, 1972.
13. Side CG, Gosling RG: Nonsurgical assessment of cardiac function. Nature 232:335, 1971.
14. Matsumoto M, Oka Y, Lin YT, Sonnenblick EH, Frater RMW: Transesophageal echocardiography. New York State Med 79:19, 1979.
15. Wells MK, Histand MB, Reeves IT, Sodal IE, Adamson H: Ultrasonic transesophageal measurements of hemodynamic parameters in humans. ISA Transactions 18:57, 1979.
16. Matsuzaki M, Matsuda Y, Ikee Y, Takahashi Y, Sasaki I, Toma Y, Ishida K, Yorozu T, Kumada T, Kusukawa R: Esophageal echocardiographic left ventricular anterolateral wall motion in normal subjects and patients with coronary artery disease. Circul 63:1085, 1981.

7. CONTRAST ECHOCARDIOGRAPHY

RICHARD S. MELTZER, M.D.* AND JOS ROELANDT, M.D.

ABSTRACT

During the 1970's, contrast echocardiography was used clinically to aid 1. structure identification, 2. shunt detection or exclusion, 3. the diagnosis of complex congenital heart disease, and 4. evaluation of valvular insufficiency. Systematic analysis of contrast timing and M-mode as well as two-dimensional echocardiographic patterns can extend these applications. New developments in microbubble technology and videodensiometric processing of two-dimensional echo-contrast images may lead to important advances in the 1980's. These include the ability to attain contrast in the left heart after peripheral venous injections, the ability to better characterize and quantify intracardiac shunts and flows, and possibly a capability for measuring intracardiac pressures or myocardial perfusion.

INTRODUCTION

Ultrasound contrast was first introduced a little more than a decade ago [1, 2] and has come into widespread clinical use during the past five years [3 – 7]. In this communication we propose to comment on methodology and contrast agents, to review the current status of contrast echocardiography in clinical practice, and to point out some promising areas for future research. Contrast echocardiography is an exciting and rapidly developing field, and we entirely agree with Harvey Feigenbaum's assessment that "the full potential of this technique has not yet been realized" [8].

* Clinician-Scientist Awardee of the American Heart Association.

Roelandt, J. (ed.) The practice of M-mode and two-dimensional echocardiography
© *1983, Martinus Nijhoff Publishers. The Hague / Boston / London*
ISBN 978-94-009-6792-2.

THEORETIC BACKGROUND

Methods, microbubbles, and contrast agents

Considerable variation exists in clinical practice in the methods used to create
ultrasonic contrast. This is partly due to uncertainly about the source of the contrast effect. In Gramiak's original communications he identified the source of
contrast effect as microbubbles [1, 2] but held that these microbubbles came
mainly from cavitation at catheter tips [9].

With this thought, though not understanding the nature of cavitation [10],
many clinicians devised elaborate methods which they believed increased the
likelihood of cavitation. Thus a folklore has developed about these methods,
such as the necessity of using right-angle stopcocks, large (or small) syringes,
small (or large) needles, hefty cardiology fellows for the strongest injection possible, etc. In the last few years there is experimental evidence that the source of
contrast is microbubbles of air present in the syringe and injection apparatus
before injection, rather than cavitation occurring during injection [11, 12]
though this still remains controversial [13]. If correct, this understanding would
lead us to downplay the importance of certain methods − such as right-angle
stopcocks and different syringe sizes. It would emphasize the importance of
methods that would increase the microbubble content of the injectate − such as
agitation immediately prior to exclusion of air from the syringe [14] and a short
delay from hook-up to injection. Contrast agents that stabilize microbubbles due
to their surfactant properties, such as gelatin, indocyanine green [11] or blood,
improve the yield of satisfactory contrast studies. Rapid injection in a large
antecubital vein is also important, though not because it causes cavitation.
Rather, it flushes the bolus of microbubble-containing blood to the heart with
less chance of "margination" and resorption of gas bubbles than occurs with
more hesitant and more distal injections. Evidence for margination is the frequently seen phenomenon of contrast appearance in the heart minutes after injection but associated temporally with upper extremity vein "milking", arm or
head motion, or deep inspiration.

Contrast agents that have been investigated experimentally for their ultrasonic
contrast effect include distilled water, normal saline, 5% dextrose solution,
isopropyl alcohol, milk, blood, decholin, Diodrast, Renografin-60, Reno-
grafin-70, indocyanine green, carbonated water, carbon dioxide (CO_2), diethyl
ether, precision microbubbles in gelatin and hydrogen peroxide [11, 15, 16].
Though some of these are too toxic for clinical use, others have been used at
some time for clinical ultrasound studies [17, 18]. Preliminary work has been
reported on a non-gaseous ultrasonic contrast agent in the form of collagen [19]
or gelatin [20] microspheres.

We prefer 5% dextrose solutions for clinical use in our patients, since it is inex-
pensive and readily available. We add one or two cc of CO_2 in the occasional pa-

tient with difficult-to-achieve contrast. We do not use CO^2 if a shunt is suspected since its safety has not been established in that setting. In neonates, where volume considerations may be important, the patient's own blood − a good surfactant − is probably the contrast agent of choice.

An important current limitation in contrast echocardiographic methodology is the variability of results. It is impossible to reliably and reproducibly attain similar contrast effects on successive injections, despite similar injection technique. In this regards research on precision stabilized microbubbles in gelatin is promising [11, 21]. A reproducible contrast agent will probably be necessary in the future if the quantitative contrast techniques described later in this review are to be successful.

Systematic analysis

It is not generally realized how much physiologic information is potentially available from systemic analysis of contrast echocardiograms. For example, very little attention has been given to the slope of contrast trajectories on M-mode echocardiographic tracings, though these represent the component of the blood velocity moving in the direction of the sound beam. This is very similar information to that obtained by pulsed Doppler echocardiography, a technique which has awakened widespread interest (Table 1).

A recent article, suggests that since the main pulmonary artery is usually nearly parallel with the sound beam, slopes of contrast trajectories on M-mode recordings have a reasonable correlation with invasively measured pulmonary blood velocities in humans [23]. In other situations where the echo beam is not parallel

Table 1. M-mode contrast echo versus Doppler echo

Similarities:
− Both look at the component of blood velocity along the echo beam direction (towards or away from transducer)
− The same transducer may be used for both studies

Advantages of M-mode contrast echocardiography
− Samples many depths simultaneously (only multigate or continuous wave Doppler instruments do this)
− Not limited by distance from targets or maximum velocity that can be detected
− Uses less expensive, more generally available equipment (only M-mode instrument and intravenous line needed)
− May have higher signal-to-noise ratio

Advantages of Doppler echocardiography
− Entirely non-invasive
− Can visualize left heart structures in absence of shunt

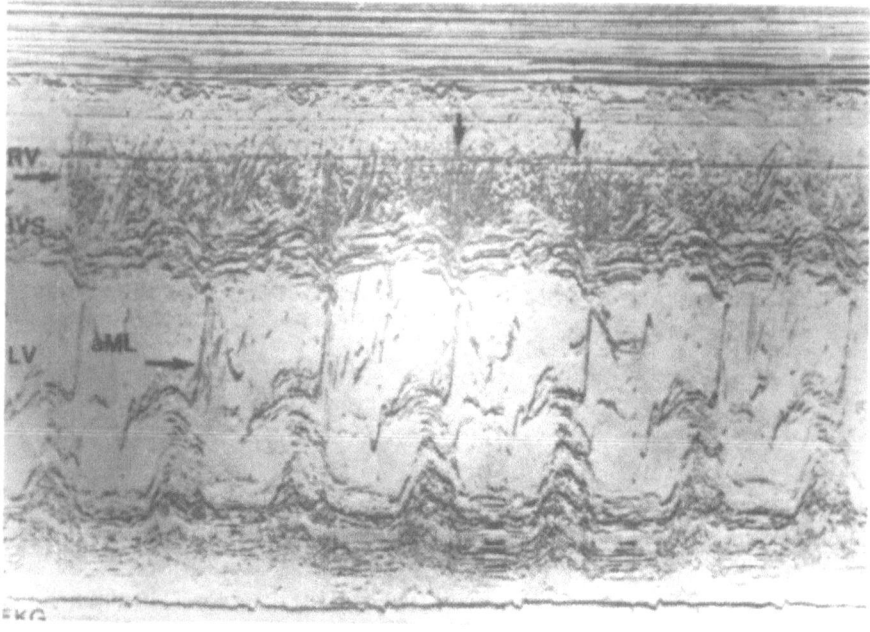

Figure 1. M-mode contrast echocardiogram in a patient with a secundum atrial septal defect. Contrast initially appears in the right ventricle (RV) during diastole and on the following cardiac cycle it appears in the left atrium, passes the anterior mitral leaflet (aML) and appears in the left ventricle (LV). Note that the contrast intensity increases in the right ventricle during inspiration (vertical arrows), while the amount of contrast passing the mitral valve decreases. Reproduced with permission from Hart Bulletin 11:164, 1980.

with the blood flow velocity, the direction rather than absolute value or magnitude of the inferior vena cava with a positive slope when the transducer is aimed superiorly is due to retrograde flow in the inferior vena cava; antegrade flow then yields a negative slope (away from the transducer).

Further, the timing of appearance, clearance, and cyclic alterations of contrast may yield important information about cardiac physiology: left heart contrast appearing within a few cycles after right heart opacification implies an intracardiac shunt, but consistent delay of more than 6 – 8 cardiac cycles suggests intrapulmonary shunting [24]. Cyclic pulmonary artery opacification in diastole after peripheral venous contrast injection suggests transposition of the great arteries with blood reaching the pulmonary artery through a patent ductus arteriosus [25]. The timing of appearance of contrast in the left heart after peripheral injection in patients with ventricular septal defects may help in the evaluation of right ventricular hemodynamics [26]. The cyclic difference of left ventricular and right ventricular opacification in a patient with an atrial septal defect is shown in Figure 1.

CONTRAST PATTERNS

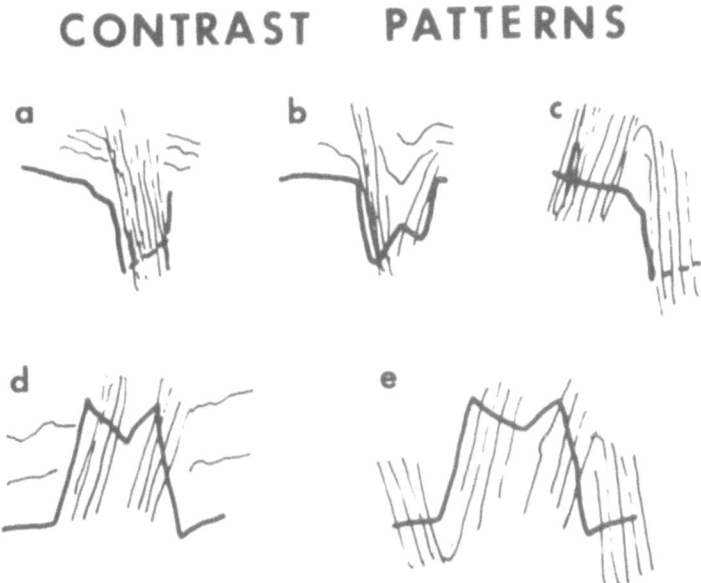

Figure 2. Some proposed M-mode contrast patterns in various right heart conditions (diagrammatic). a. Normal – there is antegrade flow and thus contrast with negative slope – motion away from the transducer – in the right ventricular outflow tract (RVOT) and proximal pulmonary artery throughout systole. b. Pulmonary hypertension. The anterograde blood flow in the RVOT occurs mainly in early systole, and retrograde flow may be seen in late systole, especially in patients with mid-systolic closure of the pulmonic valve (PV). c. In pulmonic insufficiency retrograde flow – contrast with positive slope – is seen crossing the PV in diastole. d. Normal tricuspid valve, with antegrade flow during diastole and no retrograde flow – negative slope – during systole. e. Tricuspid regurgitation, with retrograde flow – negative slope – occurring during systole.

During inspiration, there is relatively more intense right ventricular and less intense left ventricular contrast, and this effect is reversed during expiration. Patterns such as these must be sought for, perhaps on multiple injections in different views to piece together complementary bits of information. A few proposed contrast patterns in various right heart conditions are illustrated in Figure 2 [27 – 29]. These are consistent with our experience [30], but the sensitivity and specificity of these patterns has not been adequately investigated.

The type of information obtained by contrast echocardiography is fundamentally different for M-mode, two-dimensional and Doppler studies. M-mode display is best suited to analysis of timing and slopes of individual contrast trajectories. Two-dimensional display provides the spatial orientation to best define other flow characteristics shunts, vortices, filling or emptying patterns, myocardial perfusion, etc. Two-dimensional echocardiography is not well suited for the study of contrast velocity, which is best measured on M-mode tracings and perhaps in Doppler studies. Doppler contrast echocardiography has only been reported in preliminary work to date [31].

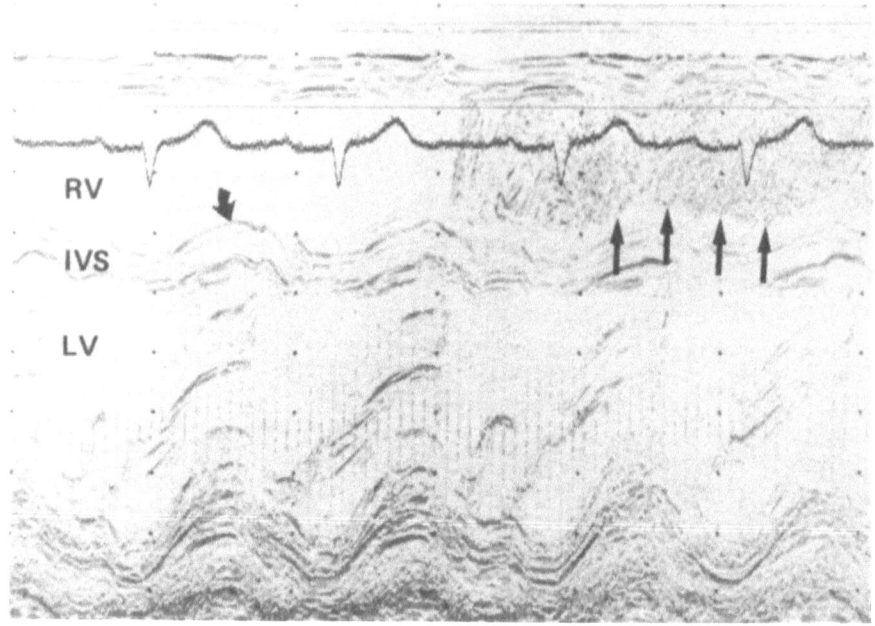

Figure 3. M-mode echocardiogram during peripheral contrast injection, showing incorrect appar‹ position of the endocardium on the right side of the interventricular septum (IVS) − curved arrow and correct position of endocardium outlined by contrast − straight arrows.

CLINICAL APPLICATIONS (Table 2)

1. Structure identification

Structure identification was the first reported use of contrast echocardiography [1, 2] and the ability to perform central or peripheral contrast injections has been an important aid to the correct interpretation of structure on both M-mode and two-dimensional echocardiography [32 − 34]. Specific structures where contrast echocardiography has aided identification or interpretation include the aortic root [1], left ventricle [32], left main coronary artery [35], the coronary sinus [36], the common pulmonary venous return [37], the inter-atrial baffle after Mustard's operation for transposition of the great arteries [38], and the pericardial space during pericardiocentesis [39]. Since these require special catheter injection, echocardiography has not advantage over conventional roentgenologic techniques, except in the rare case where there is a contraindication to ionizing radiation such as early pregnancy [40], or to angiographic contrast agents, such as allergy, renal disease or fluid overload. However, peripheral venous injections may be used to provide better identification of structures on the right side of the heart by echocardiography. This technique is helpful to correctly delineate the right side of the interventricular septum, an important clinical problem where M-mode echocardiograms may be misleading [41 − 43] (Figure 3). In normals, differentiation between the superior vena cava, pulmonary artery and aorta is aided by peripheral contrast injections using the suprasternal transducer posi-

Table 2. Clinical applications of contrast echocardiography

---

1. Structure identification and validation
   a. Peripheral injection − right heart structures
   b. Central injection via catheters − left heart structures
2. Shunt detection or exclusion
   a. Atrial septal defect, patent foramen ovale
   b. Ventricular septal defect
   c. Intrapulmonary shunt
3. Complex congenital heart disease
4. Valvular insufficiency
   a. Aortic and mitral insufficiency − aortic root or left ventricular injection necessary
   b. Tricuspid insufficiency
   c. Pulmonic insufficiency

---

tion. In transposition of the great arteries, suprasternal notch contrast echocardiography can be used to help identify the great vessels and aid diagnosis [25].

2. Shunt detection (or exclusion)

Normally the microbubbles that are the source of echocardiographic contrast are entirely removed from the circulating bloodstream by a capillary bed [44]. Thus the appearance of contrast in the left heart after peripheral venous injection is evidence for a right-to-left shunt. The timing and pattern of contrast appearance in the left heart are related to the level of the shunt and the relative pressures in the various cardiac chambers. Shunts as small as 5% can be detected by contrast echocardiography [45]. Shunts with pulmonary hypertension and Eisenmenger physiology are reliably diagnosed by peripheral contrast injections: in our series all contrast studies showed shunts in patients with ventricular septal defects and a peak right ventricular pressure half or more of systemic pressure [46]. In the absence of pulmonary hypertension, however, ventricular septal defects (VSD's) often fail to show right-to-left shunting after peripheral venous injections [26].

Occasionally a negative contrast effect of unopacified blood from the left ventricle can be noted in the right ventricle, but this sign is neither sensitive nor specific in our hands. Thus, peripheral contrast echocardiography cannot be used to rule out the presence of a VSD, and is only useful if appearance of contrast on the left side of the heart is observed. Shunts can occasionally be demonstrated during respiratory maneuvers or arrhythmias, such as ventricular premature contractions [47], even when they are not imaged at rest (Figure 4).

The situation for atrial septal defects (ASD's) is somewhat different from that for VSD's. This is due to the fact that even in ASD's uncomplicated by pulmonary hypertension, there is usually a small degree of right-to-left shunt present in early systole [48]. Thus, left sided appearance of contrast after peripheral

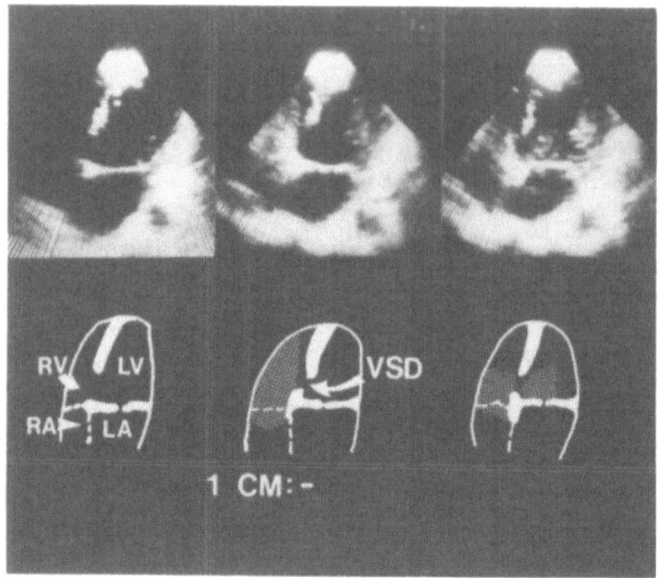

Figure 4. Apical four chamber views from pre-operative two-dimensional echocardiogram showing dropout of interventricular septal echoes in the region of a ventricular septal defect (VSD). Left panels: pre-injection. Middle panels: after peripheral 5% dextrose injection contrast opacifies the right atrium (RA) and ventricle (RV) (shading on lower middle diagram). Right panels: with a premature beat, the contrast crosses the VSD and is present in the left ventricle (LV). LA: left atrium.

contrast echocardiography is a fairly sensitive test for the presence of an ASD [46, 49 – 55] (Figure 1, page 4). In our laboratory sensitivity of contrast echocardiography for ASD diagnosis is 88%, and specificity 100%: this is superior to oximetry or nuclear medicine techniques. We find the "negative contrast effect" of unopacified blood entering the right atrium to be neither sensitive nor specific, though others have found this sign useful [55]. It is difficult to differentiate the normal "negative contrast" effect due to unopacified inferior vena cava and coronary sinus blood entering the right atrium from negative contrast due to an ASD. It is important not to call a test negative unless adequate right atrial contrast has been obtained on multiple injections from several different transducer positions, and a Valsalva maneuver should always be performed during several contrast injections before the echocardiographer can be assured that the study is indeed negative. In fact, contrast echocardiography during a Valsalva maneuver is probably "overly sensitive" to the presence of an ASD, since it may allow patent foramen ovale to be diagnosed [56, 57]. Contrast echocardiography also aids in the diagnosis of partial anomalous pulmonary venous return, a condition associated with ASD's [58].

Postoperative shunts may occasionally be seen in the early [59] or late [60] period after operative closure of an ASD. Though this may imply an unsuccessful operation, such is not always the case: a small number of patients have persistent postoperative shunts despite successful operative closure of their ASD. The mechanism for this is at present unclear.

Recent reports indicate that pulmonary wedge injections can cause left heart echocardiographic contrast [61 – 63], and that this may be used to diagnose left-to-right shunts. This procedure is potentially hazardous however [64], and is certainly experimental at present, having only been reported in humans in 2 small series by Reale et al and our own laboratory. Potential hazards include local pulmonary vascular complications [65] as well as the theoretic possibility of systemic air embolism.

3. Complex congenital heart disease

ASD's and VSD's, which are often parts of more complex malformations, are discussed above. Contrast echocardiography has been an important advance to the pediatric cardiologist, especially in the care of critically ill newborn infants with cardiac and pulmonary disease [66]. In these patients information on intracardiac flow patterns and relations is frequently of vital importance. Using the parasternal and suprasternal transducer positions, it is possible to ascertain the number and position of the great vessels and their ventricular connections [25]. Specific or suggestive contrast echocardiographic patterns have been described in atrioventricular canal defects [67], univentricular hearts [68], tricuspid atresia [69], overriding tricuspid valve and double-inlet left ventricle [5, 70]. Systematic use of the ability to evaluate flow using contrast techniques is playing an increasingly important role in pediatric cardiology. For example, the largest pediatric cardiology center in England (Newcastle-upon-Tyne) sends a cardiologist and M-mode echocardiographic instrument on its mobile intensive care unit to transport critically ill newborns back to Newcastle. The diagnosis can usually be made on the basis of clinical and contrast echocardiographic findings, allowing optimal scheduling of emergency catheterization and/or surgery upon arrival.

4. Valvular insufficiency

Demonstration of left sided valvular insufficiency requires cardiac catheterization. Kerber et al showed that echocardiographic monitoring of left ventricular or aortic root injections could detect mitral or aortic regurgitation, respectively with high sensitivity and specificity and none of the toxicity associated with angiographic dye injections [71]. Since it requires left heart catheterization, though, this technique is rarely used.

Contrast echocardiography is more useful in detecting right sided valvular insufficiency than left sided lesions. Recent work shows that contrast may be

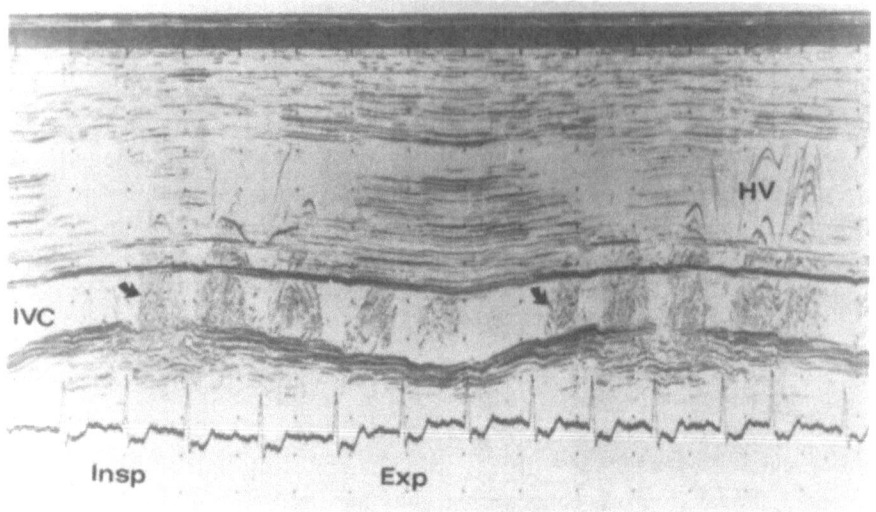

Figure 5. Inferior vena cava (IVC) echogram in a patient with tricuspid regurgitation. After injection of 5% dextrose solution in an upper extremity vein, contrast can be seen entering the IVC and hepatic vein (HV) and flowing retrograde in late systole, then reversing slope and flowing antegrade in early diastole. This effect of "v-wave synchronous" contrast is more pronounced during inspiration (insp) than expiration (exp).

observed to appear in the inferior vena cava coincident with the "v" pulsation on the right atrial pressure tracing, after upper extremity injection, in patients with tricuspid insufficiency [72 – 74] (Figure 5).

The inferior vena cava can be imaged in nearly all patients studied, since there are no "window problems" of overlying lung or bone [75]. Analysis of the timing of the contrast bolus appearance in the inferior vena cava allows the echocardiographer to diagnose tricuspid insufficiency with a fair degree of certainly – 90% sensitivity and 100% specificity to date in our laboratory. M-mode echocardiography is superior to two-dimensional techniques for this application, though inexperienced examiners will find it easier to locate the inferior vena cava with two-dimensional techniques. It is important to realize that many normals will have contrast appearing in the inferior vena cava after peripheral venous injection due to keep inspiration or Valsalva maneuver, but this will always be coincident with "a" wave. Some of the causes of false positive and false negative diagnosis of tricuspid insufficiency by contrast echocardiography are listed in Table 3.

Since no technique to diagnose tricuspid insufficiency is really ideal [76], peripheral contrast studies are a significant advance. However, they do not provide quantitative information at present. Another interesting and related technique is Doppler echocardiography, which has also been reported accurate in

Table 3. Tricuspid insufficiency: causes of false positive and false negative tests (IVC echo during contrast injections in arm)

False positive	False negative
a-wave synchronous pattern of IVC contrast appearance	insufficient central contrast
pattern of IVC contrast appearance random in cardiac cycle; not v-wave synchronous	failure to correctly identify IVC (?aorta)
deep inspiration; Valsalva maneuver, cough	failure to make repeated injections
arrhythmia (e.g., VPC) leading to IVC contrast	failure to use M-mode and exclusive reliance on 2-D echo
M-mode transducer position too superior, near right atrium	M-mode transducer position too inferior

(for further details, see reference 73)

diagnosing tricuspid regurgitation. Since microbubbles are also strong contrast agents in Doppler echocardiography [31], it is possible that contrast Doppler studies might be useful in tricuspid insufficiency.

M-mode contrast echocardiographic patterns (Figure 2, page 5) have been described in tricuspid and pulmonary insufficiency [27 – 29].

FUTURE DEVELOPMENTS

Videodensitometric techniques are being tested to obtain indicator-dilution type curves from the appearance and disappearance of contrast in two-dimensional echocardiographic studies. These may be useful in the quantitation of cardiac output [21, 77, 78], intracardiac shunts [22], and ejection fraction [79].

A unique property of echocardiographic contrast is that the motion of individual contrast particles can be followed and analyzed, in so far as they remain in the echo beam. This fact has been insufficiently utilized, though some authors are now beginning to study flow patterns in the heart, (vortices, turbulence, etc.), or quantifying one vector of the blood velocity by determining slopes of contrast trajectories on M-mode tracings.

Transmission of echocardiographic contrast through the lungs after peripheral venous injection has been achieved in experimental animals [61, 80]. If safely achieved in humans, this would enhance our ability to image left heart structures, and might particularly aid proximal coronary artery visualization.

Intra-coronary injections of a new microbubble contrast agent* have been reported to allow visualization of myocardial perfusion in experimental animals

---

* produced by Ultra Med., Inc. of Sunnyvale, California.

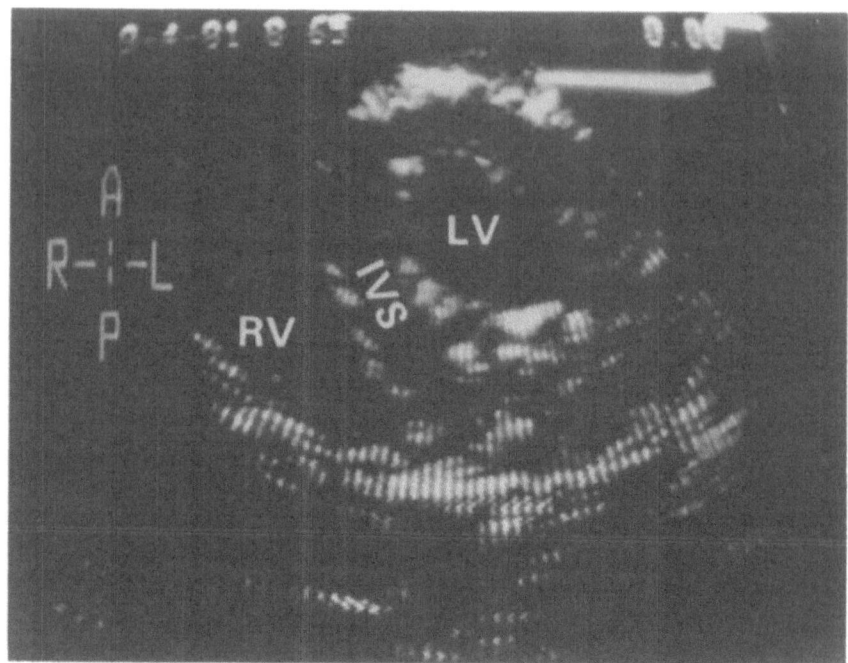

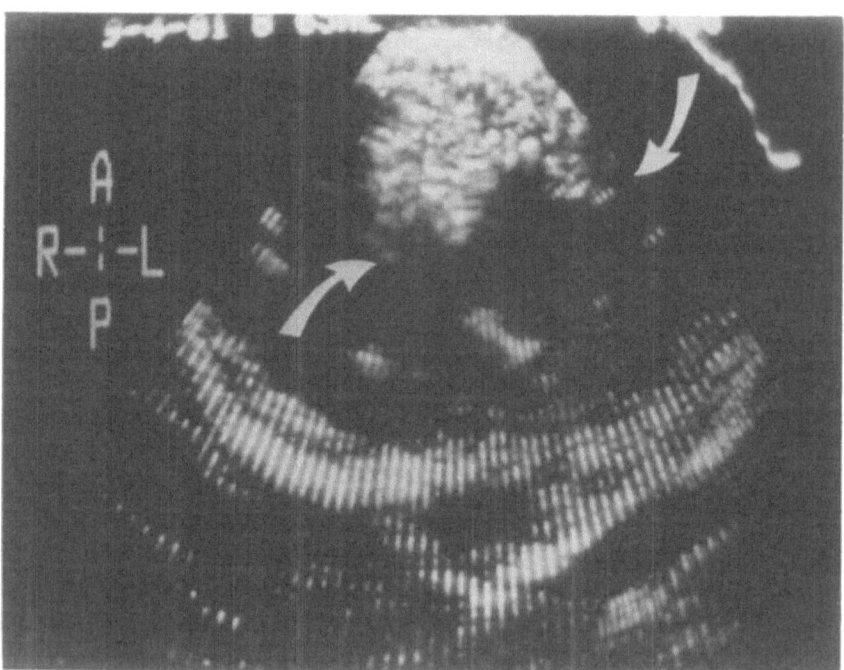

Figure 6. Stop-frame photographs from the two-dimensional echocardiogram of an openchested pig. Short axis view. Upper panel: control. Lower panel: several seconds after injection of contrast into the left anterior descending (LAD) coronary artery. Note contrast in the myocardium in the area of LAD perfusion (between the 2 arrows). Abbreviations: LV: left ventricle, RV: right ventricle, IVS: interventricular septum, A: anterior, P: posterior, R: right, L: left.

by two-dimensional echocardiography [80, 81]. An example of such a study is shown in Figure 6.

Another exciting possibility is that intracardiac pressure measurement may become available using resonant frequency analysis of precision microbubbles [82 – 84]. Precision microbubbles may also be used in the future to provide a contrast agent with a more reliable, reproducible and quantifiable contrast effect. Possibly non-gaseous contrast agents such as aggregated collagen or gelatin spheres may be employed [19, 20]. Better understanding of the phenomenon of "spontaneous contrast" on the left [85 – 87] or right [88, 89] side of the heart is needed: this might shed light on whether cavitation is ever present in human circulation. Ultrasonic studies on microbubbles may provide a method of removing small bubbles from heart-lung machines by a method known as "rectified diffusion" [90]. Contrast techniques have been used to study experimental [91] and human [92] decompression, and there is room for more work in this direction.

Microbubbles are very strong contrast agents for Doppler ultrasonic studies. Their use in this field, one of the most rapidly expanding areas in echocardiography, has just begun.

REFERENCES

1. Gramiak R, Shah PM: Echocardiography of the aortic root. Invest Radiol 5:356 – 66, 1968.
2. Gramiak R, Shah PM, Kramer DH: Ultrasound cardiography: contrast studies in anatomy and function. Radiology 92:939 – 48, 1969.
3. Seward JB, Tajik AJ, Spangler JC, Ritter DG: Echocardiographic contrast studies. Initial experience. Mayo Clin Proc 50:164 – 92, 1975.
4. Hagemeijer F, Serruys PW, Van Dorp WG: Contrast echocardiology. In Bom N (ed), Echocardiology, Martinus Nijhoff, The Hague, pp. 147 – 58, 1977.
5. Seward JB, Tajik AJ, Hagler DJ, Ritter DG: Peripheral venous contrast echocardiography. Am J Cardiol 39:202 – 12, 1977.
6. Tajik AJ, Seward JB: Contrast echocardiography. In Kotler MN and Segal BL (editors), Clinical Echocardiography, F.A. Davis, Philadelphia, 1978.
7. Nanda NC: Contrast echocardiography. In Yu PN and Goodwin JF (editors), Progress in Cardiology 8, Lea and Febiger, Philadelphia, pp. 133 – 45, 1979.
8. Feigenbaum H: Echocardiography. In Braunwald E (ed), Heart Disease, Saunder, Philadelphia, pp. 96 – 146, 1980.
9. Kremkau FW, Gramiak R, Carstensen EL, et al: Ultrasound detection of cavitation at catheter tips. Am J Roentgenology 110:177 – 83, 1979.
10. Plessett MS, Prosperetti A: Bubble dynamics and cavitation. Ann Rev Fluid Mechanics 9:145 – 85, 1977.
11. Meltzer RS, Tickner EG, Popp RL: The source of ultrasonic contrast effect. J Clin Ultrasound 8:121 – 7, 1980.
12. Barrera JG, Fulkerson PK, Rittgers SE, Nerem RM: The nature of contrast echocardiographic "targets". Circulation 58 (suppl II):II – 233, 1978.
13. Kremkau FW, Gramiak R, Carstensen EL: Letter to the editor. J Clin Ultrasound 9:A – 30, 1981.
14. Schiller NB, Goldstein JA: Methodology in contrast echocardiography. In Meltzer RS and

Roelandt J (editors), Contrast Echocardiography, Martinus Nijhoff, The Hague, pp. 47 – 50, 1982.

15. Ziskin MC, Bonakdarpour A, Weinstein DP: Contrast agents for diagnostic ultrasound. Invest Radiol 7:500 – 05, 1972.

16. Wang X, Wang J, Huang Y, Cai C: Contrast echocardiography with hydrogen peroxide. I: Experimental study. Chinese Med J 92:595 – 99, 1979.

17. Wang X, Wang J, Chen H, Lu C: Contrast echocardiography with hydrogen peroxide. II: Clinical application. Chinese Med J 92:693 – 702, 1979.

18. Meltzer RS, Serruys PW, Hugenholtz PG, Roelandt J: Intravenous carbon dioxide as an echocardiographic contrast agent. J Clin Ultrasound 9:127 – 131, 1981.

19. Ophir J, Gobuty A, McWhirt RE, Maklad NF: Ultrasonic backscatter from contrast producing collagen microspheres. Ultrasonic Imaging 2:67 – 77, 1980.

20. Ophir J, Maklad NF, Gobuty A, McWhirt RE: Progress in the development of sonographic contrast agents. Proc of Ultrasonic Imaging Conf, Cannes, France, 1980 (abstract).

21. Bommer W, Lantz B, Miller L et al: Advances in quantitative contrast echocardiography: recording and calibration of linear time-concentration curves by videodensitometry. Circulation 59 – 60 (Supple II):II – 18, 1979.

22. Hagler DJ, Tajik AJ, Seward JB, Mair DD, Ritter DG, Ritman EL: Videodensitometric quantitation of left-to-right shunts with contrast sector echocardiography. Circulation 57 – 58 (Suppl II):II – 70, 1978.

23. Shiina A, Kondo K, Nakasone Y, Tsuchiya M, Yaginuma T, Hosada S: Contrast echocardiographic evaluation of changes in flow velocity in the right side of the heart. Circulation 63:1408 – 16, 1981.

24. Shub C, Tajik AJ, Seward JB, Dines DE: Detecting intrapulmonary right-to-left shunt with contrast echocardiography. Mayo Clin Proc 51:81 – 82, 1976.

25. Mortera C, Hunter S, Tynan M: Contrast echocardiography and the suprasternal approach in infants and children. Eur J Cardiol 19:437 – 54, 1979.

26. Serwer GA, Armstrong BE, Anderson PAW, Sherman D, Benson DW jr, Edwards SB: Use of contrast echocardiography for evaluation of right ventricular hemodynamics in the presence of ventricular septal defects. Circulation 58:327 – 36, 1978.

27. Koizumi K, Umeda T, Machii M: Estimation of the flow pattern and velocity in the main pulmonary artery studied by simultaneous cross-sectional and M-mode echocardiography combined with contrast technique. Proc 2nd meeting of World Federation of Ultrasound in Med and Biol, Miyazaki, Japan, p. 71, 1979.

28. Gullace G, Savoia M, Locatelli V, Schubert F, Ranzi C: Evaluation of linear contrast echo on pulmonary valve echogram. International Meeting on bidimensional echocardiography, Milan, Italy, pp. 72 – 73, 1980.

29. Bonzel T, Fassbender D, Bogunovic N, Trieb G, Gleichmann U: Analysis of right heart blood flow from contrast patterns on the echocardiogram. In: Rijsterborgh H (ed), Echocardiology, Martinus Nijhoff, The Hague, pp. 255 – 62, 1981.

30. Meltzer RS, Valk N, Ten Cate FJ, Roelandt J: Contrast echocardiography in pulmonary hypertension: observations helping to explain the early closure sign. (Submitted to Amer Heart J).

31. Goldberg SJ, Valdez-Cruz LM, Carnahan Y, Hoenecke H, Sahn D: Comparison of microbubble detection by M-mode echocardiography and two-dimensional echo/Doppler techniques. In Rijsterborgh H (ed), Echocardiology, Martinus Nijhoff, The Hague, pp. 263 – 67, 1981.

32. Feigenbaum H: Identification of ultrasound echoes from the left ventricle by use of intracardiac injections of indocyanine green. Circulation 41:615 – 21, 1970.

33. Sahn D: The validity of structure identification for cross-sectional echocardiography. J Clin Ultrasound 2:201 – 16, 1975.

34. Gramiak R, Nanda NC: Structure identification in echocardiography. In Gramiak R and Waag RC (editors), Cardiac Ultrasound, C.V. Mosby, St. Louis, pp. 29 – 36, 1975.

35. Weyman AE, Feigenbaum H, Dillon JC, Johnston KW, Eggleton RC: Noninvasive visualization of the left main coronary artery by cross-sectional echocardiography. Circulation 54:169 – 74, 1976.

36. Snider RA, Ports TA, Silverman NH: Venous anomalies of the coronary sinus: Detection by M-mode, two-dimensional and contrast echocardiography. Circulation 60:721 – 27, 1979.

37. Paquet M, Gutgesell H: Echocardiographic features of total anomalous pulmonary venous connection. Circulation 51:599 – 665, 1975.

38. Nanda NC, Stewart S, Gramiak R, Manning JA: Echocardiography of the intra-atrial baffle in dextro-transposition of the great vessels. Circulation 51:1130 – 35, 1975.

39. Chandraratna PAN, Langevin E, O'Dell R: Echocardiographic contrast studies during pericardiocentesis. Ann Int Med 87:199 – 200, 1977.

40. Meltzer RS, Serruys PW, McGhie J, Hugenholtz PG, Roelandt J: Cardiac catheterization under echocardiographic control in a pregnant women. Am J Med 71:481 – 84, 1981.

41. Allen JW, Kim SJ, Edmiston WA, Venkatamaran K: Problems in ultrasonic estimates of septal thickness. Am J Cardiol 42:89 – 96, 1978.

42. Fowles RE, Martin RP, Popp RL: Apparent asymmetric septal hypertrophy due to angled interventricular septum. Am J Cardiol 46:386 – 92, 1980.

43. Ten Cate FJ, Hugenholtz PG, Van Dorp WG, Roelandt J: Prevalence of diagnostic abnormalities in patients with genetically determined asymmetric septal hypertrophy. Am J Cardiol 43:731 – 37, 1979

44. Meltzer RS, Tickner EG, Popp RL: Why do lungs clear ultrasonic contrast? Ultrasound in Med & Biol 6:263 – 69, 1980.

45. Pieroni DN, Varghese J, Freedom RM, Rowe RD: The sensitivity of contrast echocardiography in detecting intracardiac shunts. Cathet Cardiovasc Diagn 5:19 – 29, 1979.

46. Roelandt J, Serruys PW: Real-time cross-sectional contrast echocardiography. In Bleifeld W, Effert S, Hanrath P, Mathey D (editors), Evaluation of cardiac function by echocardiography, Springer-Verlag, Berlin, pp. 152 – 160, 1980.

47. Meltzer RS, Schwartz J, French J, Popp RL: Ventricular septal defect noted by two-dimensional echocardiography. Chest 76:455 – 57, 1979.

48. Levin AR, Spach MS, Boineau JP: Atrial pressure-flow dynamics in atrial septal defect (secundum type). Circulation 37:476 – 88, 1968.

49. Serruys PW, Van den Brand M, Hugenholtz PG, Roelandt J: Intracardiac right-to-left shunts demonstrated by two-dimensional echocardiography after peripheral vein injection. Brit Heart J 42:429 – 37, 1979.

50. Fraker TD, Harris PJ, Behar VS, Kisslo JA: Detection and exclusion of interatrial shunts by two-dimensional echocardiography and peripheral venous injections. Circulation 59:379 – 84, 1979.

51. Kronik G, Slany J, Moesslacher H: Contrast M-mode echocardiography in diagnosis of atrial septal defects in acyanotic patients. Circulation 59:372 – 78, 1979.

52. Valdez-Cruz LM, Pieroni DR, Roland JMA, Varghese PH: Echocardiographic detection of intracardiac right-to-left shunts following peripheral vein injection. Circulation 54:558 – 62, 1976.

53. Bourdillon PDV, Foale RA, Richards AF: Identification of atrial septal defects by cross-sectional contrast echocardiography. Brit Heart J 44: 401 – 5, 1980.

54. Serruys PW, Hagemeijer F, Bom AH, Roelandt J: Echocardiologie de contrast en deux dimensions et en temps réel. 2: Applications cliniques. Arch Mal Coeur 71:611 – 26, 1978.

55. Weyman AE, Wann S, Caldwell RL, Hurwitz RA, Dillon JC, Feigenbaum H: Negative contrast echocardiography: a new technique for detecting left-to-right shunts. Circulation 59:498 – 505, 1979.

56. Kronik G, Moesslacher H, Schmoliner R, Hutterer B: Kontrastechokardiographie bei Patienten mit kleinen interatrialen Kurzschlussverbindungen (offenes Foramen Ovale). Wien Klin Wochenschrift 92:290 – 93, 1980.

57. Kronik G: Contrast echocardiography in patent foramen ovale. In Meltzer RS and Roelandt J (editors), Contrast Echocardiography, Martinus Nijhoff, The Hague, pp. 137 – 152, 1982.

58. Danilowicz D, Kronzon I: Use of contrast echocardiography in the diagnosis of partial anomalous pulmonary venous connection. Am J Cardiol 43:248 – 52, 1979.

59. Valdez-Cruz LM, Pieroni DR, Roland JA, Shematek JP: Recognition of residual postoperative shunts by contrast echocardiographic techniques. Circulation 55:148 – 52, 1977.

60. Santoso T, Meltzer RS, Serruys PW, Castellanos S, Roelandt J: Small shunts may persist after atrial septal defect repair. Eur Heart J (submitted for publication).

61. Bommer WJ, Mason DT, DeMaria AN: Studies in contrast echocardiography: development of new agents with superior reproducibility and transmission through lungs. Circulation 60 (suppl II):II – 17, 1979.

62. Reale A, Pizzuto F, Gioffré PA et al: Contrast echocardiography: transmission of echoes to the left heart across the pulmonary vascular bed. Eur Heart J 1:101 – 06, 1980.

63. Meltzer RS, Serruys PW, McGhie J, Verbaan N, Roelandt J: Pulmonary wedge injections yielding left sided echocardiographic contrast. Brit Heart J 44:390 – 94, 1980.

64. Meltzer RS, Sartorius OEH, Lancée CT et al: Transmission of echocardiographic contrast through the lungs. Ultrasound in Med & Biol 7:377 – 84, 1981.

65. Meltzer RS, Kint PP, Simoons M: Hemoptysis after flushing Swan-Ganz catheters in the wedge position. New Engl J Med 304:1171, 1981 (letter to the editor).

66. Sahn DJ, Allen HD, George W, Mason M, Goldberg SJ: The utility of contrast echocardiographic techniques in the care of critically ill infants with cardiac and pulmonary disease. Circulation 56:959 – 68, 1977.

67. Hagler DJ, Tajik AJ, Seward JB, Mair DD, Ritter DG: Real-time wide-angle sector echocardiography: atrioventricular canal defects. Circulation 59:140 – 50, 1979.

68. Seward JB, Tajik AH, Hagler DJ, Giuliani ER, Gau GT, Rotter DG: Contrast echocardiography in common (single) ventricle: angio-graphic-anatomic correlation. Am J Cardiol 39:217 – 25, 1977.

69. Seward JB, Tajik AJ, Hagler DJ, Ritter DG: Echocardiographic spectrum of tricuspid atresia. Mayo Clin Proc 53:100 – 12, 1978.

70. Kato H, Yoshioka F: Echocardiographic approach fro atrioventricular malalignment and related conditions. J Cardiography 8:521 – 30, 1978.

71. Kerber RE, Kioschos JM, Lauer RM: Use of an ultrasonic contrast method in the diagnosis of valvular regurgitation and intracardiac shunts. Am J Cardiol 34:722 – 27, 1974.

72. Lieppe W, Behar VS, Scallion R, Kisslo JA: Detection of tricuspid regurgitation with two-dimensional echocardiography and peripheral vein injections. Circulation 57 – 128 – 32, 1978.

73. Meltzer RS, Van Hoogenhuyze DCA, Serruys PW, Haalebos MMP, Hugenholtz PG, Roelandt J: The diagnosis of tricuspid regurgitation by contrast echocardiography. Circulation 63:1093 – 99, 1981.

74. Wise NK, Myers S, Fraker TD, Stewart JA, Kisslo JA: Contrast M-mode ultrasonography of the inferior vena cava. Circulation 63:1100 – 03, 1981.

75. Meltzer RS, Roelandt J: Inferior vena cava echocardiography. J Clin Ultrasound 10 – 47 – 51, 1982.

76. Pepine CL, Nichols WW, Selby JH: Diagnostic tests for tricuspid isufficiency: how good? Cathet Cardiovasc Diagn 5:1 – 6, 1979.

77. Bommer W, Neef J, Neumann A, Weinert L, Lee G, Mason DT, DeMaria AN: Indicator-dilution curves obtained by photometric analysis of two-dimensional echo contrast studies. Am J Cardiol 41:370, 1978 (abstract).

78. DeMaria AN, Bommer W, Rasor J, Tickner EG, Mason DT: Determination of cardiac output by two-dimensional contrast echocardiography. In Meltzer RS and Roelandt J (editors), Contrast Echocardiography, Martinus Nijhoff, The Hague, pp. 289 – 297, 1982.

79. Bastiaans OL, Roelandt J, Piérard L, Meltzer RS: Ejection fraction from contrast echocardiographic videodensity curves. Clinical Research 29:176A, 1981 (abstract).

80. Meltzer RS, Rasor J, Vermeulen HWJ, Valk NK, Verdouw PD, Lancée CT, Tickner EG,

Roelandt J: New echocardiographic contrast agents: transmission through the lungs and myocardial perfusion imaging. Ultrasound in Med & Biol (in press).

81. DeMaria AN, Bommer WJ, Riggs K, Dagee A, Keown M, Kwan OL, Mason DT: Echocardiographic visualization of myocardial perfusion by left heart and intracoronary injection of echo contrast agents. Circulation 62 (suppl III):III – 143, 1980.

82. Fairbank WK, Scully MO: A noninvasive technique for cardiac pressure measurements: resonant scattering of ultrasound from bubbles. IEEE Transactions on Biomedical Engineering. Vol BME – 24, March 1977.

83. Tickner EG, Rasor NS: Noninvasive assessment of pulmonary hypertension using bubble ultrasonic resonance pressure (BURP) method. NIH report HR – 62817 – 2A, Bethesda, National Institutes of Health, June, 1978.

84. Tickner EG: Precision microbubbles for right side intracardiac pressure and flow measurements. In Meltzer RS and Roelandt J (editors), Contrast Echocardiography, Martinus Nijhoff, The Hague, pp. 313 – 324, 1982.

85. Schuchmann H, Feigenbaum H, Dillon JC, Chang S: Intracavitary echoes in patients with mitral prosthetic valves. J Clin Ultrasound 3:107 – 10, 1975.

86. Gramiak R, Nanda NC: Structure identification in echocardiography. In Gramiak R and Waag RC (editors), Cardiac Ultrasound, C.V. Mosby, St. Louis, pp. 29 – 46, 1975.

87. Preis LK, Hess JP, Austin JL, Craddock GB, McGuire LB, Martin RP: Left ventricular microcavitations in patients with Beall valves. Am J Cardiol 45:402, 1980.

88. Finberg HJ: Ultrasonic visualization of in vivo flow phenomena without injected contrast material. In Proceedings of the 25th Meeting of the American Institute of Ultrasound in Medicine, New Orleans, p. 17, 1980.

89. Meltzer RS, Lancée CT, Swart GR, Roelandt J: "Spontaneous" echo contrast on the right side of the heart. J Clin Ultrasound, in press.

90. Higashiizumi T, Tashiro H, Sakamoto K, Kanai H: The new ultrasonic method for the elimination of the micro-airbubbles in the extracorporal circulation. Proceedings of the 2nd Meeting of the World Federation of Ultrasound in Medicine and Biology, Miyazaki, Japan, p. 372, 1979.

91. MacKay RS, Rubissow GJ: Decompression studies using ultrasonic imaging of bubbles. IEEE Transactions on Biomedical Engineering, vol BME – 25:537 – 44, 1978;

92. Wise NK, Stewart JA, Meyers S, Casella R, Von Ramm O, Vann R, Kisslo JA: Post decompression two-dimensional echocardiographic detection of spontaneous gas phase emboli. Circulation 60 (suppl II):II – 194, 1979.

8. CONTRAST ECHOCARDIOGRAPHY IN THE NEONATE

STEWART HUNTER AND GEORGE SUTHERLAND.

INTRODUCTION

One of the major problems of neonatal medicine is the differentiation of complex congenital heart disease from severe lung disease. The neonatologist faces three potential diagnostic groups; 1. the critically ill child with a congenital cardiac lesion who requires early catheterisation and surgical intervention; 2. the child with complex congenital heart disease who does not require emergency cardiac catheterisation or immediate surgical intervention, and 3. the child with severe respiratory or systemic disease and a structurally normal heart in whom medical supportive therapy is indicated. The signs and symptoms of respiratory disease, metabolic derangement, sepsis and other neonatal ailments may mimic exactly those of congenital heart disease and great difficulty can be encountered in reaching a correct diagnosis. If, after clinical examination, chest X-ray, 12 lead electrocardiogram, blood gas estimation in air and high oxygen concentration, the diagnosis is still uncertain, cardiac catheterisation has in the past been mandatory despite its small but important risk. Frequently, these critically ill infants are in Neonatal Units which may be distant geographically from Regional Cardiothoracic Services, and they do not travel well. Thus, a reliable method which can be taken to the infants and which can identify the cardiac cases for transfer is obviously of great value. Echocardiography has a very exciting and valuable application in this situation. It can provide anatomic information enabling the first two groups to be accurately diagnosed and with the help of chamber measurement and contrast echocardiography, it can play a significant role in all three groups in determining the cardio-respiratory pathology.

Most of the data we shall present will concern M-mode echocardiography, which is still the cheapest and most universally available from of ultrasound in neonatal units.

CONTRAST ECHO TECHNIQUE

Since first described in the sixties, the technique has gained wide acceptance. Although initially used at cardiac catheterisation to detect intracardiac shunting,

Roelandt, J. (ed.) The practice of M-mode and two-dimensional echocardiography
© *1983, Martinus Nijhoff Publishers. The Hague / Boston / London*
ISBN 978-94-009-6792-2.

we confine its use to peripheral venous injections in the Intensive Care Unit. The contrast effect occurs when an ultrasound beam is reflected by microbubbles produced by an injection of fluid into the circulation. Cavitation in the fluid results from a sudden drop in pressure following injection which allows gases dissolved in the liquid to escape in the form of microbubbles, which are opaque to ultrasound. Many forms of medium have been used, including blood, indocyanine green, dextrose and normal saline. The microbubble effect is transient and disappears in a matter of seconds when the gases go back into solution, but in infants the effect persists through several cardiac cycles and can be followed through the circulation, until the bubbles are filtered off in the lungs and disappear. Our normal practise is to use 5% dextrose which is safe and cheap. The contrast studies are carried out in the Intensive Care Unit with injection into a peripheral systemic vein. The intravenous line is set up in the arm or leg and the scalp is avoided, as the children tend to move because of the discomfort of the injection. A small polythene cannula facilitates rapid injection, and dextrose is introduced through a 2 ml syringe in boluses of ½-1 ml. Small and rapid injections produce a better echo effect. Several cardiac cycles are recorded before the injection so that initial opacification can be seen and timed against the electrocardiogram, and the recording is continued until the contrast effect has disappeared. Hand injections, of course, vary greatly and it is thus impossible to compare opacification between one injection and another. The intensity and persistence of opacification of a chamber of vessel can, however, be compared with the opacification of other structures during the same injection.

The contrast studies are carried out following full echocardiographic assessment. Parasternal, subcostal and suprasternal views are recorded during separate contrast injections. The subcostal view is valuable for looking at the atrial septum and the atrioventricular junction (Sutherland et al 1981), and the suprasternal approach has major anatomical advantages in the assessment of contrast patterns in the great arteries (Mortera et al 1979). The suprasternal approach allows in all but a handful of cases visualisation of both great arteries before contrast, although occasionally the presence of endotracheal tube in a sick infant on the ventilator may make siting of the transducer difficult. In our experience failure to identify more than one great artery strongly suggests single outlet of the heart – pulmonary stresia, aortic atresia or persistent truncus arteriosus.

The usefulness of contrast echocardiography depends on its ability to recognise with great accuracy and sensitivity the presence of right to left shunting. A validatory study carried out in our unit in infants who went on to cardiac catheterisation, showed no false positives using the technique. In addition to demonstrating a right to left intracardiac shunt, the technique is also able to site the level of right to left shunting. Right to left atrial shunting is frequently present in complex congenital heart disease. In neonatal lung disease most of the right to left shunting is stated to be at ductal level. In our experience this is not true and in all cases of severe respiratory distress syndrome, there is significant

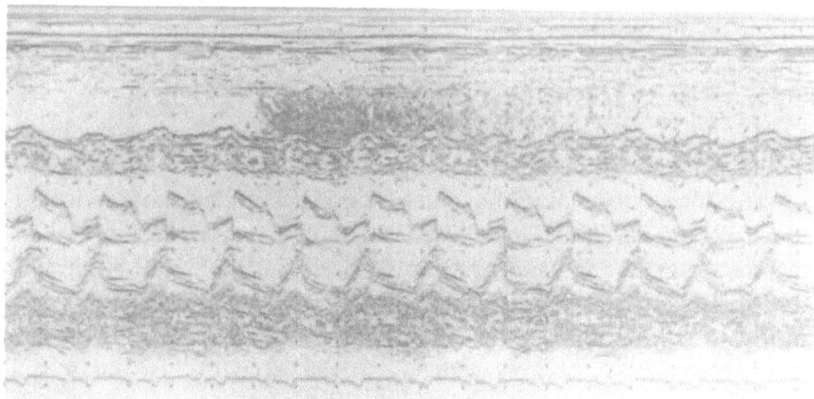

Figure 1. Contrast echocardiogram with normal haemodynamics. Contrast fills the right ventricular outflow tract but spares the left ventricle and mitral valve.

right to left atrial shunting which disappears with improvement in the lung disease.

1. Detection of right to left atrial shunting

Such shunting can be demonstrated easily and accurately using either parasternal, sub-costal or suprasternal techniques. In the parasternal view M-mode cuts across the mitral valve, right ventricle and left ventricle, and through the aorta and left atrium are used. In the structurally normal heart and in the absence of lung disease opacification only occurs in the right ventricle (Figure 1).

With right to left atrial shunting, contrast is also seen in the left atrium, left ventricle and aorta. The contrast usually passes into the left atrium during mid-diastole and through the mitral valve in later diastole, leaving the mitral valve opening non-opacified in early diastole (Figure 2).

In the presence of right to left atrial shunting it is, unfortunately, impossible usually to state whether further right to left shunting occurs at ventricular level through a VSD, or at great artery level through a ductus.

Differentiation clinically between obstructed total anomalous pulmonary venous drainage and severe hyaline membrane disease is notoriously difficult. A different pattern of mitral valve opacification occurs in total anomalous pulmonary venous drainage which is however pathognomonic. In this situation all the blood entering the left atrium is admixed with contrast and no unopacified pulmonary venous blood enters directly into that chamber. As a result, as soon as the mitral valve opens contrast will pass through it in the first opacified cycle (Figure 3).

The diagnosis of total anomalous pulmonary venous drainage will be an-

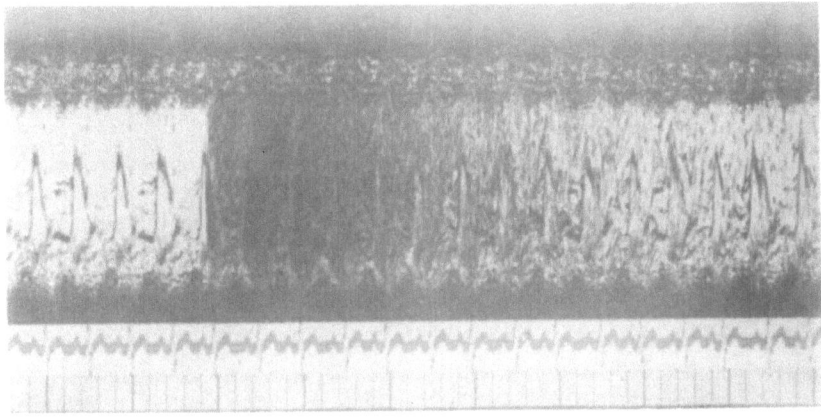

Figure 2. A case of univentricular heart with absent right atrioventricular connection. Contrast passes from right atrium to left atrium and through the mitral valve during mid to late diastole.

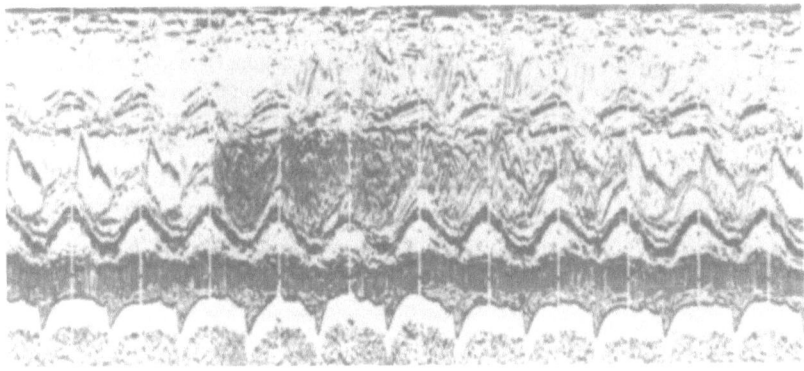

Figure 3. Contrast parasternal study in total anomalous pulmonary venous drainage. Contrast passes across the mitral valve as soon as it opens. Contrast is also seen in the right ventricular outflow tract.

ticipated before the contrast study by the experienced echocardiographer. The left atrium is always small, the right ventricle is always large and the left ventricle may be somewhat reduced in size. It is frequently possible both with the M-mode and the realtime technique to demonstrate the presence of an abnormal venous channel lying posterior to the left atrium. Using realtime echo, it is now possible in many cases to identify accurately the site of drainage and the confluence of the pulmonary veins, (Smallhorn et al 1981). However, using an M-mode echo the contrast pattern through the mitral valve and the echocardiographic assessment of chamber size can allow the diagnosis of total anomalous pulmonary venous drainage to be made and a reliable differentiation to be made from respiratory distress syndrome.

132

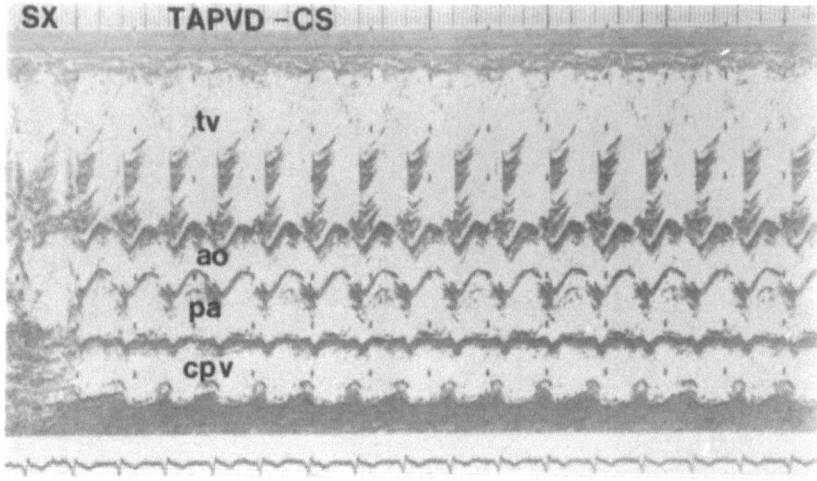

Figure 4. Subcostal M-mode echocardiogram. Right ventricle is enlarged. Behind the right ventricle lies the ascending aorta, the right pulmonary artery and finally an echo-free space proven at catheterisation to be a common anomalous pulmonary venous channel draining to coronary sinus. Abbreviations: SX : subxiphoid, TAPVD : total anomalous pulmonary venous drainage, CS : coronary sinus, Ao : aorta, PA : pulmonary artery, CVP : common pulmonary vein.

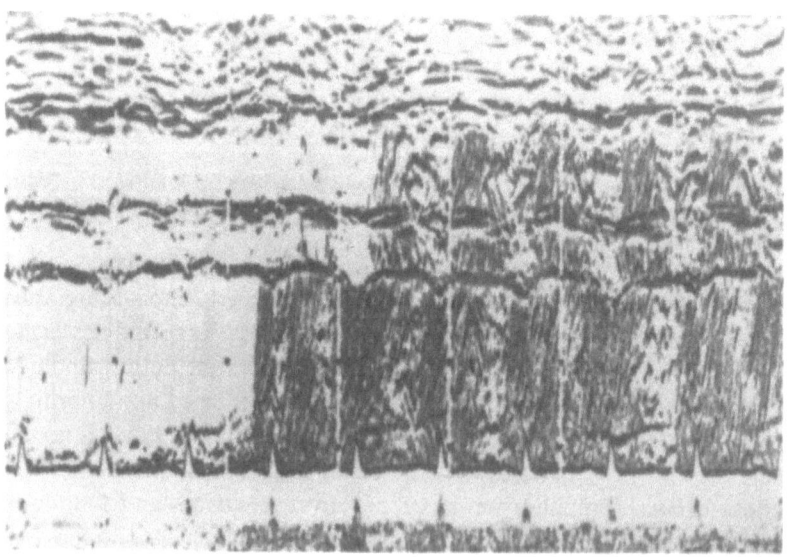

Figure 5. Suprasternal contrast echocardiogram with right to left atrial shunting. The left atrium opacifies early with both great arteries opacifying equally.

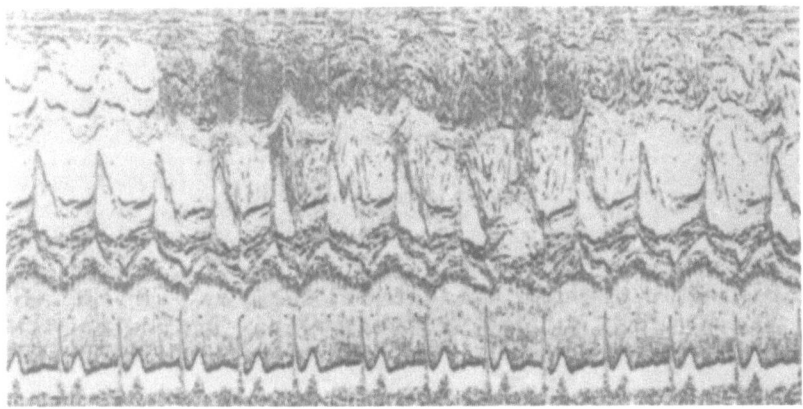

Figure 6. Parasternal contrast echocardiogram. The right ventricular outflow tract opacifies mitrally. Contrast fills the space between the mitral valve and the ventricular septum, sparing the mitral valve opening.

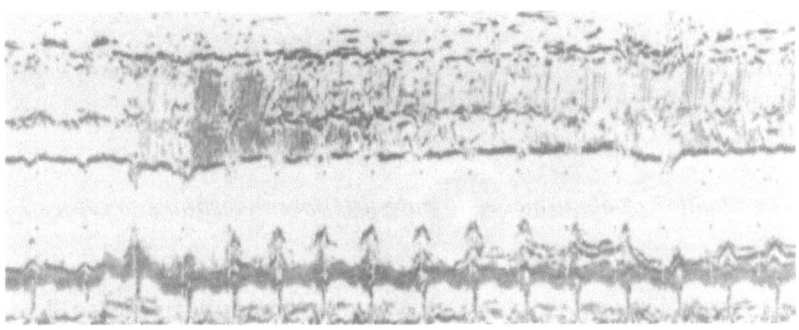

Figure 7. Suprasternal contrast echocardiogram. Contrast appears with cyclical variation in both great arteries but spared the left atrium – indicating right to left ventricular shunting.

From the suprasternal approach, right to left atrial shunting is demonstrated by early left atrial opacification in diastole followed by opacification of both great arteries. Again, it is not possible to infer an additional right to left ventricular shunt under these circumstances (Figure 5).

2. Detection of right to left ventricular shunting

From the parasternal and sub-costal approaches, right to left ventricular shunts are recognized by early right ventricular opacification with an absence of contrast appearing through the mitral valve opening. Contrast appears between the anterior mitral valve leaflet and the interventricular septum (Figure 6). In the

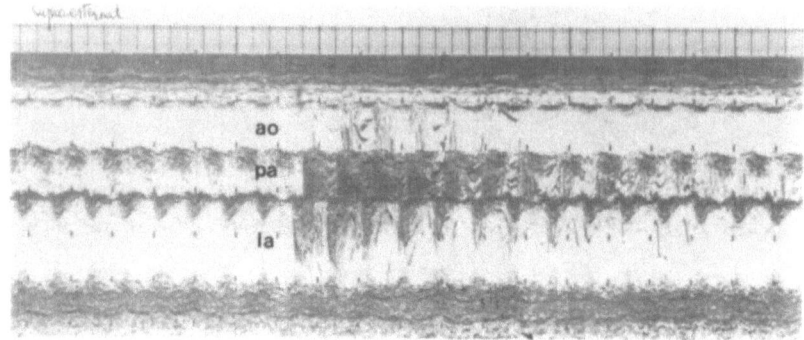

Figure 8. Suprasternal contrast echocardiogram with right to left atrial shunting. The left atrium opacifies first. Subsequently both aorta and pulmonary artery opacify, though the pulmonary artery opacifies more persistently and intensely, suggesting that it receives most of the systemic venous return – normal ventriculo-arterial connection.

suprasternal view, both great arteries opacify in systole with no left atrial opacification (Figure 7). Our correlative study has shown this to be a very sensitive technique, and very minor degrees of right to left shunting at ventricular level can be accurately demonstrated in small infants.

3. Determination of abnormal ventriculo-arterial connection as a cause of severe cyanosis

This diagnostic problem exists for all M-mode echocardiographers. Because of potentially variable cardiac anatomy and spacial relationships, it is not possible to make an accurate diagnosis of transposition of the great arteries, or double outlet right ventricle using the M-mode method alone. With 2-dimensional echo, the definition of ventriculo-arterial connections can be made with considerable reliability, based on identification of the appropriate branching patterns of the great arteries, something which is not available to the M-mode echocardiographer. The contrast technique, does however help the M-mode echocardiographer, if he sticks to the suprasternal approach, as described from our department, (Mortera et al 1979). The anatomical certainty of the suprasternal approach allows definite identification of the great artery by the M-mode technique. With the rare exception of ventricular invertion, therefore, if the pulmonary artery alone opacifies in the suprasternal view, then the ventriculo-arterial connections are normal, the systemic venous return passing in its entirety to the pulmonary artery. Even with right to left shunting at atrial or ventricular level, it is usually possible to assess ventriculo-arterial connections. When most of the systemic venous return goes to the pulmonary artery, this vessel opacifies more intensely and persistently than the aorta (Figure 8).

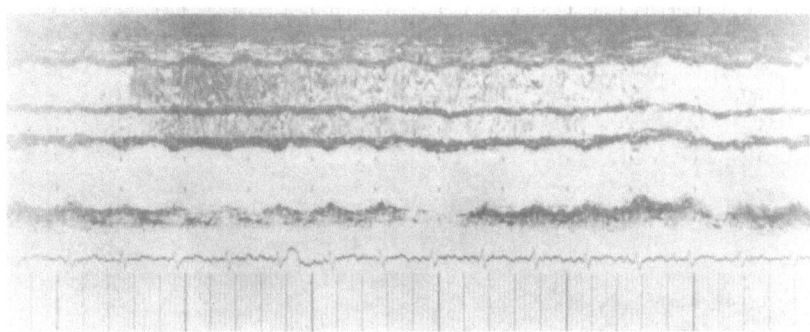

Figure 9. Suprasternal contrast echocardiogram. Contrast appears early in systole in aorta and thereafter shows cyclical variation, more intense opacification in systole. Contrast arrives late in main pulmonary artery and thereafter shows a flat opacification pattern.

Occasionally, in gross right to left shunting particularly through ventricular septal defects, the differential opacification of the two great arteries is so similar that assessment of connections cannot be made. Initially, the contrast appears in systole and thereafter becomes more intense during each succeeding systole, indicating that the great artery is connected to the heart by a semi-lunar valve. In pulmonary atresia with a persistent ductus or with bronchial collateral supply, the aorta still shows systolic intensification but the pulmonary artery which has no direct communication to the heart, gets contrast via the pulmonary communication and opacifies late with a non-cyclical patterns (Figure 9).

The most important abnormal ventriculo-arterial connection, however, in the blue sick neonate is complete transposition of the great arteries (atrioventricular concordance and ventriculo-arterial discordance). The M-mode contrast suprasternal pattern is totally different in transposition from anything so far described (Mortera et al 1979). The aorta receives most of the systemic venous return and, therefore, opacifies more persistently and more intensely. (Figure 10)

Sometimes, in the very young neonate there is so little intercirculatory communication that virtually no opacification is seen in the left atrium or in the pulmonary artery. Following balloon atrial septostomy the amount of contrast in the left atrium and pulmonary artery is increased. This pattern is characteristic in our experience of transposition of the great arteries and never seen in any other cardio-respiratory lesion. It is possible, however, in transposition and ventricular septal defect that the intercirculatory communication is so great, that virtually identical opacification occurs in both great arteries. Under these circumstances, the abnormal connection may not be diagnosed, and the aortic saturation is usually greater than 60% and with less than a 10% difference between aortic and pulmonary artery oxygen saturation. The relative opacification of the aorta and pulmonary artery can be used to predict approximate aortic saturation. In transposition the smaller the intracardiac shunting, the less is the effective

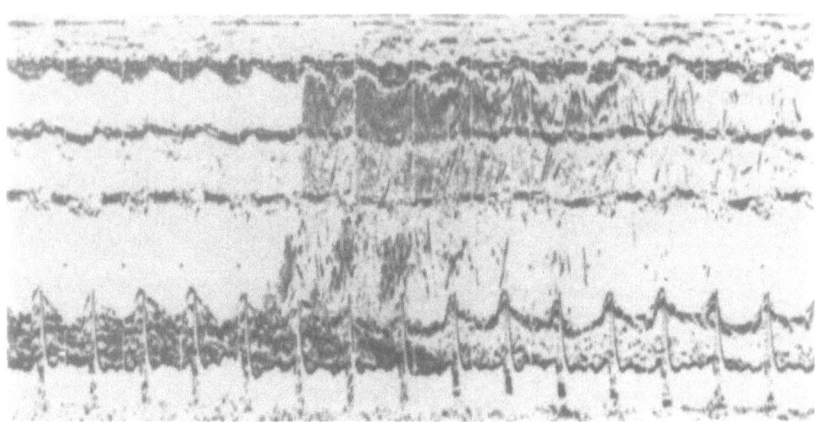

Figure 10. Suprasternal contrast echocardiogram in a case of transposition of the great arteries. Left atrial opacification is followed by opacification of both great arteries, the aorta opacifying more intensely and persistently than the pulmonary artery, suggesting that it receives most of the systemic venous return.

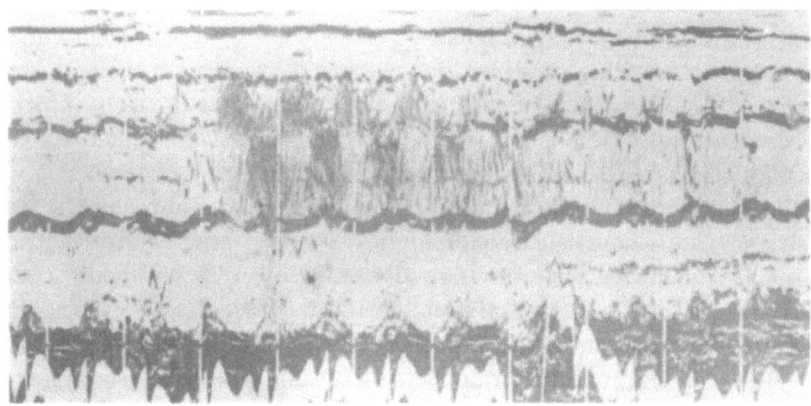

Figure 11. Suprasternal contrast echocardiogram with opacification of both great arteries. The aorta is more intensely opacified in systole and the pulmonary artery in diastole. This finding is unique to transposition of the great arteries with persistent ductus arteriosus.

pulmonary blood flow and the bluer is the infant. Conversely, with a bigger intercirculatory communication, the effective pulmonary blood flow is larger and the infant is pinker. When oxygen saturation in the aorta is less than 40%, it is our experience that the aorta opacifies more than twice as many cycles as the pulmonary artery, and when the aortic saturation is between 40 and 60% the ratio of aortic is pulmonary artery cycle opacification is between 1½ to 2.

We have also described in the past a unique pattern of opacification in the presence of transposition of the great arteries and persistent ductus arteriosus (Figure 11).

Under these circumstances, the aorta receives most of the systemic venous return and opacifies cyclically in systole. The pulmonary artery, on the other hand, has only a small amount of contrasted blood and receives most of its contrast through the duct from the aorta. The timing of this pulmonary artery opacification is, therefore, not in systole but in diastole and this alternating pattern is unique. Following ligation or spontaneous closure of the ductus, this pattern disappears.

4. Right to left shunting in lung disease

Neonates may present in the neonatal period with a combination of lung and cardiac disease. Under these circumstances, it can be extraordinarily difficult to separate out the various causes for right to left shunting. When faced with a blue baby with dyspnoea, tachypnoea and tachycardia, our first move is always to attempt, using M-mode and realtime echocardiography, to demonstrate cardiac structural normality. With practise the M-mode echocardiographer should be able to locate two ventricles, the left atrium, two semi-lunar valves, the aorta and the pulmonary artery. Absence of one of these structures strongly supports the diagnosis of complex congenital heart disease. The size of the individual chambers may also be a help, as previously described in total anomalous pulmonary venous drainage. However, there are many lesions in the neonatal period which produce enlargement of the right ventricle with a relatively small left ventricle.

Pulmonary hypertension from any cause tends to increase the size of the right ventricle, as in total anomalous pulmonary venous drainage, and diffuse lung disease such as respiratory distress syndrome. Many children with coarctation, persistent ductus arteriosus and ventricular septal defect, will also have large right ventricles and normal or even slightly small left ventricles. The size of the left atrium becomes crucial under these circumstances. In total anomalous pulmonary venous drainage, it is abnormally small. In the premature infant with lung disease and a persistent ductus arteriosus the left atrium is usually enlarged.

We are frequently left with a blue, dyspnoeic infant, in whom echocardiographically the heart appears to be structurally normal, but the right ventricle is enlarged. Using the methods already described, the M-mode echocardiogram can under these circumstances rule out transposition, pulmonary atresia or total anomalous pulmonary venous drainage. Persistent fetal circulation and diffuse lung disease remain the two likeliest non-cardiac lesions. In severe neonatal lung disease there is extensive right to left atrial shunting with the sort of pattern already described. Sequential contrast echo studies during treatment shows a diminution in the amount of right to left shunting as the pulmonary function returns to normal. However, it is incontrovertibly true that estimation of blood gases under these circumstances is probably as useful a method and undoubtedly less expensive.

138

REFERENCES

1. Sutherland GR: Praecordial and sub-xiphoid M-mode echocardiography in analysis of the atrioventricular junction. In − Echocardiography 1980. Eds. Hunter S and Hall R. Churchill Livingstone, pp. 192−212, July 1982.
2. Mortera C, Hunter S, Tynan M: Contrast echocardiography and the suprasternal approach in infants and children. European Journal of Cardiology, 9/6, 437−454, 1979.
3. Smallhorn JF, Sutherland GR, Tommasini G, Hunter S, Anderson RH, Macartney, FJ: Assessment of total anomalous pulmonary venous connection by two-dimensional echocardiography. British Heart Journal, Vol. 46, No. 6, pp. 613−623, 1981.

IV. APPLICATION AND VALIDITY OF M-MODE AND TWO-DIMENSIONAL ECHOCARDIOGRAPHY IN COMMON CARDIAC DISORDERS

The combined use of M-mode and two-dimensional echocardiography provides an extremely accurate method for the diagnosis of various cardiovascular disorders. Of course, no diagnostic method has a perfect sensitivity and specificity. Within the field of imaging techniques, however, echocardiography is certainly the most informative for the analysis of patients suspected of or having a pericardial effusion (chapter 9), an intracardiac mass lesion (chapters 10 and 11) or a cardiomyopathy (chapter 12). Dr. Cikes in chapter 9 describes how the risk of a diagnostic and therapeutic pericardiocentesis, a precedure with considerable risk to the patient, can now be minimized and how a pericardial percutaneous biopsy can be performed by guiding the needle by two-dimensional echocardiography.

While invasive studies will undoubtedly continue to be useful in the diagnosis of valvular and congenital heart disease, it appears at present that routine cardiac catheterization is being displaced from its dominant role for the preoperative assessment of such patients. It has been demonstrated in several studies that appropriate and successful valve replacement without cardiac catheterization can be performed in a large number of selected patients. The potential of echocardiography for the assessment of patients with mitral and aortic valve disease is discussed in chapters 13 and 14.

Sutherland and Hunter describe in chapter 15 the usefulness of two-dimensional echocardiography for a correct identification and classification of ventricular septal defects.

Roelandt, J. (ed.) The practice of M-mode and two-dimensional echocardiography
© *1983, Martinus Nijhoff Publishers. The Hague / Boston / London*
ISBN 978-94-009-6792-2.

9. NEW ASPECTS OF ECHOCARDIOGRAPHY FOR THE DIAGNOSIS AND TREATMENT OF PERICARDIAL DISEASE

IVO CIKES AND ALEXANDER ERNST

A number of articles have confirmed the usefulness of echocardiography in the diagnosis of pericardial effusion [1 – 18]. Because of its noninvasive nature, high sensitivity, possibility of bedside examination and repeatability it has become a method of choice in evaluating patients with pericardial effusion.

The echographic hallmarks of pericardial effusion are separation of epicardium from the parietal pericardium and poor or absent parietal pericardium motion (Figure 1).

Although a conclusive diagnosis may be obtained in a few minutes, to avoid false positive and false negative diagnosis, some technical and anatomical pitfalls must be recognised [14 – 19]. An improper diagnosis of pericardial effusion may result in improper drug therapy, in unwarranted and hazardous pericardiocentesis or even more aggressive surgical procedure. Tables 1 and 2 summarize potential sources of false-positive and false-negative diagnosis of pericardial effusion as described in the literature (Figure 2). With the considerable experience and skill of the examiner, the incidence of false positive and false negative studies is extremely low.

With its good axial resolution M-mode echocardiography is superior in qualitative diagnosis (pericardial thickening, small effusion, constrictive hemodynamics). Two-dimensional echocardiography provides multiple cross section planes of the entire pericardial sac and surrounding structures (Figure 3).It is superior in assessing the amount, distribution and loculation of pericardial fluid and particularly in avoiding diagnostic pitfalls.

Neither M-mode nor two-dimensional echocardiography provide reliable criteria for the diagnosis of cardiac tamponade and constrictive pericarditis (Figure 3). They still remain clinical and hemodynamic diagnoses [15, 19, 20]. In spite of the many echocardiographic signs of tamponade and constriction described, they are only suggestive (Table 3 and 4).

Until recently echocardiographic diagnosis of pericardial diseases was limited to the detection of pericardial effusion and rough semiquantitation of the pericardial fluid. As mentioned, its role in the diagnosis of cardiac tamponade and constrictive pericarditis is rather limited. Recently it was shown that echocardiography can be used not only for the diagnosis of pericardial effusion, but also to improve our understanding of the pathology of pericardial lesions and for the

Roelandt, J. (ed.) The practice of M-mode and two-dimensional echocardiography
© *1983, Martinus Nijhoff Publishers. The Hague / Boston / London*
ISBN 978-94-009-6792-2.

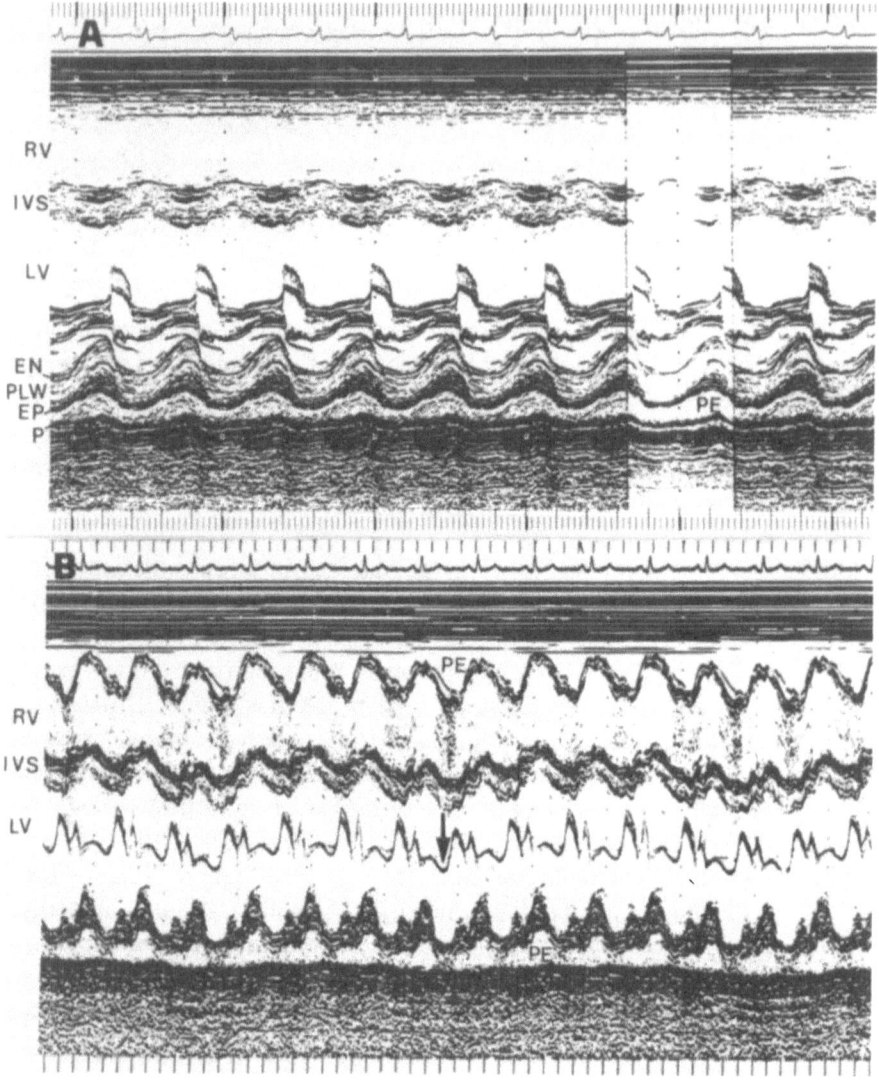

Figure 1. A. In small pericardial effusion an echo-free space appears behind the posterior left ventricular wall (PLW). B. In large pericardial effusion the anterior and posterior pericardial effusion is present. Motions of cardiac walls are exaggerated and the pseudo-prolapse pattern of the mitral valve are seen (arrow). RV : right ventricle, IVS : interventricular septum, LV : left ventricle, MV : mitral valve, EN : endocardium, EP : epicardium, P : pericardium, PE : pericardial effusion.

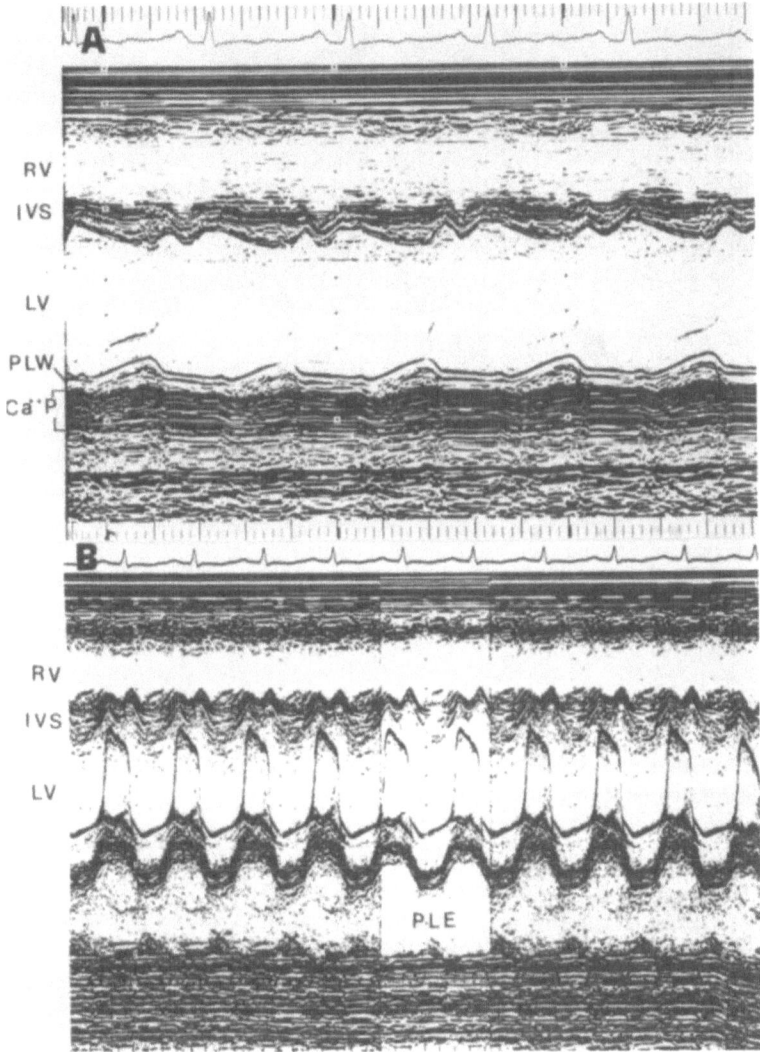

Figure 2. A. Patient with constrictive pericarditis and thickened calcified pericardium behind left ventricular posterior wall (PLW) proven at surgery. A band of dense echoes in the region of the posterior pericardium can be seen. Posterior left ventricular wall shows flat motion in mid- to late diastole. RV : right ventricle, IVS : interventricular septum, LV : left ventricle, Ca⁺⁺P : calcified pericardium. B. Large posterior echo-free space in pleural effusion (PLE) could be misinterpreted as pericardial effusion, but it is not accompanied by an anterior echo-free space, MV : mitral valve.

management of patients with pericardial disease [20, 47 – 54]. Echocardiography has thus become the main method for making decisions about patients with pericardial disease.

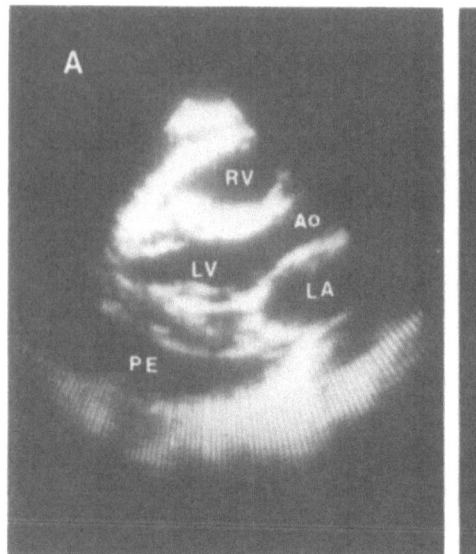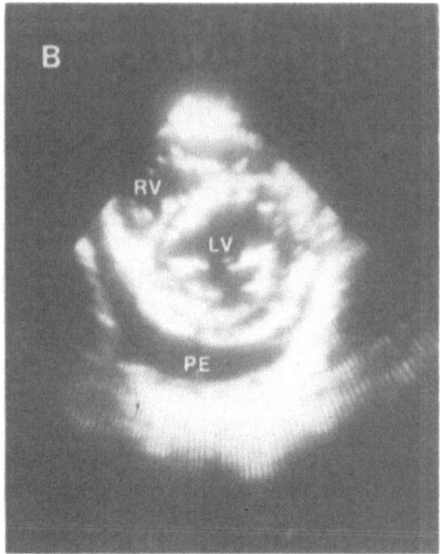

Figure 3. Long (panel A) and short axis (panel B) two-dimensional echocardiograms from a patient with a moderate pericardial effusion. The pericardial effusion accumulates posteriorly, toward cardiac apex and laterally. RV : right ventricle, LV : left ventricle, Ao : aorta, LA : right atrium, PE : pericardial effusion.

Table 1. Potential sources of false-positive diagnosis of pericardial effusion

---

A. Faulty technique
- Inadequate gain setting [14 – 16, 18 – 21]
- Improper transducer location or direction [14 – 16, 18, 21]
- Inadequate scanning of the heart [14 – 16, 18, 21]

B. False-positive anterior effusion
- Subepicardial fat [29]
- Cysts, tumors [24 – 30]
- Foramen Morgagni hiatus hernia [32]
- Indwelling right heart catheter [16, 31]
- Interventricular septum mistaken for right ventricular anterior wall [16]

C. False-positive posterior effusion
- Pleural effusion [14 – 16, 18, 19, 29a]
- Cysts, tumors [24 – 30]
- Inferior left pulmonary vein [16]
- Thoracic aorta [15]
- Coronary sinus [15, 33]
- Coronary arterial aneurysm [34]
- Giant left atrium [35]
- Portion of the right ventricule [15]
- Left ventricular pseudoaneurysm [36]
- Mitral annulus calcification [37]
- Thickened or calcified chordae tendineae [16]
- Papillary muscle mimicking left ventricular posterior wall [16]
- Collapsed lung, consolidation [10]
- Reverberation artifacts [21]

Table 2. Potential sources of false-negative diagnosis of pericardial effusion

- Faulty technique [14 – 16, 18, 21]
- Loculation of pericardial fluid [16]
- Cloth hemopericardium [38]
- Pulsatile pericardium in hyperdynamic circulation [38]

Table 3. Echocardiographic signs described in cardiac tamponade

- Reciprocal changes in right and left ventricular dimensions with the respiratory cycle [42]
- Right ventricular compression/end-respiratory diameter <7mm/ [40]
- Diminishing left posterior wall motion [2, 3]
- Swinging heart [4, 41]
- Early systolic notch of right ventricular epicardial echo [13]
- Posterior motion of right ventricular wall during diastole [43]
- Decreased D-E amplitude and E-F slope of the mitral valve [13, 42]

Table 4. Echocardiographic signs described in constrictive pericarditis

- Fluttering of the mid- and late diastolic motion of left ventricular wall [3, 15]
- Abrupt cessation or "freezing" motion of ventricules during mid- and late diastole on 2-D echocardiography [44]
- Paradoxical septal motion [45]
- Parallel moving dense bands in pericardial region [53]
- Pericardial thickening [45]
- Rapid E-F slope of the mitral leaflet [15]
- Premature opening of the pulmonary valve [46]

INTRAPERICARDIAL MASSES

So far intrapericardial structures such as pericardial adhesions, pericardial fibrinous deposits and tumorous infiltration have been exclusively findings at autopsy or cardiac surgery. Using two-dimensional echocardiography it was shown that echo-producing structures within the pericardial sac could be visualised [20, 45 – 54]. In four series 18 out of 39 described patients had surgical or autopsy findings which corresponded well to those described by echocardiography [20, 48, 50 – 54].

Over the last four and a half years we have found intrapericardial masses in 19 patients with pericardial effusion of various etiology [20, 47, 49, 51, 52, 54]. They were presented as bridging bands extending from the epicardium to the pericardium, freely vibrating bands attached to the pericardium or epicardium and shaggy or lumpy structures on the epicardial and/or pericardial surface

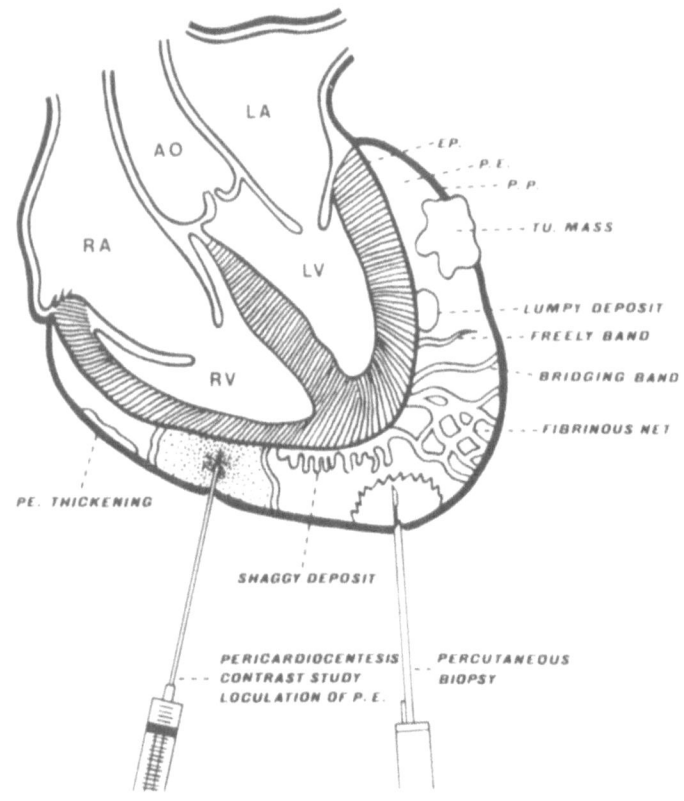

Figure 4. Schematic presentation of echo-producing structures within pericardial sac detected by two-dimensional echocardiography. EP : epicardium, P.P. : parietal pericardium, P.E. : pericardial effusion, Ao : aorta, LA : left atrium, RA : right atrium, RV : right ventricle, LV : left ventricle.

(Figures 4 and 5). Tumorous masses in patients with primary or metastatic pericardial tumors were presented as cauliflower-like or bizarre masses protruding from the pericardium into the pericardial sac (Figure 6). In patients with bridging intrapericardial bands suggested loculation of pericardial fluid can be confirmed by the lack of postural fluid redistribution or by contrast study [19, 52].

The echocardiographic finding of intrapericardial masses may be relevant for solving clinical problems in patients with pericardial effusion. It provides some new data on the pathology of underlying pericardial disease. On the basis of echocardiographic-pathologic correlations obtained so far, large cauliflower-like or bizarre pericardial masses are strongly suspect to be tumors, band-like structures indicate pericardial adhesions, while lumpy and shaggy epicardial or pericardial echoes speak in favour of fibrinous deposits. In some patients this echocardiographic finding may suggest effusive-constrictive forms of pericarditis

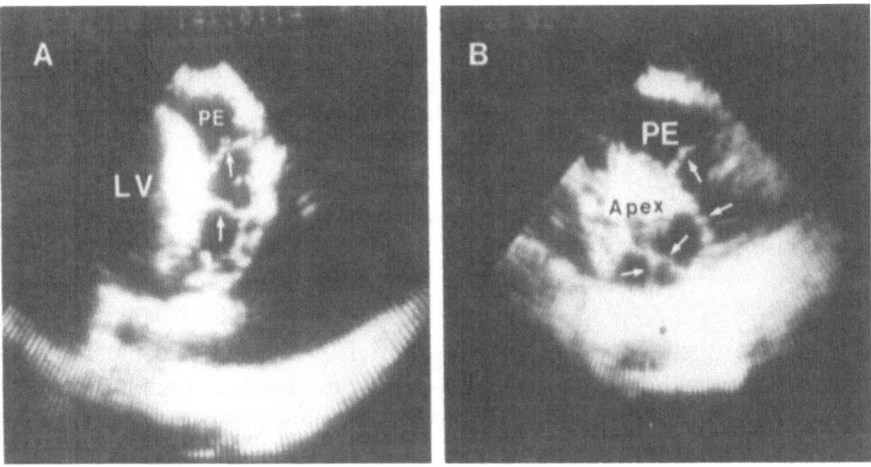

Figure 5. A. Two-dimensional echocardiogram from a patient with pericardial effusion showing bridging bands extending from epicardium to parietal pericardium (arrows). PE : pericardial effusion, LV : left ventricle, B. Short axis two-dimensional echocardiogram at the level of cardiac apex with multiple bands within the pericardial sac.

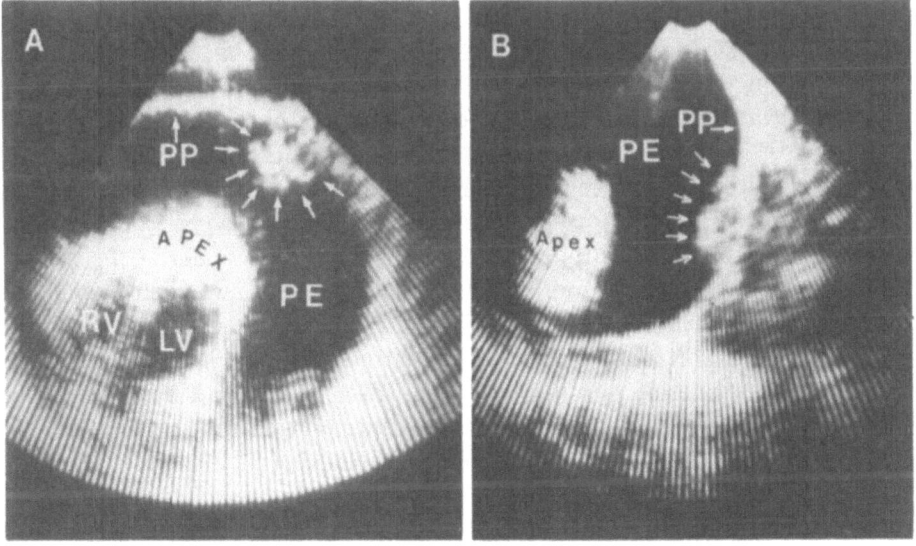

Figure 6. Two-dimensional echocardiogram from a patient with pericardial mezothelioma showing cauliflower-like tumorous masses on the thick parietal pericardium (PP). RV : right ventricle, LV : left ventricle, PE : pericardial effusion.

[48, 50]. A definite etiological diagnosis can be obtained by pericardiocentesis or percutaneous pericardial biopsy guided by two-dimensional echocardiography. Target biopsy of imaged masses can be performed under echocardiographic control. Recognition of loculated effusion is important when planning pericardiocentesis.

PERICARDIOCENTESIS

Although pericardiocentesis has been used since 1840 [55] it is still a procedure with a high risk of morbidity and mortality. It is difficult to compare the few studies dealing with the risks involved in pericardiocentesis because of the differences in diagnostic criteria of pericardial effusion, the environment in which pericardiocenteses were performed, the site of the pericardiocentesis, steps taken to minimize the hazards (ECG, plastic catheters replacing the needle, echoguidance), the hemodynamic status of patients, the duration of the study and follow-up of patients [56 – 59].

The complications reported include cardiac chamber puncture, with or without tamponade, laceration of coronary vessels, ventricular fibrillation and other ventricular or atrial arrhythmias, cardiac arrest, pneumothorax, vasovagal reactions, infection, bleeding, perforation of the stomach and non-productive pericardiocentesis [56, 59]. It is believed that the number of non-registered cardiac chamber punctures is higher than those registered. The seriousness of the problem is illustrated by Kotte and McGuire [57] who reported that 18 of 21 cardiologists and surgeons experienced in pericardiocentesis had seen at least one fatality during this procedure.

There have been several attempts to diminish the potential risk of pericardiocentesis (Figure 7). Fluoroscopic guiding of the needle for pericardiocentesis is not a reliable method, because it can not differentiate pericardial effusion from cardiac mass. In 1956 Bishop and co-workers [60] applied the pericardiocentesis needle as an exploring electrode to detect the injury currents during the contact of the electrode tip with the heart. This technique became unwarrantedly popular because it gave a spurious feeling of safety. It usually registers already existing injury. In 1966 a soft plastic catheter was introduced to replace the needle or guidewire after entering into the pericardial space. Plastic catheters may be introduced over or through the needle or guidewire [61 – 65].

Probably the most important advance in minimizing the hazards of pericardiocentesis was the introduction of echocardiography in routine diagnosis of pericardial effusion. Besides the reliable diagnosis of pericardial effusion, it also provides other data important for the safety or pericardiocentesis, such as semiquantitation, distribution and loculation of pericardial fluid. It is therefore essential for the selection of patients and the choosing of the optimal puncture site for pericardiocentesis. In 1972 Goldberg and Pollock [66] used a special

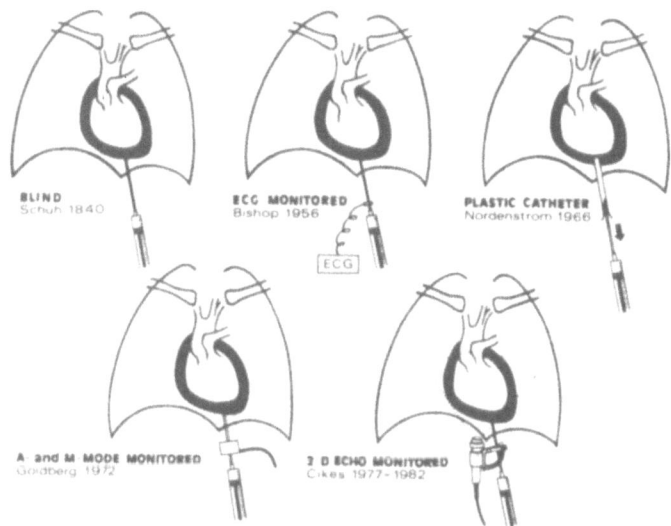

Figure 7. Historical development of the technique of pericardiocentesis.

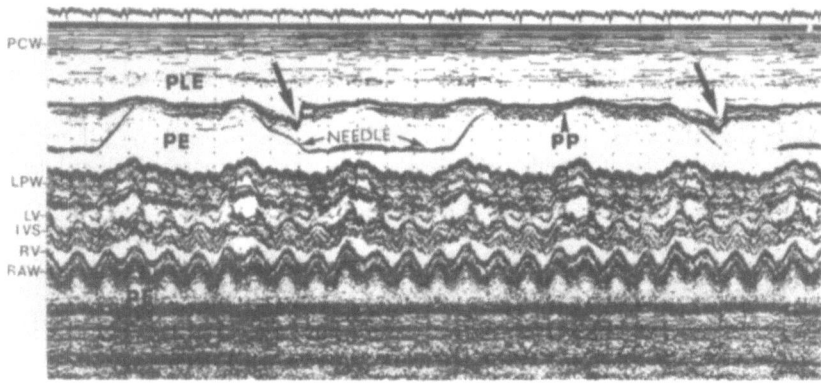

Figure 8. M-mode echocardiogram from left posterior thoracic wall during pericardiocentesis in a patient with concommitant pleural (PLE) and pericardial (PE) effusion. The needle from pleural space enters the pericardial space. Fatt arrows point the moment of invagination of parietal pericardium (PP) by needle tip. PCW : posterior chest wall, LPW : left posterior wall, LV : left ventricle, IVS : interventricular septum, RV : right ventricle, RAW : right ventricular anterior wall.

transducer with the hole in the center to direct the needle during pericardiocentesis under A- and M-mode echocardiographic control. The needle tip was seen in the A- and M-mode display as an echo arising at the needle tip – fluid interface. In one out of six patients in whom the procedure was performed, there was ventricular puncture. As is seen from the literature, this method was of no further interest in cardiology. The main disadvantage of pericardiocentesis guided under the control of A- and M-mode is the lack of spatial orientation (Figure 8).

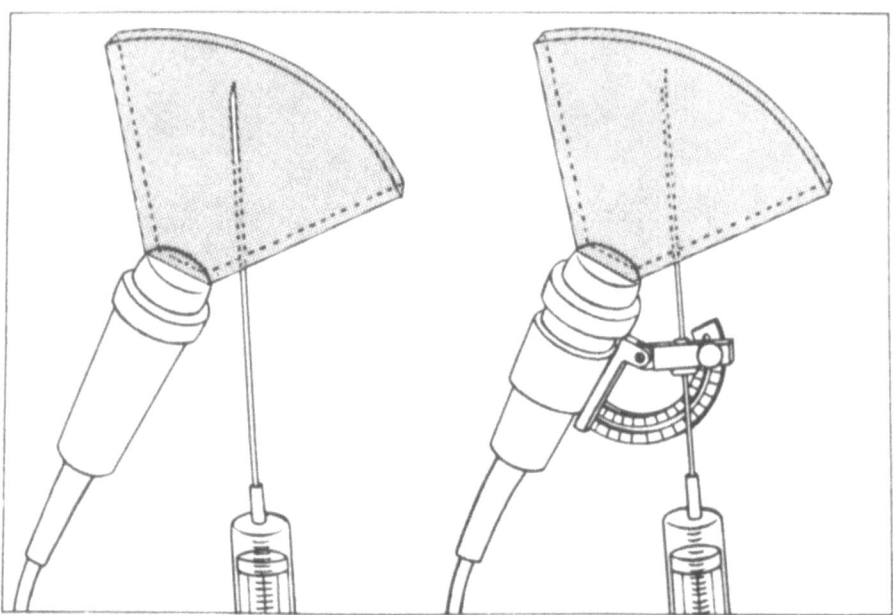

Figure 9. For safe pericardiocentesis it is essential to position the needle in the scanning plane. If the position of the needle is out of the scanning plane (left drawing) a part of the needle body could be misinterpreted as the needle tip. The further advance of such an imaged "tip" could be fatal. The drawing on the right shows a puncture or biopsy adaptor mounted to the phased array sector scan transducer. It ensures that the position of the needle is always in the scanning plane and the needle guidance at an adjustable angle to the transducer.

With a view to performing safe therapeutic or diagnostic pericardiocentesis we have, over the last four years, been guiding the introduction of the needle for pericardiocentesis using two-dimensional echocardiography in 17 patients with pericardial effusion [20, 47, 49, 51, 52, 54]. All the patients had semiquantitatively moderate to large pericardial effusion. For safe pericardiocentesis it is essential to position the needle in the scanning plane. If a portion of the needle is out of the scanning plane part of the needle body could be misinterpreted as the needle tip, as illustrated in Figure 9. The position of the needle tip can be confirmed by a contrast study — instillation of 2-5 ml of sterile normal saline or pericardial fluid through the needle. If a contrast jet appears at the presumed needle tip, it may be considered as the true tip (Figure 10). Besides the classical subxyphoid approach (Figure 11) [67], in patients with concomitant pleural effusion we performed pericardiocentesis through the posterior or lateral thoracic wall (Figure 12A). We found this approach to be most convenient provided large pleural effusion assures a large echo-free corridor toward the parietal pericardium. In addition the largest amount of pericardial fluid usually collects behind the left ventricular posterior wall and the cardiac apex moves away from the needle in systole lowering the risk of cardiac damage. After entering the pericardial sac the needle

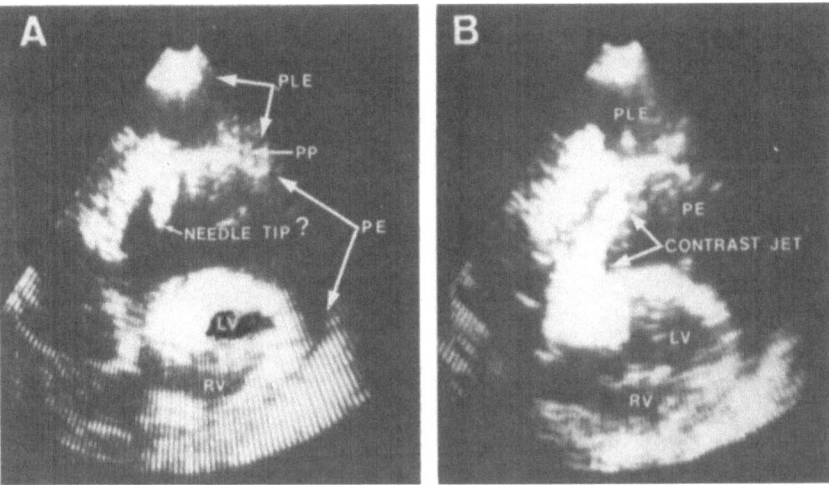

Figure 10. The position of the needle tip during pericardiocentesis may be confirmed by contrast study. Panel A shows presumed needle tip in the pericardial effusion (PE). The patient had concomitant pleural effusion (PLE) and puncture was performed by posterior thoracic approach through pleural effusion. If contrast jet appears at presumed needle tip it may be considered a true tip (panel B). LV : left ventricle, RV : right ventricle, PP : parietal pericardium.

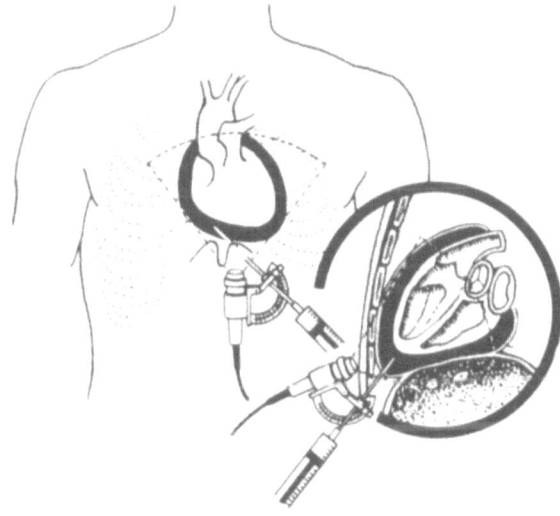

Figure 11. Schematic presentation of subcostal approach for pericardiocentesis guided by two-dimensional echocardiography.

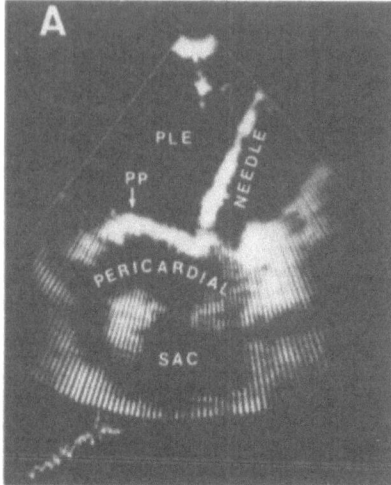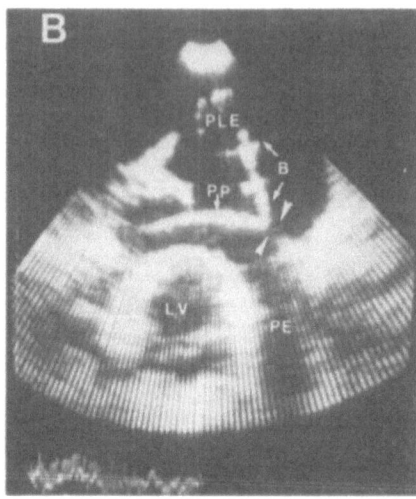

Figure 12. A. The entire length of the needle for pericardiocentesis passing through the large pleural effusion (PLE) to the parietal pericardium (PP) and pericardial sac. B. Bioptom (B) and the window (arrows) in the parietal pericardium created during pericardial biopsy. PE : pericardial effusion, LV : left ventricle.

should be replaced by a plastic catheter. The position of the needle or replacement catheter could be monitored continuously during the procedure and repositioned if found necessary. In 1 out of 17 patients from our study group a complication – ventricular puncture with intrapericardial bleeding – occurred, requiring immediate thoracotomy. In this patient the apical approach was used because an enlarged nodular liver thwarted the subxyphoid approach.

Recently, for the purpose of guiding the needle, we constructed a special puncture or biopsy adaptor mounted to the phased array sector scan transducer (see Figure 9). The needle is introduced through the guide channel in the adaptor and advances to the desired target under direct monitoring on the oscilloscope. The puncture adaptor ensures the needle guidance and needle position is always in the scanning plane, thus eliminating the possibility of misinterpretation of the needle tip. The needle can be positioned in the scanning plane at an adjustable angle by means of a flexible guide channel holder. Because the puncture needle is angled relative to the ultrasound beam, the entire length of the needle in the scanning plane is imaged. If a transducer with a central lumen is used only the needle tip is visualized, because the echo arises at the needle tip – fluid interface.

Manual adjustment of the needle in the scanning plane without an adaptor is time consuming. Attention should be devoted to preparing the patient, the adequate sterilisation of instruments and to electrical safety precautions. We believe that the technique described could eliminate the risk of the most serious complication in pericardiocentesis – that of cardiac damage.

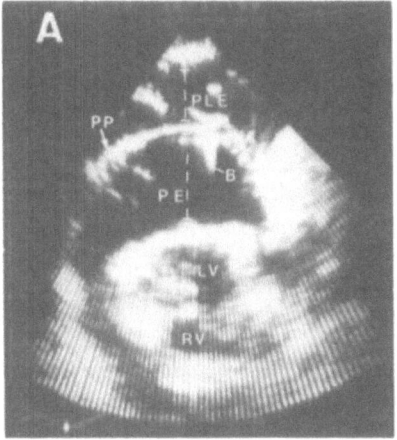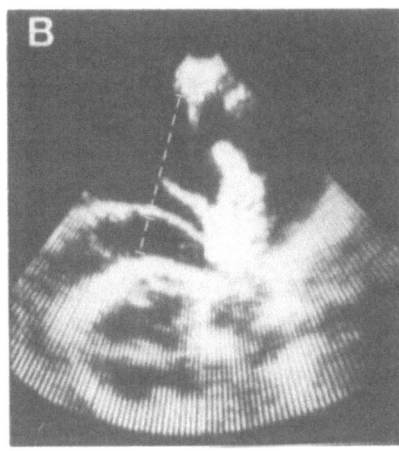

Figure 13. After pericardial biopsy and fenestration large pericardial fluid under high pressure drained into the pleural space. As a consequence a large pericardial effusion (PE) (A) diminished in favour of small pleural effusion (PLE) which became large (B). PP : parietal pericardium, B : bioptom, LV : left ventricle, RV : right ventricle.

PERCUTANEOUS PERICARDIAL BIOPSY AND FENESTRATION

Diagnostic pericardiocentesis enables etiologic diagnosis in less than one third of patients with pericardial effusion [68]. Thus in many cases of pericardial effusion thoracotomy with pericardial biopsy remains the definitive diagnostic solution. In recurrent pericardial effusion with tamponade during thoracotomy a pericardial window can be created and pericardial fluid drained into the pleural space.

In an attempt to avoid thoracotomy and general anesthesia for histologic diagnosis of pericardial lesion in patients with pericardial effusion we introduced a new technique of percutaneous pericardial biopsy and pericardial fenestration under two-dimensional echocardiographic guidance [52, 69]. The same technique as described for pericardiocentesis was used. Pericardial biopsy was performed in six patients, while pericardial window was created in two patients. In patients with concomitant left pleural effusion, the posterior or lateral thoracic approach was preferred as in pericardiocentesis (Figure 12B). A disposable Trucut Travenel biopsy needle with a 15.2 cm cannula length and 20 mm specimen notch was used. In patients with coexistent left pleural effusion after the pericardial specimen was taken the remaining window was enlarged and pericardial fluid drained into the pleural space under high pressure (Figure 13). Pericardial window created during pericardial biopsy for pericardial decompression could save repeated pericardiocentesis in recurrent pericardial effusion with tamponade. In all patients an adequate tissue specimen for histological analysis was obtained and proper histological diagnosis was made. So far no complications have been

154

observed. However, a larger series of patients is necessary to determine the safety of the described procedure. It is believed that in the future the new adaptor described above will refine and hasten the biopsy technique and improve its safety.

REFERENCES

1. Edler I: Diagnostic use of ultrasound in heart disease. Acta Med Scand 152 (Suppl 308):32, 1955.
2. Feigenbaum H, Waldhausen JA, Hyde LP: Ultrasound diagnosis of pericardial effusion. JAMA 191:711, 1965.
3. Feigenbaum H, Zaky A, Waldhausen JA: Use of ultrasound in the diagnosis of pericardial effusion. Ann Int Med 65:443, 1966.
4. Feigenbaum H, Zaky A, Grabhorn LL: Cardiac motion in patients with pericardial effusion: a study using reflected ultrasound. Circulation 34:611, 1966.
5. Moss AJ, Bruhn F: The echocardiogram: an ultrasound technique for the detection of pericardial effusion. N Engl J Med 274:380, 1966.
6. Feigenbaum H, Zaky A, Waldhausen JA: Use of reflected ultrasound in detecting pericardial effusion. Am J Cardiol 19:84, 1967.
7. Soulen RL, Dapayowker MS, Gimenez JL: Echocardiography in the diagnosis of pericardial effusion. Radiology 86:1047, 1966.
8. Rothman J, Chase NE, Kricheff II, Mayoral R, Beranbaum ER: Ultrasonic diagnosis of pericardial effusion. Circulation 35:358, 1967.
9. Pate JW, Gardner HC, Norman RS: Diagnosis of pericardial effusion by echocardiography. Ann Surg 165:826, 1967.
10. Goldberg BB, Ostrum BJ, Isard HJ: Ultrasonic determination of pericardial effusion. JAMA 202:103, 1967.
11. Klein JJ, Segal BL: Pericardial effusion diagnosed by reflected ultrasound. Am J Cardiol 22:57, 1968.
12. Feigenbaum H: Ultrasonic cardiology: diagnostic ultrasound as an aid to the management of patients with pericardial effusion, Chest 55:59, 1969.
13. Vignola PA, Pohost GM, Surfamn GD, Myers GS: Correlation of echocardiographic and clinical findings in patients with pericardial effusion. Am J Cardiol 37:701, 1976.
14. Tajik AJ: Echocardiography in pericardial effusion. Am J Med 63:29, 1977.
15. Feigenbaum H: Echocardiography, 3rd ed., Lea & Febiger, Philadelphia, 1981.
16. Nanda NC, Gramiak R: Clinical Echocardiography. C.V. Mosby Company, Saint Louis, 1978.
17. Horowitz MS, Schultz CS, Stinson EB, Harrison DC, Popp RL: Sensitivity and specificity of echocardiographic diagnosis of pericardial effusion. Circulation 50:239, 1974.
18. Roelandt J: Practical Echocardiology, Research Studies Press, Forest Grove, Oregon, 1977.
19. Martin RP, Rakowski H, French J, Popp R: Localisation of pericardial effusion with wide angle phased array echocardiography. Am J Cardiol 42:904, 1978.
20. Cikes I: Two-dimensional echocardiography in the diagnosis of pericardial effusion and adhesive pericarditis. In: Recent Advances in Ultrasound Diagnosis 2, pp. 306–316 (ed. A. Kurjak), Excerpta Medica, Amsterdam-Oxford-Princeton, 1980.
21. Walinsky P: Pitfalls in the diagnosis of pericardial effusion. In: Clinical Echocardiography, pp. 111–112 (ed. M.N. Kottler and B.L. Segal), F.A. Davis Company, Philadelphia, 1978.
22. Popp RL, Rubenson DS, Tucker CR, French JW: Echocardiography: M-mode and two-dimensional methods. Ann Intern Med 93:844, 1980.
23. Feigenbaum H: Echocardiographic diagnosis of pericardial effusion. Am J Cardiol 26:475, 1970.
24. Foote WC, Jefferson CM, Price HL: False-positive echocardiographic diagnosis of pericardial

effusion: result of tumor encasement of the heart simulating constrictive pericarditis. Chest 71:546, 1977.

25. Lin TK, Stech JM, Eckert WG, Lin JJ, Farha SJ, Hagan CT: Pericardial angiosarcoma simulating pericardial effusion by echocardiography. Chest 73: 881, 1978.

26. Chandraratna PAN, Littman BB, Serafini A, Whayne T, Robinson H: Echocardiographic evaluation of extracardiac masses. Br Heart J 40:741, 1978.

27. Millman A, Meller J, Motro M, Blank HS, Horowitz I, Herman MV, Teichholz LE: Pericardial tumor or fibrosis mimicking pericardial effusion by echocardiography. Ann Int Med 86:434, 1977.

28. Child JS, Abbasi AS, Pearce ML: Echocardiographic differentiation of mediastinal tumors from primary cardiac disease. Chest 67:108, 1975.

29. Tingelstad JB, McWilliams NB, Thomas CS: Confirmation of a retrosternal mass by echocardiogram. J Clin U 4:129, 1976.

29a. Greene DA, Kleid JJ, Naidu S: Unusual echocardiographic manifestation of pericardial effusion. Am J Cardiol 39:112, 1977.

30. Felner JM, Fleming WH, Franch RH: Echocardiographic identification of a pericardial cyst. Chest 68:386, 1975.

31. Reeves WC, Nanda NC, Barold SS: Echocardiographic evaluation of intracardiac pacing catheters: M-mode and two-dimensional studies. Circulation 58:1049, 1978.

32. Popp RL, Harrison DC: Echocardiography. In: Noninvasive Cardiology (ed. AM Weisler) Grune & Stratton, New York, 1974.

33. Cohen BE, Winer HE, Kronzon I: Echocardiographic findings in patients with left superior vena cava and dilated coronary sinus. Am J Cardiol 44:158, 1979.

34. Come PC, Riley MF, Fortuin NJ: Echocardiographic mimicry of pericardial effusion. Am J Cardiol 47:365, 1981.

35. Ratshin RA, Smith MK, Hood WP: Possible false-positive diagnosis of pericardial effusion by echocardiography in presence of large left atrium. Chest 65:112, 1974.

36. Roelandt J, Van Den Brand M, Vletter WB, Nauta J, Hugenholtz PG: Echocardiographic diagnosis of pseudo-aneurysm of the left ventricle. Circulation 52:466, 1975.

37. D'Cruz IA, Cohen HA, Prabhu R, Bisla V, Glick G: Clinical manifestations of mitral annulus calcification, with emphasis on its echocardiographic features. Am Heart J 94:367, 1977.

38. Kerber RE, Payvandi MN: Echocardiography in acute hemopericardium: production of false-negative echocardiograms by pericardial cloths. Circulation (suppl 3) 56:24, 1977.

39. Cassarella WJ, Schneider BO: Pitfalls in the ultrasonic diagnosis of pericardial effusion. Am J Roentgenol Rad Ther Nucl Med 110:760, 1970.

40. Schiller NB, Botvinick EH: Right ventricular compression as a sign of cardiac tamponade: an analysis of echocardiographic ventricular dimensions and their clinical implications. Circulation 56:774.

41. Gabor GE, Winsberg F, Bloom HS: Electrical and mechanical alteration in pericardial effusion. Chest 59, 341, 1971.

42. D'Cruz IA, Prabhu R, Cohen HC, Glick G: Potential pitfalls in quantification of pericardial effusions by echocardiography. Br Heart J 39:529, 1977.

43. Shina S, Yaginuma T, Kondo K, Kawai N, Hosoda S: Echocardiographic evaluation of impending cardiac tamponade. J Cardiogr 9:555, 1979.

44. Parisi AF, Tow DE: Pericardial Disease. In: Noninvasive Approaches to Cardiovascular Diagnosis (ed. AE Parisi, DE Tow), Appleton-Century-Crofts, New York, pp. 167 – 180, 1979.

45. Gibson TC, Grossman W, McLaurin LP: Echocardiography in patients with constrictive pericarditis. Circulation 49 & 50 (suppl 3):86, 1974.

46. Nishimoto M, Tanaka C, Oku H, Ikuno Y, Kawai S, Furukawa K, Takeuchi K, Shiota K: Presystolic pulmonary valve opening in constrictive pericarditis. J Cardiogr 7:55, 1977.

47. Cikes I, Cikes N, Pustisek S: Dvodimenzionalni echokardiografski prikaz fibrinoznog perikar-

156

ditisa i perikardijalnih adhezija u bolesnice sa sistemskim lupus eritematodesom, Zbornik radova kardioloskih sekcija SLD i ZLH, Zlatar, 1979.

48. Chang S, Chang JK: Cross-sectional echocardiography and progressive constrictive pericarditis. In: Recent Advances in Ultrasound Diagnosis 2 (ed. A Kurjak), Excerpta Medica, Amsterdam-Oxford-Princeton, pp. 317 – 322, 1980.

49. Cikes I, Cikes N, Ivancic R: Two-dimensional echocardiography in the diagnosis of pericardial and pleuropericardial adhesions. In: Proceedings of the International Congress on Echocardiography, Rome, 1980.

50. Martin RP, Bowdan R, Filly K, Popp RL: Intrapericardial abnormalities in patients with pericardial effusion: findings by two-dimensional echocardiography. Circulation 61:568, 1980.

51. Cikes I, Cikes N, Drinkovic N, Jelic I, Pustisek S: Two-dimensional echocardiography in the detection of intrapericardial masses in pericardial effusion (abstract), 4th Symposium on Echocardiography, Rotterdam, p. 6, 1981.

52. Cikes I, Ernst A: New possibilities in echocardiographic diagnosis of pericardial diseases. In: Recent Advances in Ultrasound Diagnosis 3, (ed. A Kurjak, A Kratochwil), Excerpta Medica, Amsterdam-Oxford-Princeton, pp. 377 – 386, 1981.

53. Chandraratna PAN, Aronow S: Detection of pericardial metastases by cross-sectional echocardiography. Circulation 63:19, 1981.

54. Cikes I: Echocardiography in pericardial disease. In: Progress in Medical Ultrasound 3 (ed. A Kurjak), Excerpta Medica, Amsterdam-Oxford-Princeton, 1982.

55. Schuh F: Erfahrungen über die Paracentese der Brust und des Herzbeutels. Med. Jarhb.d.k.k. Oster-Staates Wien (Neuste Folge 24) 33:388, 1841.

56. Wong B, Murphy JA, Chang CJ, Hassenein K, Dunn M: The risk of pericardiocentesis, Am J Cardiol 44:1110, 1979.

57. Kotte JH, McGuire J: Pericardial paracentesis, Mod Conc Cardiovasc Dis 20:102, 1979.

58. Kilpatrick ZN, Chapman CG: On pericardiocentesis. Am J Cardiol 16:722, 1965.

59. Krikorian JG, Hancock EW: Pericardiocentesis. Am J Med 65:808, 1978.

60. Bishop LH, Estes EH, McIntosh HD: The electrocardiogram as a safeguard in pericardiocentesis. JAMA 62:264, 1956.

61. Nordenstrom B: Percutaneous catheterization of the pericardium. Acta Radiol 4:662, 1966.

62. Glancy DL, Richter MA: Catheter drainage of the pericardial space. Cathet Cardiovasc Diagn 2:311, 1975.

63. Masumi RA, Rios JC, Ross AM, Ewy GA: Technique for insertion of an indwelling intrapericardial catheter. Br Heart J 30:333, 1968.

64. Owens WC, Schaefer RA, Rahimtoola SH: Pericardiocentesis: Insertion of a pericardial catheter. Cathet Cardiovasc Diagn 1:317, 1975.

65. Wei JY, Taylor GJ, Aschuff SC: Recurrent cardiac tamponade and large pericardial effusions: Management with an indwelling pericardial catheter. Am J Cardiol 42:281, 1978.

66. Goldberg BB, Pollock HM: Ultrasonically guided pericardiocentesis. Am J Cardiol 31:490, 1973.

67. Marfan AB: Ponction du péricarde par l'épigastre. Ann Méd chir inf 15:529, 1911.

68. Hancock EW, Krikorian JG: Benefits and risks of pericardiocentesis, 1970 – 1976. Proceedings of the Association of University Cardiologists, Phoenix, Arizona, 1977.

69. Ernst A, Cikes I, Persic T, Cepelja Z: Percutaneous pericardial biopsy and fenestration guided by echocardiography, Abstracts, 4th European Congress in Ultrasonics in Medicine, Dubrovnik, Excerpta Medica, Amsterdam, p. 67, 1981.

10. ECHOCARDIOGRAPHY OF THE CARDIOMYOPATHIES: CONGESTIVE, HYPERTROPHIC AND RESTRICTIVE TYPES

F.J. ten Cate and J. Roelandt

INTRODUCTION

Echocardiography has revolutionized our ability to diagnose, classify and study the natural history and effects of therapeutic interventions in patients with cardiomyopathy. These commonly present with symptoms of chest pain, dyspnea, palpitations, syncope and/or abnormal signs on their electrocardiogram or chest X-ray. With the introduction of echocardiography the diagnosis often is made fortuitously during a routine echocardiographic examination in patients with minor complaints.

Cardiomyopathies are heart muscle disease of unknown cause (primary or idiopathic cardiomyopathy) and are divided into dilated (or congestive), hypertrophic, and restrictive types [1]. Since both the etiologic and pathophysiologic classification of cardiomyopathies based on hemodynamics, pathologic findings or clinical grounds are limited we propose an echocardiographic classification which is most useful in clinical practice.

Abnormalities of structure and function are mainly related to the left ventricle (LV) in these patients. Therefore the echocardiographic analysis and classification is based on abnormalities of the left ventricle (Table 1). Hemodynamic changes are reflected in mitral valve motion and in left atrial and right ventricular size [2].

Table 1. Echocardiographic classification of the cardiomyopathies

- Dilated LV cavity with normal walls and decreased function
  - Dilated (congestive) cardiomyopathy
- Normal LV cavity with thickened walls and normal function
  - Symmetric hypertrophy
    Restrictive (infiltrative) cardiomyopathy
  - Asymmetric hypertrophy
    Hypertrophic cardiomyopathy (HCM)
    Hypertrophic obstructive cardiomyopathy (HOCM)

Roelandt, J. (ed.) The practice of M-mode and two-dimensional echocardiography
© *1983, Martinus Nijhoff Publishers. The Hague / Boston / London*
ISBN 978-94-009-6792-2.

DILATED CARDIOMYOPATHY

The heart in these patients is overweight and shows dilatation of all cardiac chambers while the myocardium is pale and flabby. LV wall thickness is normal, although some degree of hypertrophy may occasionally be present. The endocardium is usually thickened and a mural thrombus is found in 60% of the cases at necropsy. Coronary arteries are usually normal. Although a viral cause has been proposed for this condition no definite proof is available and its etiology may well be multifactorial. Causes of the secondary types of dilated cardiomyopathy of which the clinical manifestation is similar to the primary type are listed in Table 2.

Table 2. Secondary causes of dilated cardiomyopathy

- Ischemic heart disease
- End-stage valvular heart disease
- Infective
- Metabolic
- General systemic disease
- Inherited musculoskeletal disease
- Sensitivity or toxic reaction to drugs
- Postpartum

Hemodynamic abnormalities in patients with dilated cardiomyopathy result from loss of myocardial contractile function (pump failure). Consequently there is a severely dilated LV with low ejection fraction and a high end-diastolic pressure. In some cases biventricular failure is present.

ECHOCARDIOGRAPHIC MANIFESTATIONS

Echocardiographically, an increased LV cavity dimension and a low fractional shortening (< 25%) are found. The LV acquires a globular shape and its outflow tract is wide (Figures 1 and 2). Fractional thickening and the amplitude of motion of the LV walls are reduced. Mean and peak velocities of dimensional shortening and lengthening are low. The duration of the rapid filling period is short as compared to normal.

In the dilated LV the mitral valve apparatus tends to remain close to the LVPW and the aML therefore can be at a level distinctly posterior to the posterior aortic wall. Systolic motion of the mitral valve is normal but additional linear echoes are often seen draped over the mitral valve configuration, spanning its peaks from cycle to cycle. They probably result from superimposition of echoes originating from different areas of the mitral valve apparatus (sound beam width artifact). Because of the LV dilatation, the mitral valve apparatus is

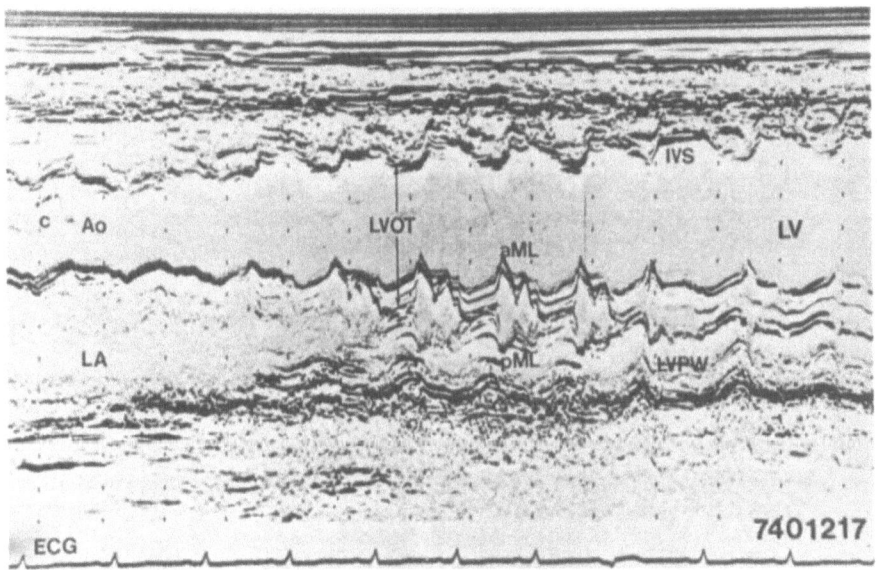

Figure 1. M-mode scan of a patient with dilated cardiomyopathy. The left ventricular (LV) cavity dimension, the left atrial (LA) cavity and left ventricular outflow tract (LVOT) are enlarged. Mitral valve motion shows a "B" notch and multiple systolic echoes. Ao : aorta, c : valve cusps of aorta, IVS : interventricular septum, aML : anterior mitral valve leaflet, pML : posterior mitral valve leaflet. (With permission from Roelandt J., Practical Echocardiology, Research Studies Press, Forest Grove, 1977).

stretched to an extent that valve mechanics is altered.

This together with the higher heart rate results in a "double-diamond" diastolic mitral valve pattern in which, because of reduced mobility, the anterior and posterior mitral leaflets have amplitudes of motion which are almost equal.

The decreased amplitude of opening (less than 20 mm) is further a result of the low cardiac output. An increased end-diastolic pressure is usually present and this may be reflected on the mitral valve echogram as a shortened PR-AC interval (< 50 msec) interrupted by a "B-notch". The elevated end-diastolic pressure and mitral regurgitation when present lead to left atrial enlargement. A decreased systolic opening amplitude on the aortic valve is present when cardiac output is low. Right ventricular dilatation occurs late in the stage of illness. Mural thrombi often complicate dilated cardiomyopathy and are best detected with two-dimensional echocardiography. Salient echocardiographic features of dilated cardiomyopathy are listed in Table 3.

The echocardiographic syndrome of "dilated cardiomyopathy" does not always correspond with the clinical diagnosis of a primary cardiomyopathy. It is also found in patients with severe LV dysfunction due to end-stage valvular heart disease (e.g. aortic stenosis) or with coronary heart disease being the two most common conditions seen in clinical practice. Valvular heart disease is readily

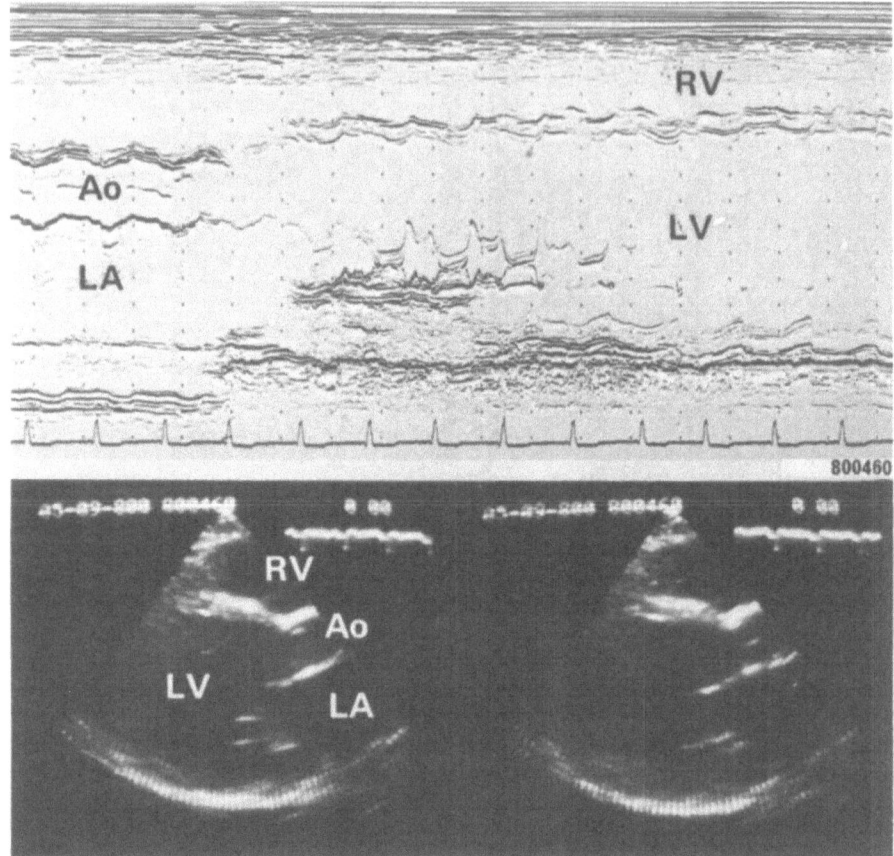

Figure 2. M-mode scan (top) and stop-frames of two-dimensional parasternal long axis (PSLAX) views (bottom) at early systole (left) and early diastole (right). Note the hypocontractile dilated left ventricle (LV) with a wide outflow tract (LVOT). The globular shape is apparent on the PSLAX views. Ao : aorta, LA : left atrium, RV : right ventricle.

Table 3. Echocardiographic findings of dilated cardiomyopathy

Left ventricle

cavity diameter ↑
outflow tract ↑
globular LV shape
systolic function ↓

Mitral valve

"double diamond" pattern
PR-AC interval < 50 msec
"B" notch

Associated findings

LA dilatation
RV dilatation

diagnosed or excluded by studying the valves. Diffuse wall motion abnormalities are in favor of a primary dilated cardiomyopathy, whereas segmental abnormalities more often occur in coronary artery diasease. The clinical context is further helpful in differentiating between primary and secundary cardiomyopathy.

HYPERTROPHIC CARDIOMYOPATHY (HCM)

The most striking structural abnormality in hypertrophic cardiomyopathy resides in the interventricular septum (IVS) which is nearly always thicker than the left ventricular free wall (about 5% of the patients with this condition have symmetric hypertrophy). The thickest portion of the IVS is usually located about midway between the aortic valve and left ventricular apex. Occasionally, the hypertrophy is more confined to the upper third and exceptionally to the lower third of the IVS.

Anterior displacement of the antero – lateral and postero – medial papillary muscles and the peculiar deformity of the LV cavity are highly characteristic. A fibrotic endocardial lesion just below the aortic valve on the IVS may be present. Coronary arteries are normal. Although histologic findings of fibre disarray of cardiac muscle excised at cardiac surgery or at necropsy have been proposed to be diagnostic, it has recently been shown that a combination of abnormalities rather than this single isolated feature make the diagnosis of HCM. Fibre disarray may indeed be seen with other disorders such as coronary artery disease, hypertension, hyperthyreoidism, in patients on chronic hemodialysis treatment and in infants of diabetic mothers (Table 4). Cardiac function is impaired by a combination of normal systolic function and abnormal diastolic relaxation and compliance. In some patients a functional obstruction to LV outflow may be present: hypertrophic obstructive cardiomyopathy "HOCM" or idiopathic hypertrophic subaortic stenosis "IHSS".

The clinical manifestations are heterogenic and can range from an asymptomatic individual with echocardiographic signs of HCM to a patient with severe complaints of angina, dyspnea or syncope [1]. Sudden unexpected death may be

Table 4. Clinical conditions simulating hypertrophic cardiomyopathy

- Hypertensive heart disease
- Ischemic heart disease
- Severe aortic stenosis
- Coarctation of aorta
- Heart in acromegaly
- Heart in hyper- or hypothyreoidism
- Infants of diabetic mothers
- Chronic hemodialysis

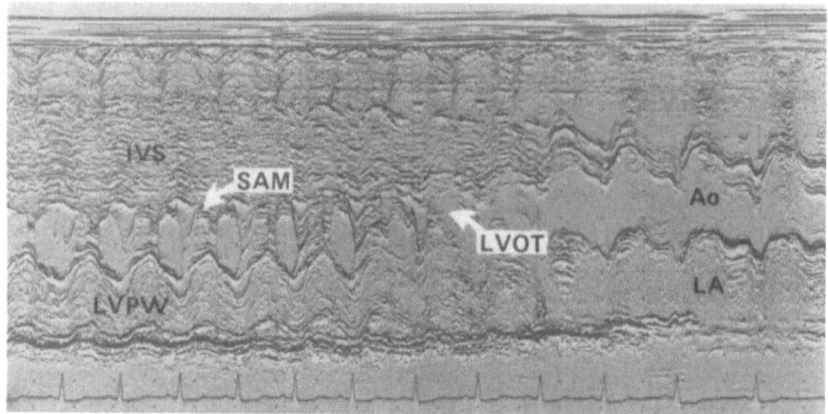

Figure 3. M-mode echocardiogram of a patient with severe hypertrophic obstructive cardiomyopathy (HOCM). Note the increased hypertrophy of the interventricular septum (IVS), which is hypokinetic, the narrow left ventricular outflow tract (LVOT) and systolic anterior motion (SAM) of the anterior mitral valve leaflet. Ao : aorta; LA : left atrium, LVPW : left ventricular posterior wall.

the first symptom of the disease and is the most common cause of sudden death in young individuals dying during active exercise.

Studies in the U.S. and Holland have demonstrated that cardiomyopathic asymmetric septal hypertrophy is usually genetically transmitted as an autosomal dominant trait [3, 4].

ECHOCARDIOGRAPHIC MANIFESTATIONS

Echocardiography is a reliable and certainly the best clinical method to detect the anatomic abnormalities of hypertrophic cardiomyopathy. A ratio of septal thickness to that of the LVPW in the posterobasal region of 1.3 or greater has been reported to be diagnostic for the condition (Figure 3). It should be emphasized that identification of the right side of the IVS may be difficult from routine echocardiograms. The isolated echocardiographic demonstration of asymmetric septal hypertrophy is a sensitive but not a specific marker for the diagnosis of primary hypertrophic cardiomyopathy and may be found in other conditions (Table 4).

The prevalence of a ratio of IVS/free wall thickness of 1.3 or greater in a general hospital population with heart disease, but without proven cardiomyopathy, is 8% [4]. Fractional and peak rates of thickening of the IVS are decreased while the same parameters of the LV free wall are increased, resulting in a normal or even above normal overall systolic LV function. The variability of the spectrum of LV dysfunction is better appreciated when diastolic function parameters are considered. Peak left ventricular filling rate is reduced (reflected in a decreased early diastolic closure rate of the aML) and the duration of the early (rapid) diastolic filling period is prolonged in some patients. Angina pectoris is common in patients with prolonged early diastolic relaxation, probably as a result of functional obstruction to inflow in otherwise normal coronary arteries.

Angina pectoris might therefore be useful as a clinical indicator of severe diastolic LV dysfunction.

Other echocardiographic features of hypertrophic cardiomyopathy are narrowing of the LVOT and the small LV size (Figure 3).

To determine the actual shape of the LV and the pattern and extent of myocardial hypertrophy in HCM, two-dimensional echocardiography is the best method [5, 6].

Four patterns of distribution of left ventricular hypertrophy can be identified when the parasternal short axis view at mitral valve level is used (Table 5) [5].

Type I: About 10% of patients have myocardial hypertrophy of the IVS confined to its anterior portion. This pattern of local hypertrophy is also seen in about 10% of patients where septal hypertrophy is equal in basal and apical regions.

Type II: In 20% myocardial hypertrophy involves both the anterior and posterior segments of the IVS whereas the LV free wall is essentially normal.

Type III: Most HCM patients (50%) have hypertrophy involving substantial portions of both the IVS and LVPW (Figure 6). Predominant regions of hypertrophy are the anterior or posterior parts of the IVS. These patients have a higher prevalence of obstruction to LV outflow.

Type IV: In this type different portions of the IVS are involved such as the posterior segment or the apical region of the LV wall. Some patients have hypertrophy only confined to portions of the antero-lateral LV free wall.

It is obvious that in patients in whom there is clinical suspicion of HCM but failure of the M-mode echocardiogram to demonstrate signs of HCM a two-dimensional echocardiographic analysis is mandatory.

Among patients with HCM, the thickness of the IVS is not dependent on the presence of LVOT obstruction at rest, and, indeed, IVS thickness is similar in patients with LVOT obstruction at rest and those without.

Examination of the basal portion of the LV free wall may permit delineation of these two groups of patients since in the non-obstructive group, the posterolateral basal portion of the LV wall behind the mitral valve is not only

Table 5. Morphologic types of myocardial hypertrophy in HCM

Type I	: Anterior portion of IVS (10%)
Type II	: Anterior and posterior portions of IVS (20%)
Type III	: Anterior and/or posterior IVS plus anterolateral wall (50%)
Type IV	: Posterior IVS and/or posterolateral wall (20%)

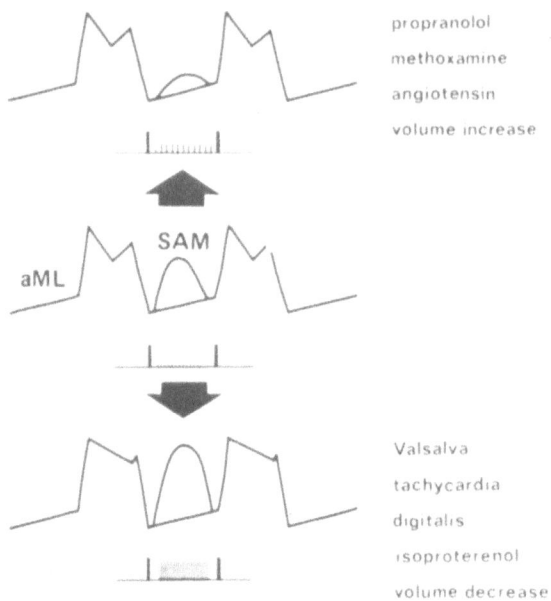

Figure 4. Diagram of systolic anterior motion (SAM) of the anterior mitral valve leaflet (aML) and heart murmur, indicating which factors can influence the magnitude of SAM and loudness of the murmur.

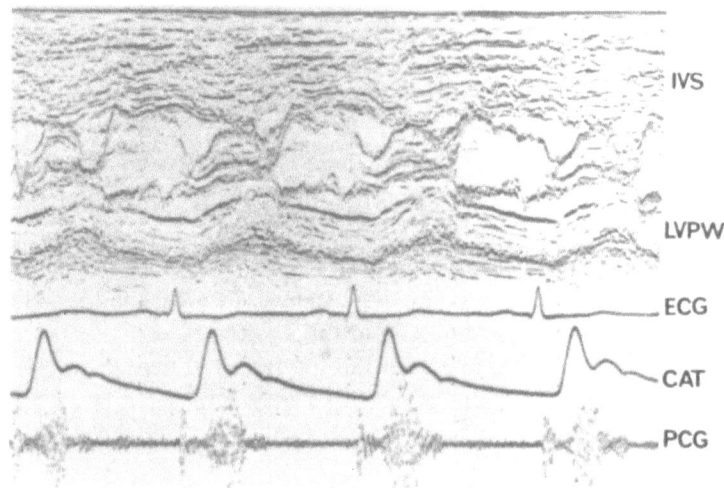

Figure 5. M-mode echocardiogram of patient with hypertrophic obstructive cardiomyopathy (HOCM), showing systolic anterior motion (SAM), appearing coincident with the characteristic mid- and late-systolic murmur (PCG : phonocardiogram) and the characteristic carotid artery tracing (CAT) with its bisferiens appearance. Observe that the rate of upstroke of SAM and systolic anterior motion of the left ventricular posterior wall (LVPW) are different indicating independent aML motion. ECG : electrocardiogram, IVS : interventricular septum.

thinner than the IVS but also thinner than the LV wall below the tips of the mitral valve. This is contrary to the normal LV and the LV of patients with hypertrophic obstructive cardiomyopathy, where this posterobasal portion of the LV wall represents the thickest part of the free wall and decreases in thickness from base to apex.

LVOT obstruction results chiefly from systolic anterior movement (SAM) of the anterior mitral valve leaflet (Figure 3). Four explanations have been offered for this SAM: 1. the mitral valve is pulled against the IVS by the contraction of the papillary muscles, which are abnormally located and oriented within the LV as a result of the asymmetric hypertrophy; 2. the mitral valve is pushed against the IVS because of its abnormal anterior position in the LVOT; 3. SAM results from an abnormal mitral valve coaptation, and 4. the aML is drawn towards the IVS because of the lower pressure that occurs as blood is ejected at a high velocity through the narrowed LVOT (Venturi effect). SAM and the abnormal bending of the papillary muscles, especially of the anterolateral one, prevents closure and is the most likely explanation for the mitral regurgitation often present in these patients.

As obstructive hypertrophic cardiomyopathy is a functional disease, SAM may be observed intermittently (e.g. in post-extrasystolic complexes) or may be evoked by amylnitrate or Valsalva maneuver (Figure 4). When the aML touches the IVS for more than 50% of systole, there is always a large outflow gradient. On two-dimensional images, SAM is best visualized in the apical long axis view. It is important to differentiate true from pseudo SAM patterns. True SAM demonstrates independent motion which cannot be related to any motion of a structure posterior to it. The aML returns to a closed position at the end of systole before the aortic valve closes (Table 6). It might therefore be helpful to have the carotid artery tracing or phonocardiogram recorded simultaneously. It should be mentioned that SAM does not always involve the middle part of the aML but may be more pronounced at the level of the chordae or even at its upper part.

SAM may be observed in other conditions than obstructive hypertrophic car-

Table 6. Echocardiographic diagnosis of SAM

True SAM pattern:
- aML reopens in systole after C point and returns to the closed position before D point
- initial slope independent of posterior structures
- occurs in HCM and in hyperkinetic circulatory states (e.g. afterload reduction)

False SAM patterns are seen in:
- large pericardial effusion ("swinging heart syndrome")
- interference of posterior aortic wall echoes with mitral valve echoes
- hyperkinetic posterior wall

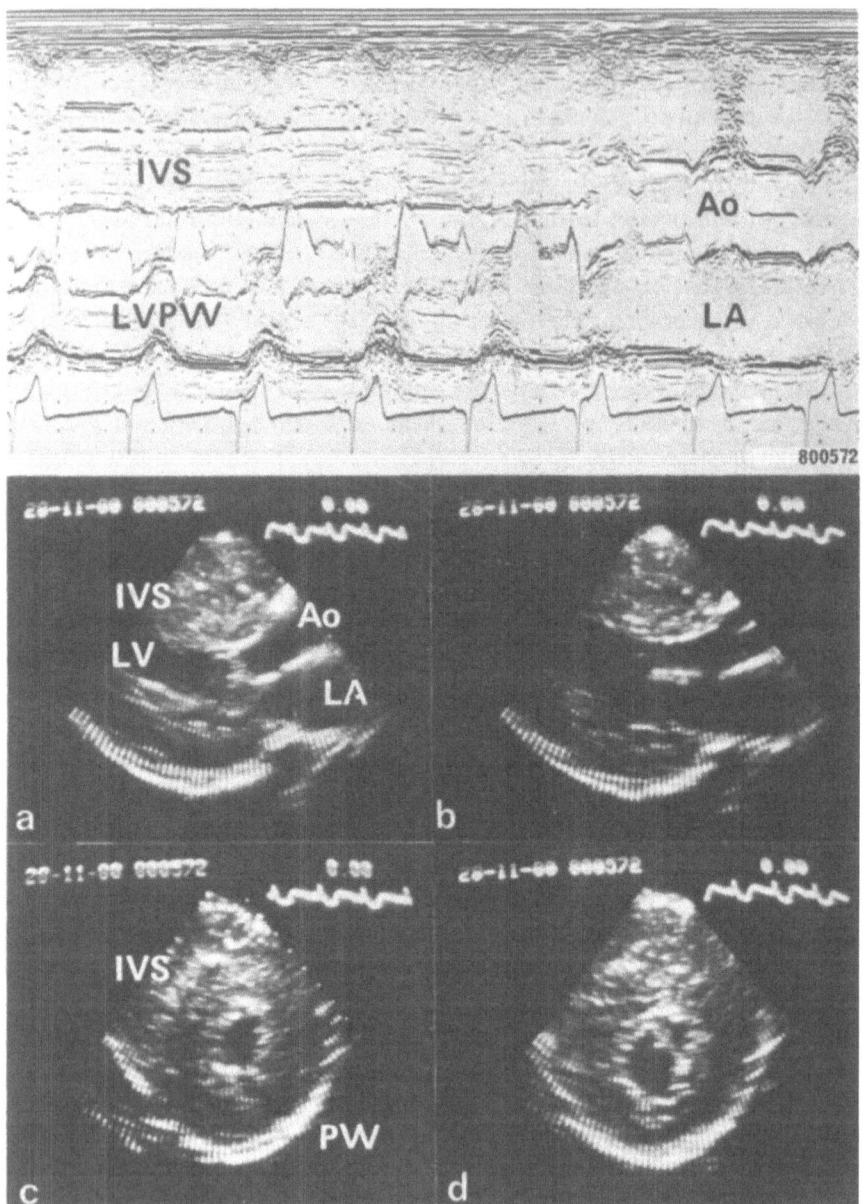

Figure 6. M-mode (top) and two-dimensional echocardiograms of a patient with hypertrophic cardiomyopathy (bottom). The parasternal long axis views (PSLAX) in systole (a) and diastole (b) and the parasternal short axis views (PSSAX) (c and d) are shown. Note that the septal (IVS) hypertrophy seen in the PSSAX views extends to the left ventricular anterolateral wall (type III HCM). An abnormal position of the aML or SAM is seen in the PSLAX view in systole and is not apparent on the M-mode echocardiogram. Ao : aorta, LA : left atrium, LV : left ventricle, PW : LV posterior wall.

diomyopathy such as aortic stenosis and incompetence, fixed subaortic stenosis, coarctation of the aorta, and in hypercontractile states especially when associated with hypovolemia. Confusing patterns may be seen in the mitral valve prolapse syndrome and in conditions with hyperactivity of the LVPW (e.g. RV volume overload). False SAM is sometimes seen with the swinging heart syndrome in large pericardial effusion.

The echo findings of ASH, a narrow LVOT and SAM are not a 100% specific for obstructive hypertrophic cardiomyopathy and may exceptionally be seen in infiltrative cardiomyopathy.

Echocardiographically, one may sometimes see an increased reflectivity of the mural septal endocardium at the level of the LVOT representing a fibrous plaque. This plaque originates at the area where the aML touches the IVS and is the anatomic equivalent of SAM. The abnormal LV cavity shape is best recognized by two-dimensional echocardiography. Other echocardiographic findings may be found: 1. increased left atrial size as a response to the impaired LV filling and mitral regurgitation; 2. partial systolic closure of the aortic valve cusps, produced by the subvalvular obstruction. A similar pattern can be seen on the pulmonary valve and is related to muscular obliteration of the right ventricular infundibulum during systole. Salient echocardiographic features of hypertrophic (obstructive) cardiomyopathy are given in Table 7.

After a myotomy-myectomy an enlarged LVOT can be demonstrated echocardiographically, and the actual excision of septal muscle is visualized in both the parasternal and apical long axis views (Figure 7). SAM does not always disappear.

Echocardiography remains the method of choice to follow patients with HCM longitudinally in the natural course of their disease and can also be used to determine the effect of therapeutic interventions, considering that a combination of echocardiographic signs rather than a single feature is diagnostic for HCM [7].

Table 7. Echocardiographic diagnosis of hypertrophic cardiomyopathy

Left ventricle

Asymmetric septal hypertrophy (ASH)
Outflow tract ↓
Abnormal cavity shape
Diastolic function ↓

Mitral valve

Systolic anterior motion (SAM)
EF slope ↓

Associated findings

LA dilatation
Mid-systolic aortic valve closure

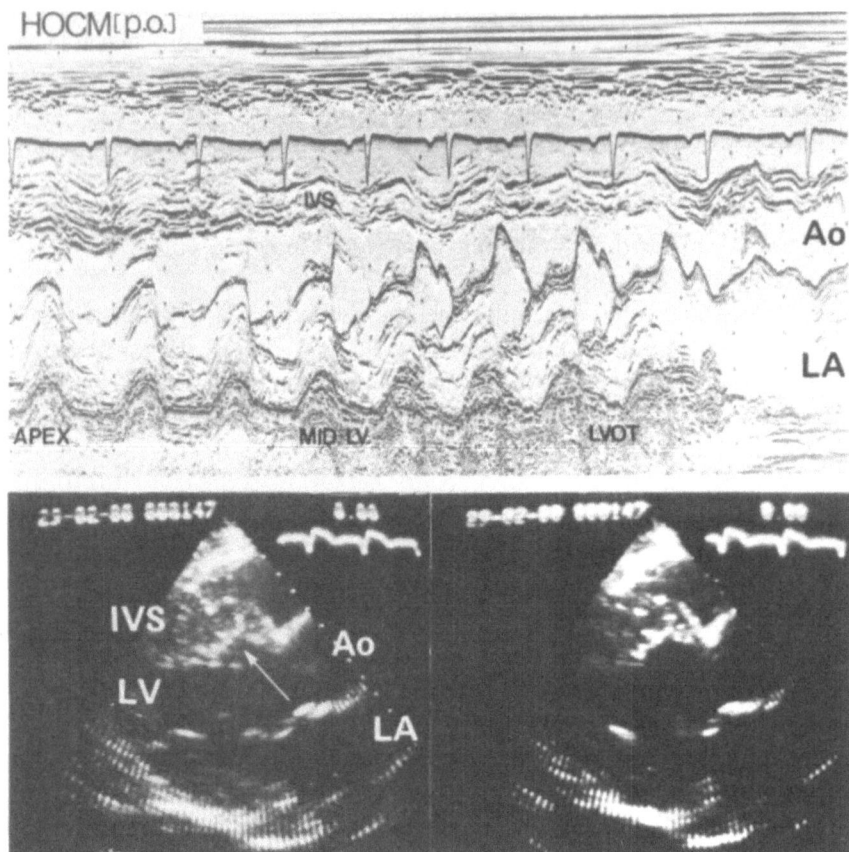

Figure 7. M-mode echocardiogram (top) and two-dimensional parasternal long axis views (bottom) of a patient who underwent myotomy-myectomy for HOCM. Note the wide LVOT as a result of the excision, on the M-mode and two-dimensional echocardiograms (arrow). Ao : aorta, IVS : interventricular septum, LA : left atrium, LV : left ventricle, LVOT : left ventricular outflow tract.

INFILTRATIVE (RESTRICTIVE) CARDIOMYOPATHY

The primary form of this condition is extremely rare. Secondary forms result from infiltration of the myocardium with either amyloid (amyloidosis), iron (hemocromatosis), neoplastic cells (eosinophilic leukemia), or glycogen. A clinical picture similar to that seen in restrictive cardiomyopathy occurs with ventricular obliteration by endomyocardial fibroelastosis and Löffler's endocarditis (Table 8).

Pathologically, there is marked hypertrophy of the LV walls with a normal or slight increase in cavity size. Clinically, the patients present with dyspnea or chest pain and signs of congestive heart failure while the heart may be normal on chest

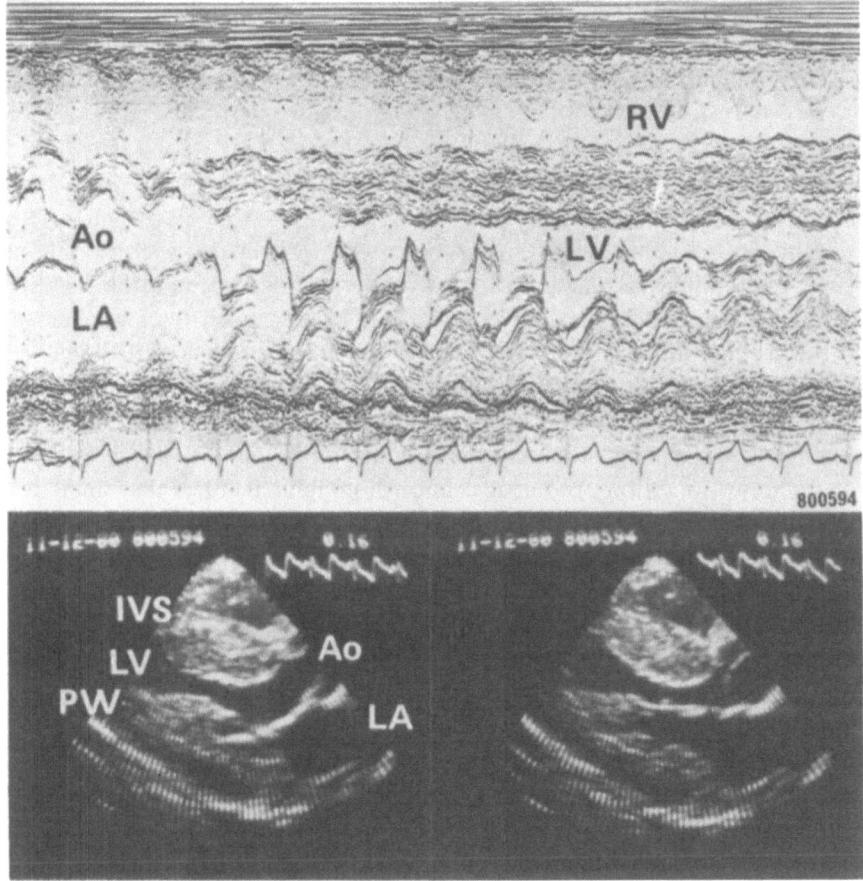

Figure 8. M-mode and two-dimensional echocardiograms of a patient with infiltrative cardiomyopathy due to amyloidosis. The symmetric hypertrophy of the interventricular septum (IVS) and left ventricular posterior wall (LVPW) and the small size of the left ventricle (LV) are apparent. Note the hypertrophy of the anterior heart wall which is typical for this condition.

Table 8. Causes of infiltrative (restrictive) cardiomyopathy

- Primary amyloidosis
- Sarcoidosis
- Scleroderma
- Hemochromatosis
- Pompe's disease
- Endomyocardial fibrosis
- Löffler endocarditis

X-ray. The disease is relatively rare. Some authors have suggested that patients with restrictive cardiomyopathy have a form of hypertrophic cardiomyopathy with predominant signs of decreased left ventricular distensibility and fibrosis.

ECHOCARDIOGRAPHIC MANIFESTATIONS

The echocardiographic findings are not specific. At an early stage, left ventricular cavity dimension may be normal as well as the motion of both IVS and LVPW. With progression of myocardial involvement wall thickness increases and thickening diminishes (30%) (Figure 9). There is a reduced EF slope of the aML indicating a reduced filling rate of the LV. A shortened PR-AC interval, indicative of an elevated end-diastolic pressure, is also found in most of these patients. Systemic hypertension may cause similar abnormalities and is in fact the most common condition producing echocardiographic features that simulate the echocardiographic patterns of restrictive (infiltrative) cardiomyopathy. Exceptionally, these echocardiographic findings are also seen in patients with coronary artery disease and in those with aortic stenosis. On real-time two-dimensional echocardiography the infiltration of the myocardium has a "sparkling" appearance. This "sparkling" is caused by different ultrasound reflection characteristics of the infiltrative material compared to normal myocardium (Figure 10).

Echocardiography, however, is of value in distinguishing restrictive cardiomyopathy from constrictive pericarditis of which the clinical picture may be quite similar. These two entities have different therapeutic and prognostic implications and are sometimes difficult to differentiate clinically and hemodynamically. Normal wall thickness, normal LVPW motion and paradoxical IVS motion are seen with constrictive pericarditis. The echocardiographic findings in infiltrative cardiomyopathy are listed in Table 9.

Table 9. Echocardiographic diagnosis of infiltrative (restrictive) cardiomyopathy

---

Left ventricle

Symmetric hypertrophy
Normal cavity diameter
Systolic and diastolic function ↓

Mitral valve

EF slope ↓
PR-AC interval < 50 msec
'B' notch

Associated findings

Increased LA cavity
Amyloid infiltration: "sparkling" sign and hypertrophy of anterior heart wall

---

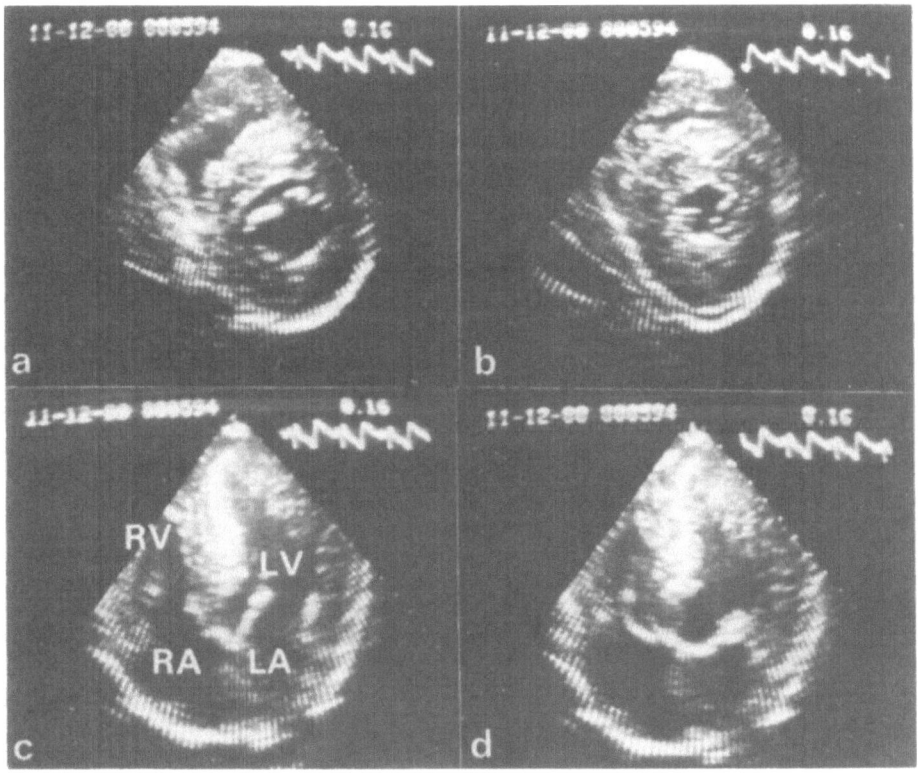

Figure 9. Parasternal short axis views (PSSAX) in diastole (a) and systole (b) and apical four chamber views (AP4C) in diastole (c) and systole (d) of a patient with amyloidosis. Note the symmetric hypertrophy of the left ventricular (LV) walls. In the AP4C views the infiltrative material gives peculiar reflective characteristics to the myocardium. LA : left atrium, RA : right atrium, RV : right ventricle.

CONCLUSION

Echocardiography is useful in evaluating a patient with a suspected cardiomyopathy. Measuring LV cavity dimensions, wall thickness and systolic function allows classification of patients into one of three categories: dilated, hypertrophic or restrictive cardiomyopathy. Echocardiography is an extremely sensitive and undoubtedly the best method to diagnose hypertrophic cardiomyopathy provided that the diagnostic complexes as described above are interpreted in clinical context.

REFERENCES

1. Goodwin JF, Oakley CM: The cardiomyopathies. Brit Heart J 34:545, 1972.
2. Roelandt J: Practical echocardiology. Research Studies Press, Forest Grove, Oregon, 1977.
3. Clark CE, Henry WL, Epstein S: Familial prevalence and genetic transmission of idiopathic hypertrophic subaortic stenosis. New Eng J of M 289:709, 1973.
4. Ten Cate FJ, Hugenholtz PG, Van Dorp WG, Roelandt J: Prevalence of diagnostic abnormalities in patients with genetically transmitted Asymmetric Septal Hypertrophy. Am J Cardiol 43:731, 1979.
5. Maron BJ, Gottdiener JS, Epstein S: Patterns and significance of distribution of left ventricular hypertrophy in hypertrophic cardiomyopathy. Am J Card 48:418, 1982.
6. DeMaria AN, Bommer W, Lee J, Mason DT: Value and limitations of two-dimensional echocardiography in assessment of cardiomyopathy. Am J Card 46:1224, 1980.
7. Grimer PF, Mayewski RJ, Mushkin AI, Greenland P: Selection and Interpretation of diagnostic tests and procedures. Ann Int Med 94 (suppl):581, 1981.
8. Siqueria-Filho AG, Cunha CLP, Tajik AJ et al: M-mode and two-dimensional echocardiographic features in cardiac amyloidosis. Circulation 63:188, 1981.
9. Child JS, Levisman JA, Abbasi AS: Echocardiographic manifestations of infiltrative cardiomyopathy: a report of seven cases due to amyloid. Chest 70:726, 1976.

11. ECHOCARDIOGRAPHY IN VEGETATIVE ENDOCARDITIS

IVO CIKES

During the past three decades the clinical, microbiological and therapeutic features of infective endocarditis have undergone striking changes. If one searched, today, for the classical diagnostic criteria – fever, changing murmur, splenomegaly, systemic embolisation and positive blood cultures – one would fail to suspect the diagnosis of infective endocarditis in as many as 90% of patients presenting with this disease process [1].

The characteristic lesion of infective endocarditis is a vegetation. It is a friable mass intimately involved with the valve leaflets microscopically consisting of fibrin, platelets, a group of polymorphonuclear leucocytes and microorganisms. With prolonged survival areas of fibrosis and calcification may occur. The usual sites are the atrial surface of the mitral valves and ventricular surface of the aortic valve. Occasionally they can be seen on the endocardium of cardiac cavities. The vegetations vary from small flat adherent nodules to large masses several centimeters in diameter, which could be sesile or pedunculated [2, 3].

Nonrational use of antimicrobial drugs resulted in high incidences of negative blood culture which make diagnosis of infective endocarditis more difficult. Early diagnosis and prompt antimicrobial therapy is essential to prevent irreversible valvular damage with subsequent acute congestive heart failure and to diminish the risk of embolisation. The need for a noninvasive method that could directly identify vegetation and other concomitant lesions in infective endocarditis was therefore manifest.

Currently, echocardiography is the only technique available (except for cardiac surgery and autopsy) that can visualize vegetation in vivo. Cardiac catheterisation may be hazardous because of the possibility of dislodgement of vegetation. Since the initial report of Schelbert and Muller [4] in 1972 many investigators have confirmed the utility of echocardiography in the diagnosis and therapy of infective endocarditis [5 – 9]. However, definitive conclusions concerning the sensitivity and specificity of these findings as well as their clinical implications in patient management and prognosis are not available. Also, there are only few comparative data available, evaluating the role of M-mode versus two-dimensional echocardiography in infective endocarditis.

Roelandt, J. (ed.) The practice of M-mode and two-dimensional echocardiography
© *1983, Martinus Nijhoff Publishers. The Hague / Boston / London*
ISBN 978-94-009-6792-2.

ECHOCARDIOGRAPHIC SIGNS OF INFECTIVE ENDOCARDITIS

The most direct echocardiographic sign of infective endocarditis is visualization of vegetations. Vegetative lesions could be found on valve leaflets, chordae of the mitral or tricuspid valve and rarely, on the mural endocardium of the cardiac chambers. The aortic and mitral valves are most frequently involved, less often the tricuspid valve and exceptionally the pulmonary valve.

Echocardiographically valvular vegetations are usually described as non-uniform leaflet thickening, a shaggy or fuzzy mass of echoes on the valve leaflet which usually do not restrict valve leaflet mobility (Figure 1). They are recorded during systole or diastole. In contrast chronic valvular lesions – fibrosis and calcification are characteristically more uniform valvular thickening impairing the leaflet motion. If vegetations develop on pre-existing valve disease such as rheumatic valvular lesions combined patterns of both lesions can be seen, which limits demonstration of characteristic patterns suggesting vegetation [5 – 8, 10].

Besides identifying vegetation, M-mode echocardiography can document leaflet destruction, rupture of chordae tendineae, diastolic fluttering of the mitral leaflet or interventricular septum, pericardial effusion, changes in chamber dimensions and contractility and hemodynamically dependent events such as premature diastolic closure of the mitral valve. However, because of the lack of spatial orientation M-mode echocardiography cannot estimate the size, morphology and exact localisation of vegetation to the specific valvular structure. In addition in some patients vizualisation of the tricuspid and pulmonic valve may be difficult [10].

It was shown that two-dimensional echocardiography with its spatial orientation may overcome the limitations of M-mode echocardiography. This technique allows estimation of vegetation size, shape and mobility and provides the possibility of detecting complications of infective endocarditis. It enables one to differentiate the sessile from pedunculated lesion. In right-sided vegetation and possibly in infected prosthetic valves the two-dimensional technique may be superior to the M-mode echocardiography [7].

Different moving patterns could be demonstrated in the real-time. Small and sessile vegetations usually show valve dependent motions. Large or pedunculated vegetations may exhibit independent motions, sometimes chaotic or flail-like, particularly when leaflet destruction occurs.

Severeal indirect signs could be helpful in assessing the severity of infective endocarditis. Hyperkinetic motion of the left ventricular walls indicates a volume overload in aortic or mitral incompetency. Excessive systolic expansion of the left atrium may be recorded in acute mitral regurgitation and mitral valve preclosure in acute aortic regurgitation. Flail mitral or aortic leaflet usually indicate destruction of valvular or subvalvular apparatus. A typical finding of rupture of chordae tendineae of the anterior or posterior mitral leaflet could be demonstrated. Fine diastolic fluttering of the anterior mitral leaflet appears in

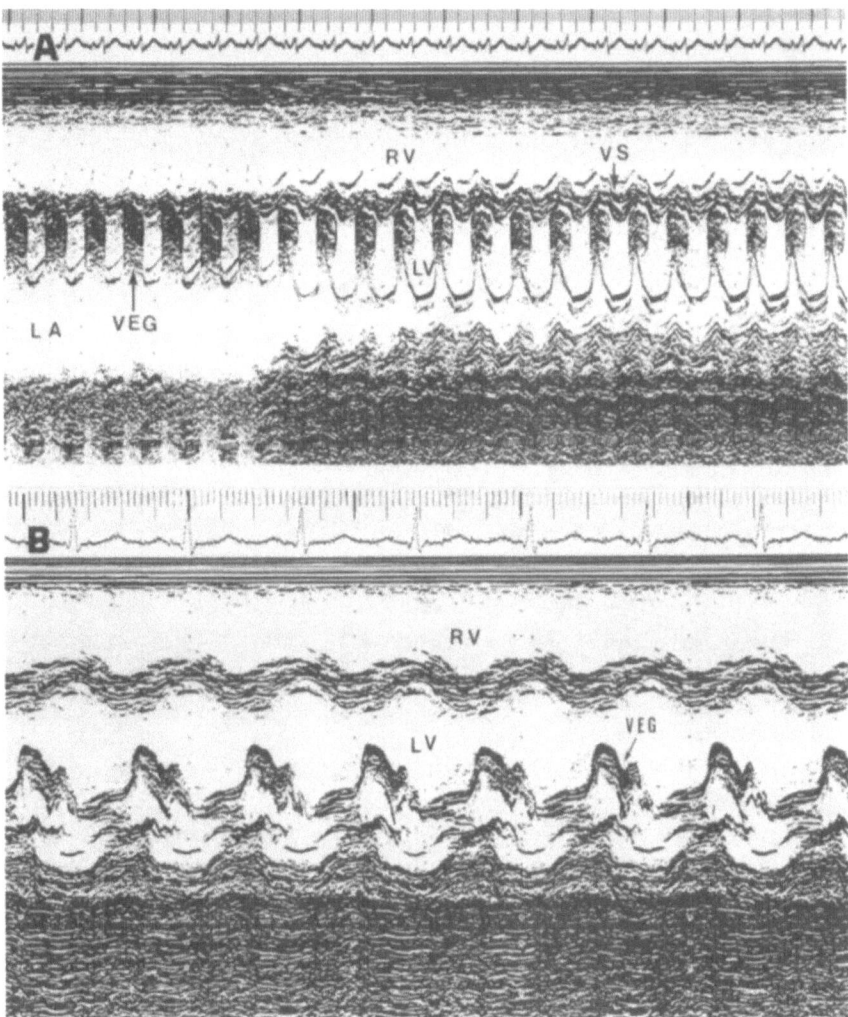

Figure 1. Echocardiogdrams from patients with infective endocarditis showing typical aortic valve (A) and mitral valve (B) vegetation (VEG). Dense echoes from vegetation present during diastole do not interfere with valve leaflet mobility. Echoes from the aortic valve vegetation are seen in the left ventricular outflow tract in diastole. RV : right ventricle, VS : ventricular septum, LV : left ventricle, LA : left atrium.

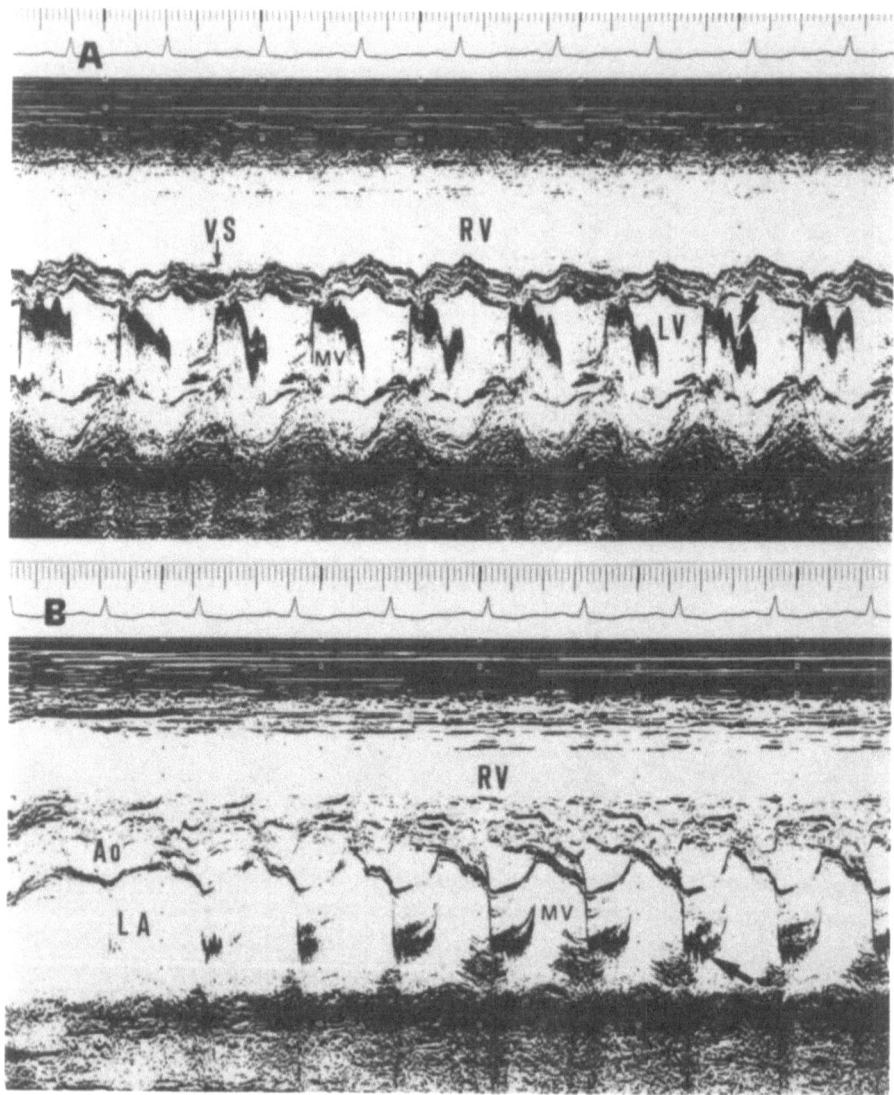

Figure 2. A. Echocardiogram from a patient with vegetations (arrow) of the mitral valve and ruptured chordae tendineae of the anterior mitral leaflet. During diastole the anterior leaflet exhibits a chaotic, coarse fluttering with diastolic motion pattern varying from beat to beat. RV : right ventricle, VS : ventricular septum, LV : left ventricle, MV : mitral valve. B. Echocardiogram from patient with vegetation of the mitral valve and rupture of chordae tendineae manifested as coarse vibrations (arrows) during systole. Ao : aorta, LA : left atrium.

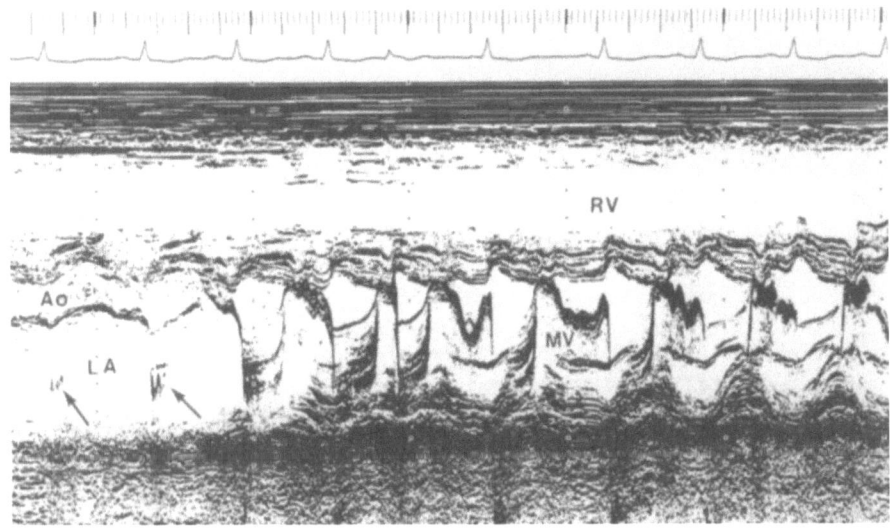

Figure 3. Vegetations of the mitral valve with rupture of the chordae tendineae, prolapsing into the left atrium during systole (arrows). RV : right ventricle, Ao : aorta, LA : left atrium, MV : mitral valve.

aortic regurgitation. Mitral valve preclosure and fine fluttering of the anterior mitral leaflet are better demonstrated with M-mode technique [10, 11, 12].

MITRAL VALVE

The shaggy or fuzzy echoes can be identified on the anterior or posterior leaflet or both. They are usually seen during diastole, rarely during systole and typically do not restrict the leaflet motion [5 – 8, 10 – 12]. Mitral valve vegetations begin on the atrial aspects of the leaflets. With subsequent extension chordae tendineae may be involved and chordal rupture may occur. Torn chordae tendineae of the anterior mitral leaflet are usually characterised by chaotic coarse diastolic, rarely systolic, fluttering of the anterior leaflet with variation of the diastolic pattern of motion from beat to beat [13], Figure 2A. Rupture of the chordae tendineae of the posterior leaflet is represented by chaotic diastolic anterior motion of the posterior leaflet [14]. Systolic fluttering is also described in torn chordae or disrupted mitral valve [15], Figure 2B. Sometimes it is impossible to distinguish torn chordae tendineae from mitral valve prolapse [10]. If rupture of chordae tendineae of both leaflets occurs, a combination of the described findings is seen. Occasionally, during systole a part of the flail mitral valve or vegetation can be seen extending into the left atrial cavity (Figure 3). With spatially oriented two-dimensional echocardiography flail mitral valve leaflet can be easily demonstrated. Flail mitral leaflet can be distinguished from mitral valve prolapse

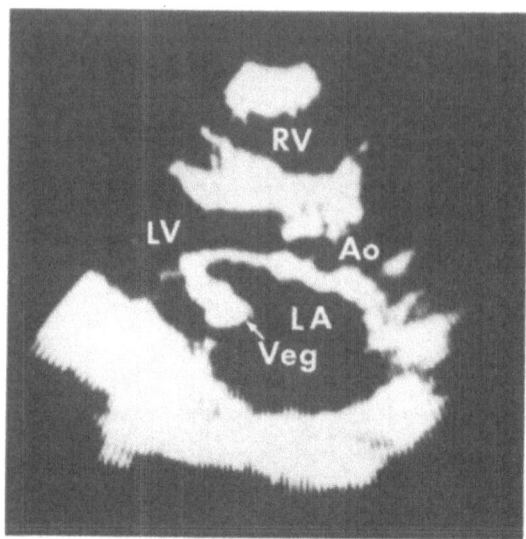

Figure 4. A long axis image of the large pedunculated vegetation (arrow) of the anterior mitral leaflet. RV : right ventricle, Ao : aorta, LV : left ventricle, LA : left atrium.

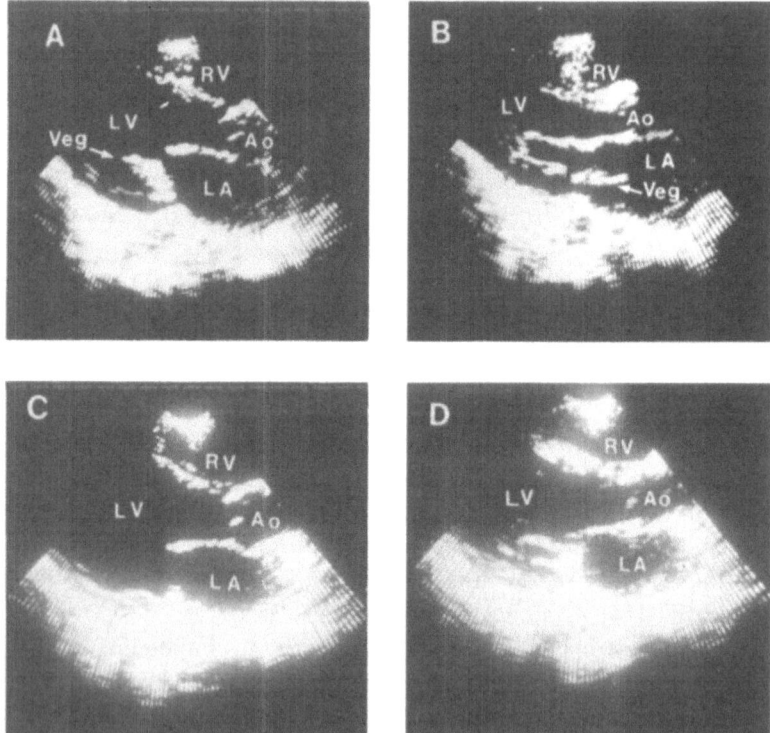

Figure 5. Band-like vegetation (arrows) is attached to the posterior mitral leaflet. During diastole (A) the vegetation band moves into the left ventricle. In systole (B) it is recorded in the left atrium. Diastolic (C) and systolic (D) frames recorded immediately after an episode of peripheral embolism show disappearance of the previously imaged vegetation band. RV : right ventricle, Ao : aorta, LV : left ventricle, LA : left atrium.

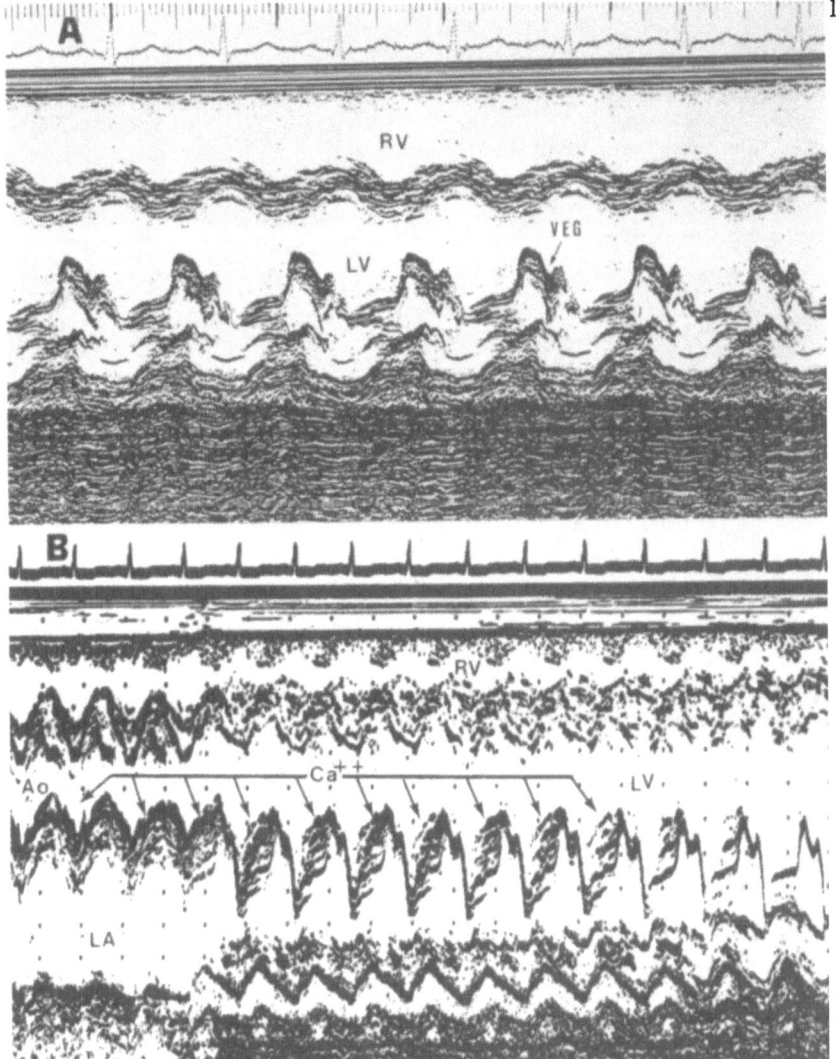

Figure 6. Two echocardiograms suggesting vegetations of the anterior mitral leaflet. True vegetation of infective endocarditis (A) can be differentiated by its attachement to the atrial aspects of the leaflet. Echocardiogram B shows calcification (arrows) of the aortic root extending to the ventricular side of the anterior mitral leaflet mimicking vegetations. During aortic valve replacement calcific mass had to be scraped from the anterior mitral leaflet. RV : right ventricle, LV : left ventricle, VEG : vegetation, Ao : aorta, LA : left atrium.

by imaging the tip of the leaflet pointing toward the left atrium, whereas in mitral valve prolapse the leaflet tip points toward the left ventricle [16], Figure 4. Two-dimensional echocardiography is more sensitive and reliable than M-mode technique in the diagnosis of flail mitral valve [17]. The flail portion of a disrupted mitral valve or vegetation can be easily demonstrated in the left atrium in systole coming back into the left ventricle in diastole.

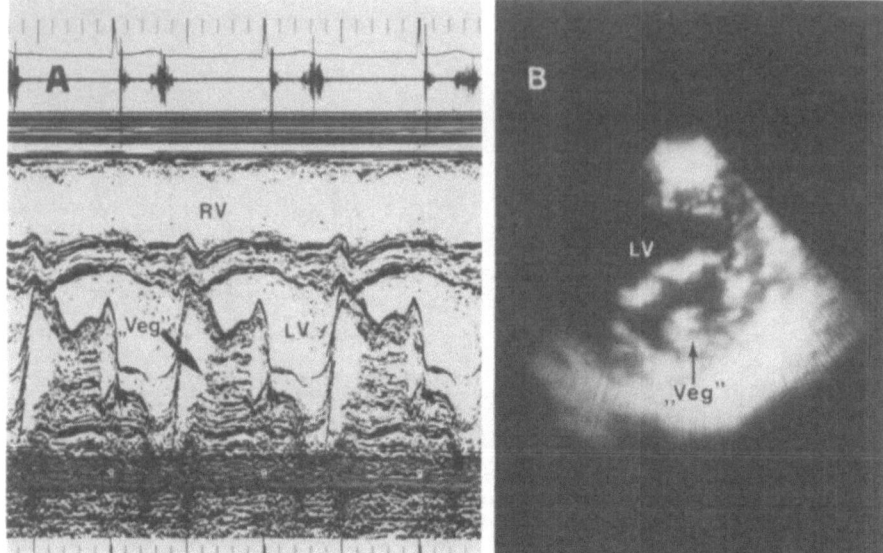

Figure 7. A. M-mode echocardiogram from the patient with mitral valve prolapse. Redundant posterior mitral leaflet mimicks vegetation (arrow). B. Short-axis section through redundant scalloped mitral leaflets shows mitral valve area with mass of echoes simulating vegetations (arrow). RV : right ventricle, LV : left ventricle.

After an episode of peripheral embolisation vegetations could diminish or disappear from the mitral valve (Figure 5). To the inexperienced observer myxomatous degeneration of the mitral valve, left atrial myxoma, flail leaflets, clot formation, calcification extending from the aorta to the anterior leaflet may present some difficulties in interpretation [10, 12, 18]. Figure 6 shows calcification of the aortic valve and posterior aortic wall extending to the anterior mitral leaflet mimicking vegetations. However, these echoes are localised on the ventricular side of the anterior mitral leaflet whereas true vegetations have their origin on the atrial side of mitral leaflets.

Echoes from myxomatous degeneration of the mitral valve are rather uniform, linear, not shaggy or fuzzy (Figure 7A). A short axis section through redundant scalloped mitral leaflets may show the mitral valve area with a mass of echoes simulating vegetations (Figure 7B). This pseudo-vegetation pattern in a two-dimensional echocardiogram was found in 17 (14.2%) of our 120 patients with mitral valve prolapse [19].

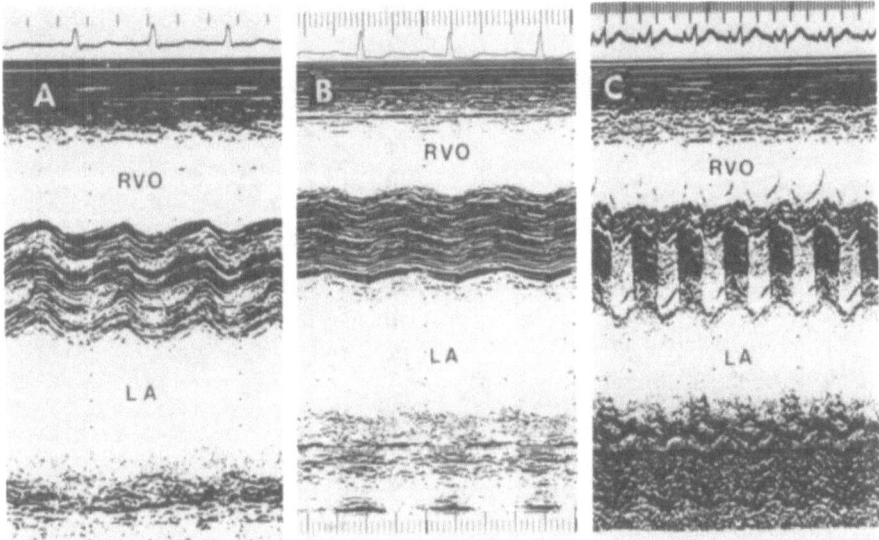

Figure 8. Echocardiographic features of fibrotic (A), calcific (B) and vegetative (C) aortic valve lesions. In patient with fibrotic aortic stenosis increased thickeness of the aortic leaflets with decreased systolic aperture is seen. In the patient with severe calcific aortic stenosis a dense band of echoes of the aortic root level makes the assessment of valve motion impossible. In the patient with vegetations of infective endocarditis a dense cloud of shaggy echoes recorded during diastole do not restrict leaflets motion. RVO : right ventricular outflow tract, LA : left atrium.

AORTIC VALVE

Vegetations are attached to the ventricular surface of the aortic leaflets. On M-mode echocardiography they appear as multiple, irregular, parallel lines or shaggy echoes. Depending on transducer position they are usually seen only during systole or diastole [5, 6, 20], Figure 8C. Echoes from a fibrotic or calcified aortic valve are more uniform, linearly extending through both systole and diastole, restricting normal motion of the leaflets (Figure 8A, B).

Flail or ruptured aortic leaflets with or without attached vegetation usually prolapse into the left ventricular outflow tract during diastole and return into the aortic root during systole (Figure 9A). A similar cluster of echoes in the left ventricular outflow tract may be seen in pedunculated corde-like vegetation [20]. Except in infective endocarditis, flail or disrupted aortic valve may be found in myxomatous degeneration of the aortic valve [21]. We have seen a similar pattern in a patient with a calcified bicuspid aortic valve partially detached from the aortic annulus (Figure 9B). Rupture of the aortic valve cusp without vegetation may be presented as a fine diastolic fluttering of the aortic valve [20].

Bulky vegetation may, although rarely does, obstruct the aortic root thus thwarting ejection into the aorta (Figure 10A). Figure 10B presents the short axis

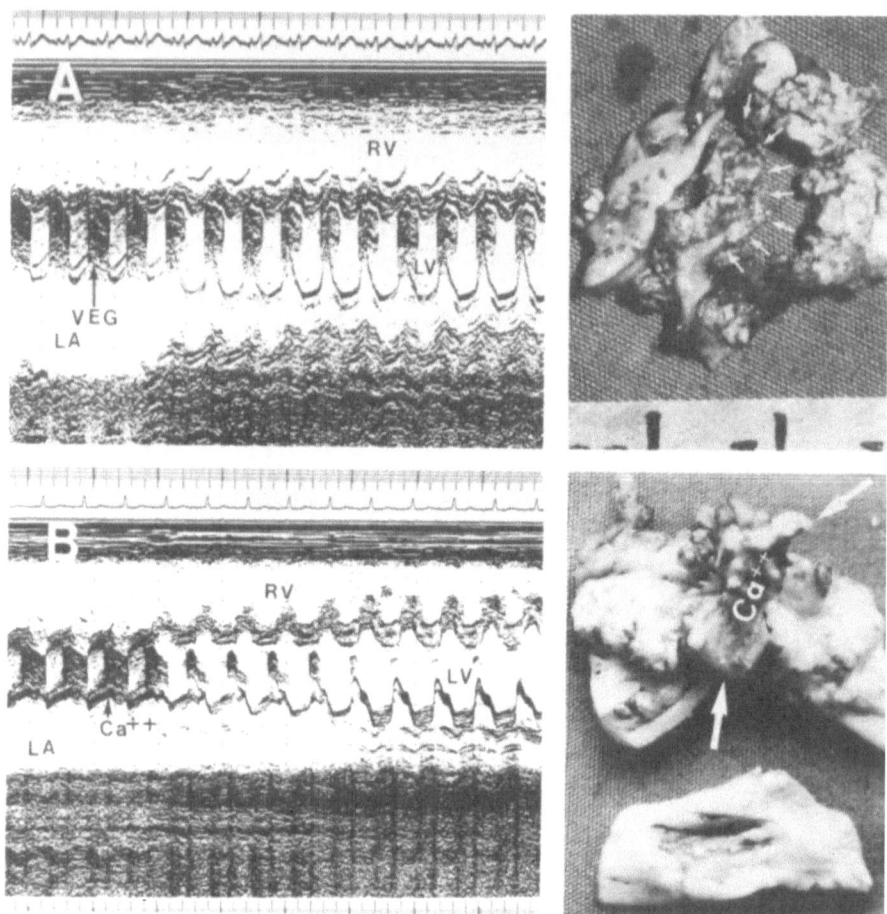

Figure 9. Two M-mode echocardiograms demonstrating possible pitfall in the diagnosis of vegetative lesion. Similar M-mode pattern with dense shaggey echoes attached to the anterior mitral leaflet are present in both patients with different underlying lesions. A. Band-like aortic valve vegetations (arrows). B. Patient with calcified bicuspid aortic valve partially dettached from the aortic annulus. Large horn-like calcification (between large arrows) moved in diastole into the left ventricular outflow tract simulating flail aortic valve or band-like vegetation. RV : right ventricle, LA : left atrium, LV : left ventricle, VEG : vegetation, Ca^{++} mass.

section of the aortic root with vegetation which obstructs the left coronary artery causing myocardial infarction. A double echo or echo-free space in the aortic wall may suggest intramural abcess of the aortic root [12, 22].

The fine diastolic fluttering of the anterior mitral valve leaflet and hyperdynamic left ventricular wall motion confirm the presence of aortic insufficiency. In accute severe aortic insufficiency left ventricular end-diastolic pressure rapidly increases, equalizes and exceeds left atrial pressure causing mitral valve preclosure. The premature closure of the mitral valve prevents the transmission

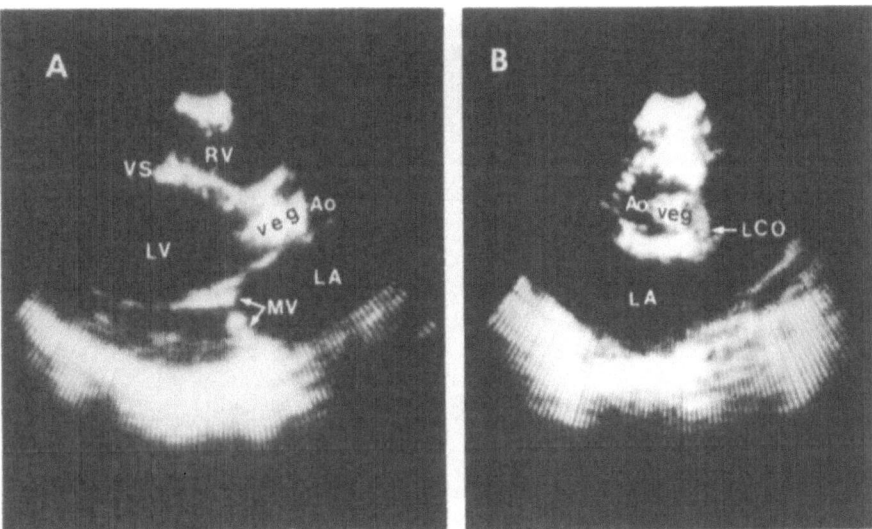

Figure 10. A. A systolic long-axis image of a large vegetative mass (Veg) located in region of right aortic valve cusp. B. A short-axis section of the aortic root with vegetative mass (Veg) obstructing the ostium of the left coronary artery (LCO) causing myocardial infarction. RV : right ventricle, VS : ventricular septum, Ao : aorta, Veg : vegetation, LV : left ventricle, LA : left atrium, LCO : left coronary ostium.

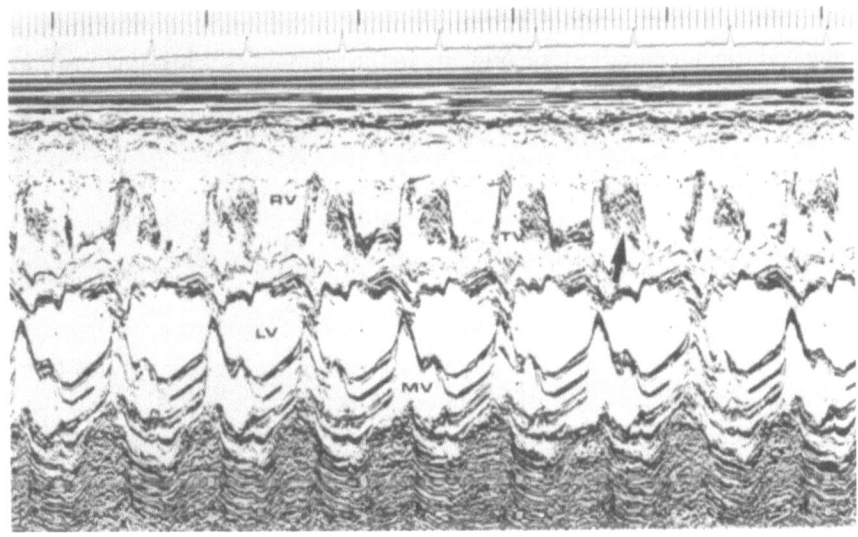

Figure 11. M-mode echocardiogram from the septic patient shows mass of echoes (arrow) moving in a pattern of tricuspid valve motion. M-mode echocardiogram in conjunction with other clinical data was compatible with infective endocarditis with vegetation of the tricuspid valve. However, two-dimensional echocardiogram disclosed large tumorous mass protruding through tricuspid valve (see Figure 12). RV : right ventricle, TV : tricuspid valve, LV : left ventricle, MV : mitral valve.

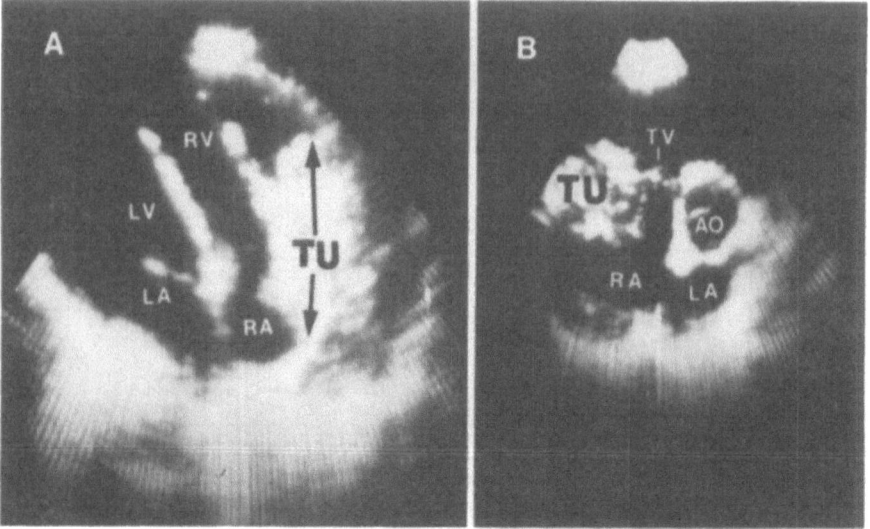

Figure 12. A. Apical two-dimensional presentation from same patient as in Figure 11 showing large tumorous mass (TU) occupying large portion of right atrial cavity extending through atrio-ventricular groove into the right ventricle. B. Tumorous mass (TU) in short-axis presentation. Histology revealed sarcoma. RV : right ventricle, LV : left ventricle, LA : left atrium, RA : right atrium, TV : tricuspid valve, Ao : aorta.

of high ventricular end-diastolic pressure to the pulmonary veins, thus preventing pulmonary oedema [23].

Severe acute aortic insufficiency may cause premature opening of the aortic valve due to pronounced elevation of left ventricular diastolic pressure that equalizes and exceeds the aortic diastolic pressure [12].

TRICUSPID AND PULMONARY VALVES

Vegetations of the tricuspid and pulmonary valves are rare and most often are seen in drug addicts. In rightsided infective endocarditis vegetations often involve the cores of the cusps and their surfaces may remain relatively smooth [24]. Echocardiographic morpholy of tricuspid and pulmonary valve vegetations ressembles that of the mitral and aortic valve. Vegetations of the tricuspid valve are usually larger than those of the mitral valve and may simulate right cavitary tumour. Conversely, tumourous masses protruding through the tricuspid valve may simulate tricuspid vegetation (Figure 11, 12), especially on M-mode presentation. Echoes from catheters and pacing electrodes, in the right ventricle can also mimic tricuspid valve vegetation [25].

SENSITIVITY AND SPECIFICITY

The exact sensitivity of echocardiography in the diagnosis of infective endocar-ditis has not been firmly established. In several studies rather low sensitivity was reported varying widely from 34 per cent to 69 per cent [5, 6, 8, 11, 12, 26]. Several factors could contribute to this low sensitivity: a difficult patient with small echocardiographic window, improper instrument setting, pre-existent valvular changes or prosthetic valve, blind areas, echocardiographic examina-tions earlier than two weeks after the onset of clinical symptoms, vegetations less than 2 mm in size. Finally, as autopsy studies have shown, vegetations may not be present (vegetations were found in only 53% of the patients dying of active in-fective endocarditis) [27, 28].

Regarding specificity, several studies have shown a good correlation of echocardiographically detected vegetation with surgical or autopsy findings [5 – 8, 11]. However, pre-existent valvular fibrosis or calcification, myxomatous degeneration of the valve, leaflets tumour, left atrial myxoma, noninfective leaflet disruption and indwelling catheters may be a potential source of false positive diagnosis to the inexperienced examiner. Some technical problems may also cause interpretation difficulties: improper gain settings, television "after im-ages" during video replaying, and spurious valve thickening in the far field [10]. With considerable experience of the examiner the incidence of false positive diagnosis is low.

CLINICAL IMPLICATIONS OF ECHOCARDIOGRAPHIC FINDINGS IN INFECTIVE ENDOCARDITIS

According to initial studies [29, 30] it was believed that almost all patients with echocardiographically detected vegetation had a high incidence of life threaten-ing complications and required surgical intervention. However, a recent prospec-tive study by Stewart and co-workers [31] has shown that 70 per cent of the pa-tients with echocardiographically detected vegetation were without significant complications and could be successfully treated medically. In this study com-plications could not be predicted by any morphological characteristic of the vegetation. Thus the echocardiographically imaged vegetation does not necessarily indicate a poor prognosis and the need for early surgical therapy [10 – 12, 31]. In several studies [9, 29] the incidence of systemic embolism was significantly higher in patients with vegetations than in those without vegeta-tions. In our 36 patients with infective endocarditis there was a 55 per cent in-cidence of emboli in patients with vegetations as opposed to 12.5 per cent in-cidence in those without vegetations.

The indications for surgical therapy in infective endocarditis are relatively well defined. Refractory congestive heart failure, persistent infection, recurrent emboli, new conduction disturbances and mycotic aneurysm are major indications for surgical intervention [32]. Echocardiography is an ideal method for following up the hemodynamic status in these seriously ill patients. It may easily identify hemodynamic deterioration and its etiology and may help in choosing appropriate therapy as well as timing of surgical intervention. The clinical significance of premature closure of the mitral valve has already been discussed. Data derived from this noninvasive technique are usually sufficient to circumvent the hazard of invasive procedures. Recurrent emboli are not always an indication for surgery. If after peripheral embolism echocardiographic examination shows that the valves are clear of vegetations and the patient is haemodynamically stable, there is no need for surgery.

Controversy still exists concerning the treatment of patients with large mobile vegetations. Their frightening, chaotic motion suggests a tendency to systemic embolism. In most of our patients large, especially pedunculated, cord-like vegetations were a source of serious, often fatal, embolism and peripheral mycotic aneurysms. Due to this experience, in cases of threatening vegetations we indicated early surgical operation irrespective of the presence of active infection. Other authors [10, 11] think that in these patients prophylactic surgery to prevent systemic emboli is not justified. More experience with a larger number of patients is necessary before definite conclusions may be reached.

In our patients with vegetative lesions surgery was most commonly performed in refractory congestive heart failure, often with premature closure of the mitral valve, in large and pedunculated cord-like vegetations, in flail leaflets and in persistent infection.

Echocardiography can directly detect or indirectly suggest almost all the described cardiovascular complications of infective endocarditis: valve destruction with resultant regurgitation, severe acute congestive heart failure, rupture of chordae tendineae, sinus Valsalva rupture with subsequent left or right shunts, perivalvular abscess, coronary ostia emboli, myocardial infarction, ventricular septal defect, "myocarditis", pericarditis, peripheral embolism, mycotic aneurysms [33]. Thus many patients suspected of having endocarditis may benefit from this noninvasive examination. However, in order to obtain maximum benefits one must be aware of many pitfalls in using this technique. As has already been discussed, there are many sources of false negative examinations and lack of direct or indirect signs of endocarditis in no way excludes the presence of infective endocarditis [10 – 12]. The mere imaging of vegetations does not indicate disease activity; it should be judged in conjunction with other clinical data. The examiner must be familiar with sources of false positive findings as well.

The detection of vegetation indentifies a subset of patients with a greater risk of complications, but it does not always indicate a poor prognosis or the need for early surgery. Conversely, the lack of detectable vegetations usually identifies a group of patients with endocarditis who have a good prognosis, usually without the need for early surgical intervention [10 – 12]. Although echocardiography may be very helpful in contributing to the diagnosis and assessment of the severity of the disease, clinical management decisions must be made individually in concert with other clinical findings.

REFERENCES

1. Weinstein L, Rubin RH: Infective endocarditis. Progr CV Dis 16:239, 1973.
2. Pomerance A, Davies MJ: The Pathology of the Heart, Blackwell Scientific Publications, Oxford, 1975.
3. Robbins SL: Pathology, W.B. Saunders Co., Philadelphia, 1969.
4. Schelbert HR, Muller OF: Detection of fungal vegetations involving a Starr-Edwards prosthesis by means of ultrasound. Vasc Surg 6:20, 1972.
5. Roy P, Tajik AJ, Guiliani ER, Schattenberg TT, Gau GT, Frye RL: Spectrum of echocardiographic findings in bacterial endocarditis. Circulation 53:474, 1976.
6. Wann LS, Dillon JC, Weyman SE, Feigenbaum H: Echocardiography in bacterial endocarditis. N Engl J Med 295:135, 1976.
7. Gilbert BW, Haney RS, Crawford F, McClellan J, Gallis HA, Johnson ML, Kisslo JA: Two-dimensional echocardiographic assessment of vegetative endocarditis. Circulation 55:346, 1977.
8. Dillon JC: Echocardiography in valvular vegetations. Am J Med 62:856, 1977.
9. Davis RS, Strom JA, Frishman W, Becker R, Matsumoto M, LeJemtel T, Sonnenblick EH, Frater RWM: The demonstration of vegetations by echocardiography in bacterial endocarditis. Am J Med 69:57, 1980.
10. Feigenbaum, H: Echocardiography. 3rd ed., Lea & Febiger, Philadelphia, 1981.
11. Stewart JA, Winsberg F, Kisslo JA: Vegetative endocarditis. In: Two-Dimensional Echocardiography, pp. 79 – 92 (ed. JA Kisslo), Churchill Livingstone, New York, 1980.
12. Gura GM, Tajik AJ: Clinical usefulness of echocardiography in infective endocarditis. In: Progress in Cardiology, pp. 73 – 84 (ed. PN Yu and JF Goodwin), Lea & Febiger, Philadelphia, 1979.
13. Duchak JM, Chang S, Feigenbaum H: Echocardiographic features of torn chordae tendineae. Am J Cardiol 29:260, (Abstr.) 1972.
14. Burges J, Clark R, Kamagaki M, Cohn K: Echocardiographic findings in different types of mitral regurgitation. Circulation 48:97, 1973.
15. Meyer JF, Frank MJ, Goldberg S, Cheng TO: Systolic mitral flutter, an echocardiographic clue to the diagnosis of ruptured chordae tendineae. Am Heart J 94:3, 1977.
16. Mintz GS, Kotler MN, Segal BL, Parry WR: Two-dimensional echocardiographic recognition of ruptured chordae tendinae. Circulation 57:244, 1978.
17. Mintz GS, Kotler MN, Parry WR, Segal BL: Statistical comparison of M-mode and two-dimensional echocardiographic diagnosis of flail mitral leaflets. Am J Cardiol 42:253, 1980.
18. Chandraratna PAN, Langevin E: Limitations of the echocardiogram in diagnosing valvular vegetations in patients with mitral valve prolapse. Circulation 56:436, 1977.
19. Cikes I: Clinical and echocardiographic study of mitral valve prolapse. Thesis. Zagreb, 1981.
20. Wray TM: The variable echocardiographic features in aortic valve endocarditis. Circulation 52:658, 1975.
21. Estevez CM, Dillon JC, Walker PD, Feigenbaum H, Chang S: Echocardiographic manifestations of aortic rupture in a myxomatous aortic valve. Chest 69:685, 1976.
22. Fox S, Kotler MN, Segal BL, Parry W: Echocardiographic diagnosis of acute aortic valve endocarditis and its complications. Arch Intern Med 137:85, 1977.
23. Kotler MN, Segal BL, Parry WR: Role of echocardiography in the diagnosis of bacterial en-

188

docarditis, cardiac tumors, Wolf-Parkinson-White syndrome, mitral annular calcification, aortic root dissection and Marfan's syndrome. In: Clinical Echocardiography, pp. 167–186 (eds. MN Kotler and BL Segal), F.A. Davis Company, Philadelphia, 1978.

24. Roberts WC: Characteristics and consequences of infective endocarditis (active or healed or both) learned from morphologic studies. In: Infective Endocarditis, pp. 55–123 (ed. SH Rahimtoola), Grune & Stratton, New York, 1978.

25. Reeves WC, Nanda NC: Echocardiographic evaluation of intracardiac pacing catheters: M-mode and two-dimensional studies. Circulation, 58:1049, 1978.

26. Thomson KR, Nanda N, Gramiak R: The reliability of echocardiography in the diagnosis of infective endocarditis. Radiology, 125:473, 1977.

27. Buchbinder NA, Roberts WC: Left-sided valvular active infective endocarditis: a study of forty-five necropsy patients. Am J Med 53:20, 1972.

28. Arnett EN, Roberts WC: Active infective endocarditis: a clinicopathologic analysis of 137 necropsy patients. Current Problems in Cardiology, Vol. 1, No. 7, 1976.

29. Young JB, Welton D, Quinones MA, Ishimori T, Alexander JK, Miller RR: Prognostic significance of valvular vegetations identified by M-mode echocardiography in infective endocarditis. Circulation (Suppl. 2), 58:41, (Abstr.), 1978.

30. Strom J, Davis R, Frishman W, Becker R, Matsumoto M, Sonnenblick E: The demonstration of vegetations by echocardiography in bacterial endocarditis: an indication for early surgical intervention. Circulation (Suppl. 2), 60:37 (Abstr.), 1979.

31. Stewart JA, Silimperi D, Harris P, Wise NK, Fraker TD, Kisslo JA: Echocardiographic documentation of vegetation of vegetative lesions in infective endocarditis: clinical implications. Circulation 61:374, 1980.

32. Okies JE, Star A: Cardiac surgery in infective endocarditis. In: Infective Endocarditis, pp. 361–377 (ed. SH Rahimtoola), Grune & Stratton, New Gork, 1978.

33. McAnulty JH, Rahimtoola SH, DeMots H, Griswold HE: Clinical features of infective endocarditis. In: Infective Endocarditis, pp. 125–148 (ed. SH Rahimtoola), Grune & Stratton, New York, 1978.

12. ECHOCARDIOGRAPHY OF INTRACARDIAC MASSES: TUMORS AND THROMBI

F.J. ten Cate and J. Roelandt

Patients presenting with clinical signs of obstruction to blood flow, embolization or constitutional alterations, in the presence of a cardiac murmur, challenge the echocardiographer to make (or exclude) the diagnosis of an intracardiac tumor. In the context of a myocardial infarction the presence of a thrombus must be suspected.

Two-dimensional echocardiography has become the technique of choice to identify intracardiac masses since the method allows the display of intracardiac structures in a spatial manner and to visualize areas of the heart which are not accessible to other non-invasive techniques. In addition multiple tomographic views of the heart can be imaged. The method is now considered as the most sensitive to detect, characterize and localize intracardiac mass lesions. In most instances, a definitive diagnosis is made and the method can replace invasive angiocardiography for preoperative assessment.

Cardiac tumors may be of primary or secondary (metastatic) types. The latter occur more frequently than primary types, are rarely seen intracavitary and most often involve the pericardium. Their characteristic echocardiographic manifestation is that of a pericardial effusion. In this chapter we will discuss the echocardiographic diagnosis of primary intracardiac tumors and intracardiac thrombi.

1. ATRIAL TUMORS

An atrial myxoma is the most common primary tumor of the heart. It originates from the endocardium and is mainly seen in adults. Approximately 75% of myxomas are located in the left atrium (LA). They are usually solitary and generally arise on a pedicle from the fossa ovalis region. They vary in size from 0.4 to 8 cm. They are clinically suspected in the presence of signs of peripheral embolization or syncope and varying auscultatory findings (see Table 1).

The M-mode echocardiographic features of a left atrial myxoma are summarized in Table 2 [1, 2]. The multi-layered appearance on the echocardiogram of a LA myxoma results from different ultrasonic energy absorption by the tumor tissue. The small echo-free space behind the anterior mitral leaflet (aML)

Roelandt, J. (ed.) The practice of M-mode and two-dimensional echocardiography
© *1983, Martinus Nijhoff Publishers. The Hague / Boston / London*
ISBN 978-94-009-6792-2.

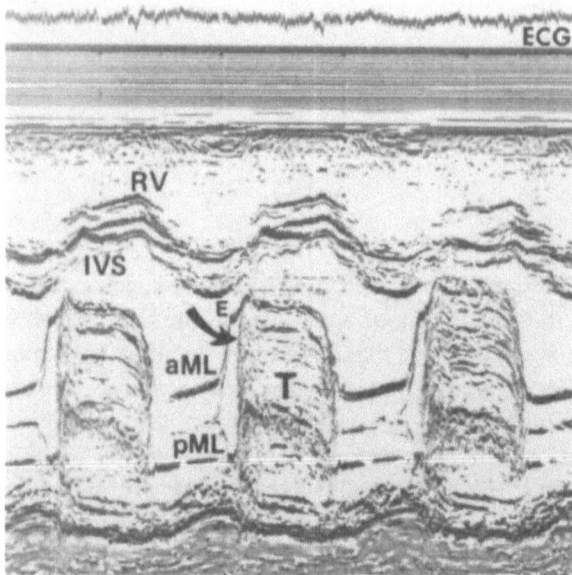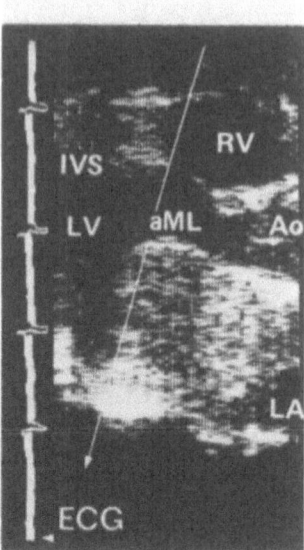

Figure 1. M-mode and two-dimensional echocardiograms of a patient with a left atrial myxoma. The two-dimensional study was performed with a linear array electronic scanner. The arrow at the bottom of the electrocardiogram (ECG) indicates the moment in diastole at which the stop-frame photograph was taken. The tumor mass fills the mitral valve orifice and largely the left atrial cavity. The arrow represents the approximate sound beam direction from which the M-mode echocardiogram was recorded. Note the interval between mitral valve opening and appearance of tumor echoes (arrow), which results in a slight additional opening of the valve after the E point. These events are difficult to appreciate from two-dimensional studies. Abbreviations: aML and pML: anterior and posterior mitral valve leaflets; Ao : aorta, IVS : interventricular septum, LA : left atrium, LV and RV : left and right ventricles. (With permission: J. Roelandt, Ultrasonics in Clinical Diagnosis, third edition. Wells PNT, Goldberg BB (editors), in press).

Table 1. Clinical manifestation of intra-cardiac mass lesions

- Peripheral embolization
- Valvular obstruction
- Mechanical hemolysis
- Biochemical effects
- Constitutional symptoms (e.g. malaise, unexplained fever)

Table 2. M-mode echocardiographic features of LA myxoma

- Multiple multi-layered echoes behind aML in diastole
- Small echo-free space following aML opening due to tumor lagging
- Reduced EF-slope of aML
- Varying systolic appearance of tumor echoes in LA dependent upon site of tumor attachment

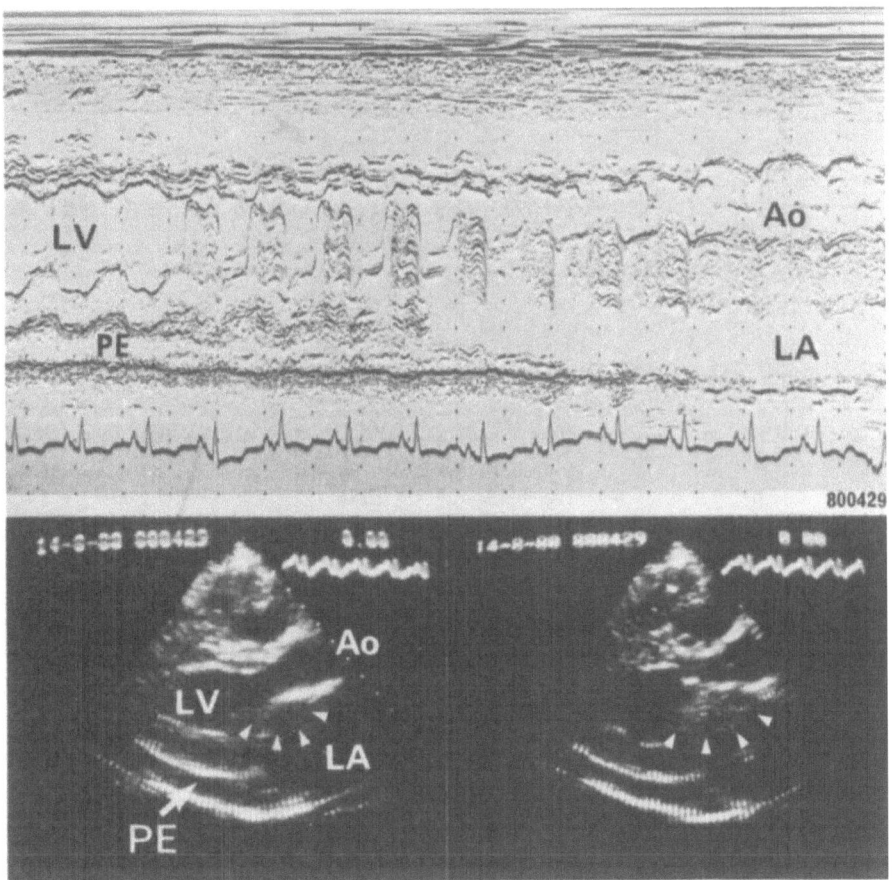

Figure 2. M-mode scan (top) and parasternal long axis views (bottom) of a patient with left atrial myxoma (see arrow heads). Note systolic appearance of tumor echoes in the left atrium (LA). Ao = aorta, LV = left ventricle.

is due to lagging of the tumor. This is a highly characteristic sign of a prolapsing mass and helps to differentiate a prolapsing LA mass, most commonly a myxoma, from vegetations on the mitral valve in bacterial endocarditis. The reduced EF-slope of the aML indicates the impaired filling rate of the LV because of obstruction of the mitral valve orifice by the tumor mass. The pattern may resemble mitral stenosis (Figures 1 and 2). The varying systolic appearance of a mass of echoes in the LA cavity close to the interatrial septum is highly suggestive for a LA myxoma. Sometimes a LA myxoma may have an atypical localization and appearance such as thick echoes behind the posterior aortic wall. Therefore the LA cavity should always be visualized from different directions. An empty cavity in different tomographic views virtually excludes an intra-atrial mass.

Two-dimensional echocardiography allows to assess the presence, location,

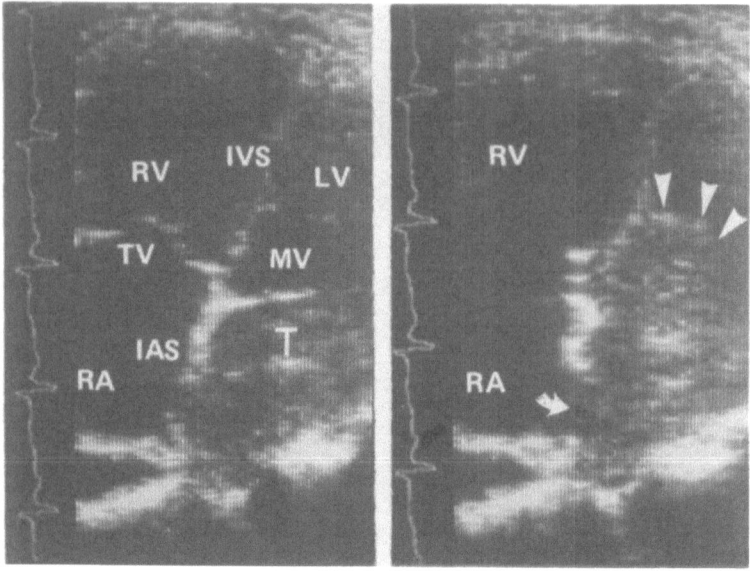

Figure 3. Two-dimensional subcostal four chamber view of a patient with a left atrial myxoma. The attachment of the tumor (T) to the inter-atrial septum is seen. During diastole, the tumor prolapses through the mitral valve orifice and pulls the interatrial septum (IAS) (see arrow). Abbreviations: IVS: interventricular septum, LA : left atrium, LV : left ventricle, RA : right atrium, RV : right ventricle.

mobility, size and shape of the tumor mass (Figure 3). The attachment of the tumor mostly by a (long) stalk on the inter-atrial septum, is best demonstrated from the apical and subcostal transducer positions.

Two-dimensional echocardiography is the best method to diagnose bi-atrial myxomas as right-sided cardiac chambers are readily visualized.

Off-axis echoes, reverberations and even normal cardiac structures which may move in and out of the echo beams can falsely mimic a tumor mass. Again this may be solved by visualizing several two-dimensional views from different transducer positions.

A right atrial (RA) myxoma may produce dense linear echoes behind the anterior tricuspid leaflet (aTL), a pattern similar to that seen behind the aML with a LA myxoma. Since the tricuspid valve and right atrium are difficult to registrate by M-mode echocardiography, the diagnosis is usually made by two-dimensional echocardiography. This is the most sensitive method especially when the parasternal long axis view of the right ventricle, subcostal and apical four chamber views are used. Right-sided prolapsing masses may have atypical appearances such as abnormal clouds of echoes in the right ventricular outflow tract. Tumors which are small, sessile or restricted in motion are always best visualized by two-dimensional echocardiography.

In children RA tumors of different histologic types have been described. Careful examination of the right atrium and inferior vena cava is always necessary for diagnosis of a right atrial mass which originates from a kidney tumor (Wilm's tumor).

2. VENTRICULAR TUMORS

Ventricular tumors are mostly of other histologic types than myxomata and originate from the myocardium (fibroma, fibrosarcoma, rhabdomyoma, rhabdomyosarcoma). They are more common in children than in adults, rhabdomyomata being the most frequent. These tumors have been reported as echomasses in the right ventricular outflow tract with or without evidence of pulmonary stenosis (Figure 4) or in the left ventricular outflow tract simulating aortic stenosis. Fibroma or papilloma of the papillary muscles have been described in the right and left ventricle. Rhabdomyomata and metastatic tumors may present as clusters of echoes in the region of the ventricular septum anterior to the mitral valve, or in the right ventricular cavity. Two-dimensional echocardiography is most useful for diagnosing ventricular tumors and the apical and subxyphoid views are most useful.

The differential diagnosis of ventricular tumors includes infective vegetations, valvular "redundancy" in mitral valve prolapse syndrome, echoes produced by prosthetic valves, and intracavitary thrombus (Table 3).

Metastatic spread of malignant tumors mostly involve the pericardium and present as pericardial effusion.

Secundary (metastatic) tumors are sometimes seen echocardiographically as an intra-mural mass or an excessive atrial or ventricular wall thickness. Two-dimensional echocardiography is the superior technique to demonstrate these localized wall abnormalities.

Table 3. Echocardiographic differential diagnosis of intracardiac masses

- Cardiac tumors
- Infective vegetations
- Valvular "redundancy" in mitral valve prolapse syndrome
- Echoes produced by prosthetic cardiac valves
- Intracavitary thrombi
- Prominent trabeculae, muscular bridges
- Papillary muscles
- Amputated chordae after valve replacement
- Spurious or phantom echoes (see chaper 3)

194

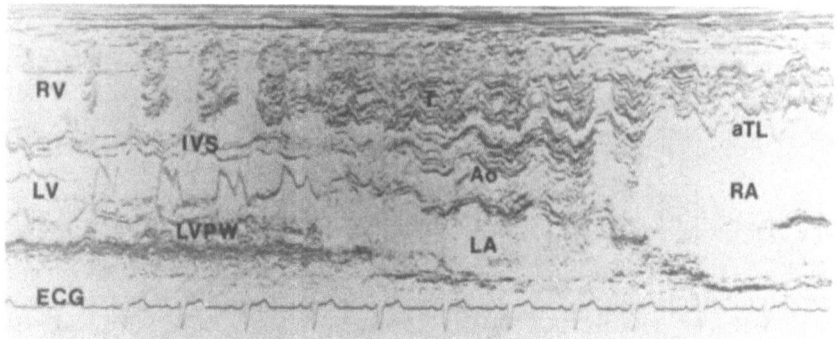

Figure 4. M-mode scan including the right (RV) and left ventricle (LV), the aorta (Ao) and anterior leaflet of the tricuspid valve (aTL). It demonstrates multiple echoes of a tumor mass (T) occupying the infundibulum and part of the dilated RV cavity. IVS : Interventricular septum, LVPW : left ventricular posterior wall, RA : right atrium. (With permission: J Roelandt et al: J Clin Ultrasound 5:191, 1976).

3. LEFT VENTRICULAR THROMBI

Intraventricular thrombi are mainly associated with myocardial infarction (especially with aneurysm formation). Other conditions are mitral stenosis (with atrial fibrillation), prosthetic valves and cardiomyopathy (Table 4) [3, 4].

Intracardiac thrombi may be the origin of neurologic disorders presenting as transient ischemic attacks or stroke. Their demonstration is thus of obvious importance for proper management of these patients. The diagnosis is mainly two-dimensionally using apical views. Several studies, however, have reported failure to visualize ventricular thrombi in a certain proportion of patients with subsequent confirmation. This emphasizes the need for caution in interpreting a negative echocardiographic study.

The echocardiographic features of left ventricular thrombus are summarized in Table 5.

Table 4. Clinical entities associated with cardiac thrombi

– Transmural myocardial infarction
– Ischemic aneurysm
– Mitral stenosis
– Prosthetic valves
– Dilated cardiomyopathy
– Neurologic disorders (TIA's and stroke)

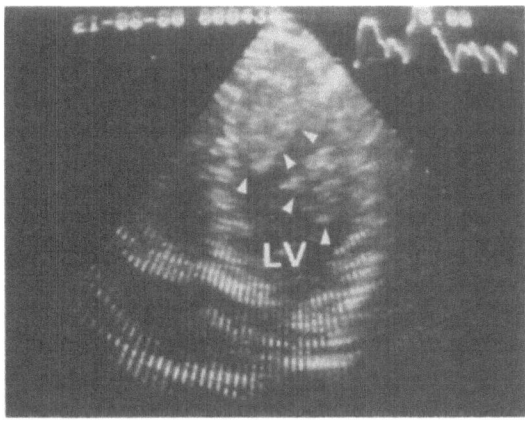

Figure 5. Apical four chamber view of a patient with two LV-clots (see arrow heads); one located in the apex of the left ventricle (LV) and one attached to the LV free wall.

Table 5. Echocardiographic features of LV thrombi

- Associated wall motion abnormality
- Frequent apical location
- Distinct thrombus margin
- Free motion of the intracavitary thrombus margin
- Acoustically distinct from underlying myocardium
- Variation noted on serial examination

(Am J Cardiol 47:145, 1981)

3.1. Wall motion abnormalities

Wall motion abnormalities adjacent to the thrombus location have been found in all studies. These abnormalities can vary from hypokinesia to dyskinesia in patients with aneurysm formation.

3.2. Thrombus location

In 90% of the cases the location of an LV thrombus is in the apical area LV thrombi will thus best detected from the apical transducer position (Figure 5).

3.3. Thrombus margin identification

It is important to identify a distinct thrombus margin. This may be difficult, however, in the presence of a mural thrombus. Attempts should always be made to identify the pericardium, endocardium and thrombus margins. In this respect, multiple gain and reject settings are helpful. In the presence of an ischemic aneurysm the walls of the aneurysm are thin. Thus, the finding of normal wall thickness in an aneurysmal segment should raise suspicion of a mural thrombus.

Another difficulty in identifying thrombus margins is related to the ultrasound beam width. The spurious echoes which may originate from myocardial scar can simulate a thrombus. The correct diagnosis requires multiple two-dimensional views.

3.4. Motion of thrombus margin

Motion of the intracavitary thrombus margin is usually limited. A swirling mass of intracavitary echoes may exceptionally been seen and is indicative of a discrete thrombus or a manifestation of early thrombus formation. This pattern is readily distinguished from chordal and papillary muscle structures.

3.5. Acoustic density of thrombi

The acoustic density of thrombi is usually greater than that of the adjacent myocardium. Protruding thrombi tend to be relatively echodense, whereas mural thrombi in general tend to be less echo-dense (Figure 5). The latter are therefore difficult to distinguish from the myocardium.

When a thrombus contains fluid it may be seen as an echo-free space. The different composition of a recently formed thrombus results in a greater echo-density than that of an older thrombus. Therefore, a thrombus is better visualized in its early stage of development after an acute myocardial infarction than in a later stage of the disease.

3.6. Thrombus variation in serial studies

Helpful in the diagnosis of a LV thrombus is its variation in size and shape which may be noted on serial studies. The complete disappearance of a mass on serial examination or the development of an echo-dense mass with the characteristics of a thrombus during acute myocardial infarction provides support for the diagnosis. It should be noted that thrombi may resolve without anti-coagulant therapy and sometimes recur during treatment.

3.7. False positive diagnosis of left ventricular thrombus (Table 6)

As a result of the limited lateral resolution and of near field artifacts false-positive diagnosis of LV thrombus may be suggested on two-dimensional echocardiographic images.

Therefore different transducer positions must be used. Real masses remain in the same anatomic position when imaged from different angles, while artifacts vary or disappear.

The identification of normal or pathological apical structures such as the medial papillary muscles, trabeculae, chordae tendinae or tangential left ventricular wall echoes can give a false-positive diagnosis of left ventricular thrombus.

Table 6. "False" positive diagnosis of LV thrombus

Due to ultrasonic technique and instrumentation

- Lateral resolution (spurious echoes)
- Near field artifact in apical views
- Reverberations (phantom echoes)

Incorrect identification of normal or pathological apical structures

- Papillary muscles
- Muscle trabeculations
- Chordal structures
- Tangential LV wall echoes

4. ATRIAL THROMBI

Although the appearance of a LA thrombus has been described in the early years of echocardiography, the diagnosis has been made more often and reliably after the introduction of two-dimensional echocardiography [5].

A left atrial thrombus is suspected to be present in a patient presenting with signs of systemic embolization who has mitral stenosis, atrial tachyarrhythmia's or after mitral valve replacement. Right atrial thrombi are extremely rare.

The typical LA thrombus is irregular, laminated, non-mobile and has a broad base of attachment to the LA wall. Many intra-atrial thrombi, however, are in the LA appendage, an area not accessible to M-mode scanning. The LA cavity is enlarged and mitral valve motion may be consistent with mitral stenosis. LA myxomata are usually ovoid, well demarcated, mobile and attached with a stalk to the inter-atrial septum. This makes the differential diagnosis between an LA myxoma and an LA thrombus possible in many cases.

To avoid false-positive diagnosis of an LA-thrombus, different gain settings and multiple tomographic views are needed and a LA thrombus is always seen in the same anatomic area.

REFERENCES

1. Pietro DA, Parisi AF: Intracardiac masses. The Med Clin of North Amer 64:239–51, 1980.
2. Kotler MN, Segal BL: Clinical echocardiography. Cardiovascular Clinics. Davis Company Philadelphia, 1978.
3. Asinger RW, Mikell FL, Sharma B et al: Observations on detecting left ventricular thrombi with two-dimensional echocardiography: emphasis on avoidance of false-positive diagnosis. Amer J Card 47:145–56, 1981.
4. Meltzer RS, Guthaner D, Rakowski H et al: Diagnosis of left ventricular thrombi by two-dimensional echocardiography. Brit Heart J 42:261–65, 1979.
5. Depace NL, Soulen RL, Kotler MN et al: Two-dimensional echocardiographic detection of intra-atrial masses. Amer J Cardiol 48:954–60, 1981.

13. ECHOCARDIOGRAPHY OF THE MITRAL VALVE: ACCURACY OF CRITERIA FOR CLINICAL DECISION-MAKING IN DAILY PRACTICE

P. HANRATH, B.A. LANGENSTEIN AND J. POLSTER

Since pulsed ultrasound was first introduced to examine the heart in the 1950s, echocardiography plays a significant role in the diagnosis and management of patients, especially those with suspected valvular heart disease. In this chapter it is described how in our opinion echocardiography has to be applied in daily practice in patients with different kinds of mitral valve disease in order to make the diagnosis, to assess the severity of the lesion and how to manage these patients.

MITRAL VALVE

Mitral valve is one of the easiest intracardiac structures which can be visualized by echocardiography and which consequently is one of the most studied structures. Normally, the diastolic pattern of the anterior mitral leaflet is registered on a time motion recording as an "M-shape" image. The motion of the posterior leaflet is smaller and a mirror image of the motion of anterior leaflet ("W-shape" image).

MITRAL STENOSIS

By M-mode echocardiography mitral stenosis is manifested by a marked thickening of the valve leaflets and a reduction of their motion (Figure 1). The movement of the posterior mitral leaflet is usually paradoxical in diastole, moving anteriorly rather than posteriorly. This phenomenon occurs in our experience in over 90% of patients with mitral stenosis and results from the large anterior leaflet pulling the small posterior leaflet with it in an anterior direction when it opens.

It is important to remember that mitral stenosis occurs as a result of scarring and fibrosis of the leaflets with fusion of the commissures. That allows this abnormal movement to occur. Due to the morphological changes the opening amplitude (D-E) and the early diastolic closing velocity (E-F) are reduced. The amplitude of the A-wave, if sinus rhythm is present, is also diminished. However, because flattening of the E-F slope may be seen in other conditions (cases with reduced left ventricular compliance) as well, we hesitate to make the

Roelandt, J. (ed.) The practice of M-mode and two-dimensional echocardiography
© *1983, Martinus Nijhoff Publishers. The Hague / Boston / London*
ISBN 978-94-009-6792-2.

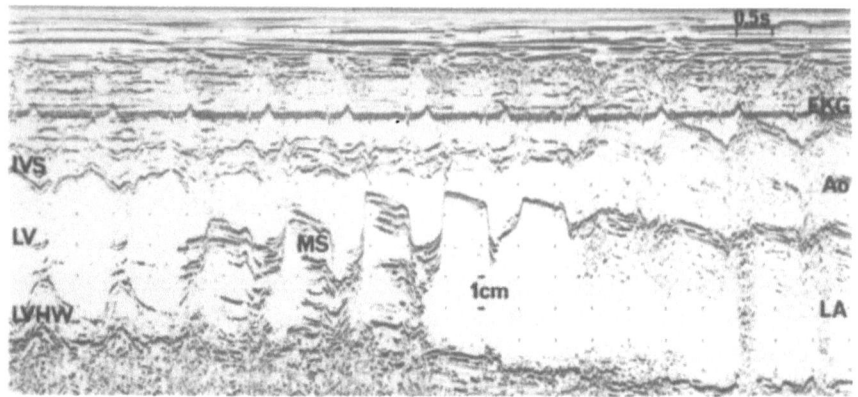

Figure 1. M-mode sweep from the aortic root into the left ventricle in a patient with mitral stenosis. Ao : Aorta, IVS : interventricular septum, MI : mitral leaflets, LA : left atrium, LVPW : left ventricular posterior wall

diagnosis of mitral stenosis if the above-mentioned leaflet thickening or anterior diastolic motion of the posterior leaflet is missing.

Other findings, such as left atrial enlargement and the echocardiographic stigmata of pulmonary hypertension with or without secondary tricuspid regurgitation may be a secondary effect of mitral valve disease, but they are of little help in either making the diagnosis or in the assessment of the severity of mitral valve stenosis.

Early reports on the use of M-mode echocardiography put great emphasis on the measurement of the rate of reduction in the E-F slope as an index of severity of mitral stenosis. The greater the reduction in the slope, the more the severity of the stenosis. Although formerly accepted as clinically useful, the more recently performed re-evaluation of this parameter in comparison with the valve area derived from the Gorlin formula showed that this index is no longer useful for the evaluation of the severity of mitral valve stenosis [1]. The limitation of the "slope technique" from M-mode recordings is caused by the small spatial orientation of this technique. Depending on which part of the anterior leaflet is within the ultrasound beam, different slopes can be measured. The relative immobility of the anterior leaflet tip and the diastolic forward bowing of the midportion of the anterior leaflet make this possible. It is generally accepted that the two-dimensional echocardiogram adds little over M-mode to the primary diagnosis of rheumatic mitral valve disease. But there is no doubt that the two-dimensional approach is so far superior in assessing the severity of mitral stenosis. The improved spatial orientation of two-dimensional echocardiography allows clear visualization and measurement of the mitral valve orifice. The orifice is measured in the parasternal short axis view at the level of the leaflet tips. The image with the whole mitral valve area should be frozen during rapid filling at the time of maximal valve opening, which however, in practice is difficult to achieve, probably due to rapid motion of the valve apparatus during this phase of the heart cycle. An accurate echocardiographic image is however important for planimetry. The short axis view through the narrowest orifice near the leaflet tips must be obtained. If not, the results of planimetry will produce a value artificially to high, often observed in patients with combined mitral annulus calcification, due to poor lateral resolution. Gain setting must be reduced to eliminate sound reverberations produced by the leaflets, thus underestimating the real valve area.

When compared with direct measurements made at surgery or indirect measurements made by the Gorlin formula, this approach for assessing mitral valve orifice has been shown to be accurate and reproducible in literature [2 – 4]. In general the valve area can be measured within 0.3 cm^2 of the area determined at cardiac catheterization or surgery. This needs however a computer device and is somewhat time consuming. The percentage of error is greatest in patients with very small valve areas. From the practical clinical standpoint of view important is however that we can reliably differentiate patients with critical mitral stenosis (valve area < 1 cm^2) from those with mild stenosis or normal valve areas (> 1.5 cm^2) by this technique.

If one keeps in mind the above-mentioned pit falls, two-dimensional echocardiography has distinct advantages over cardiac catheterization in the assessment of the severity of mitral valve stenosis. The two-dimensional approach provides a non-invasive, risk-free means of studying the mitral valve repeatably and allows direct measurements of the mitral valve area. The formula of Gorlin, however, which is used in the hemodynamic calculation of the valve area, assumes an idealized orifice and was not derived to express flow through a funnel-shaped opening. Furthermore, whereas the Gorlin formula loses accuracy in the presence of mitral regurgitation, the echocardiographic estimation of mitral valve area does not depend on flow measurements and therefore does not lose accuracy in the presence of a combined stenotic and regurgitant lesion.

MITRAL REGURGITATION

The role of echocardiography in the evaluation of patients with mitral regurgitation is not as well defined as in patients with mitral stenosis. At present the diagnosis of mitral regurgitation and the assessment of its severity are better made clinically and angiographically than by one- or two-dimensional echocardiography. Echocardiographic findings suggesting mitral incompetence include excessive mitral valve motion, left atrial and left ventricular dilatation, prominent pulsation of the dilated left ventricular walls or left atrial wall, early systolic closure of the aortic valve and a steep mitral E-F slope. These parameters, however, are not specific for the presence of mitral regurgitation and are therefore not very useful in clinical practice.

Despite these limitations, echocardiography has a role in the management of

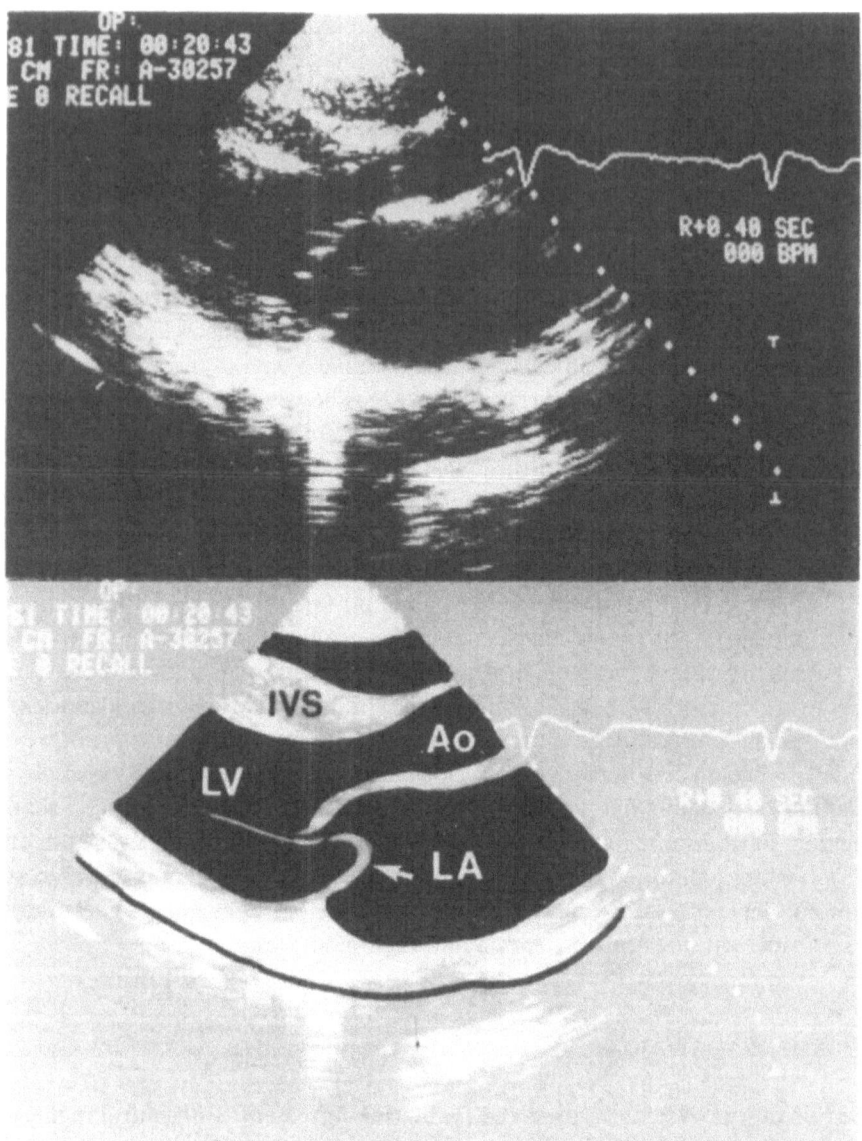

Figure 2. Parasternal long axis view of a patient with posterior mitral leaflet prolapse. Ao : aorta, IVS : intraventricular septum, LA : left atrium, LV : left ventricle.

patients with mitral regurgitation. It is a most useful tool for delineating the etiology of mitral regurgitation. For example, in patients with mitral regurgitation and left ventricular failure the question arises whether a primary disease of the mitral leaflet has led to mitral regurgitation and following left heart failure or whether myocardial disease has led to left ventricular failure and secondary

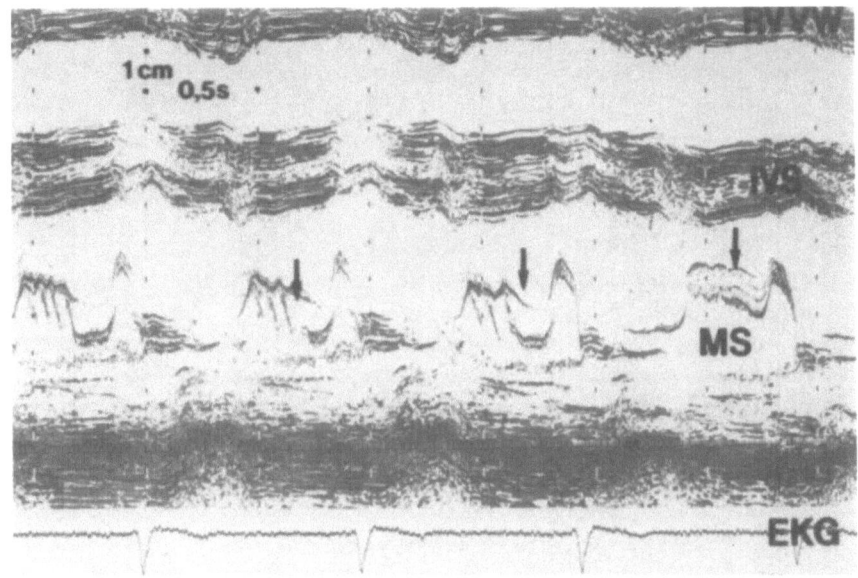

Figure 3. Abnormal diastolic oscillation of the anterior mitral leaflet due to partial rupture of the chordae tendineae. IVS : interventricular septum, ML : mitral leaflets, RVAW : right ventricular anterior wall.

mitral ring dilatation with consecutive incompetence. This clinically important question can often be answered non-invasively by echocardiography.

Depending on whether the mitral valve apparatus is involved in this disease we differentiate between primary and secondary forms of mitral regurgitation. Primary forms are rheumatic mitral valve disease, mitral valve prolapse (Figure 2), ruptured chordae tendineae (Figure 3, 4), calcification of the mitral valve annulus, valvular masses and congenital abnormalities of the mitral valve. They can often be identified by the combined use of M-mode and 2-D echocardiography. The recognition of the echocardiographic stigmata of these different causes of mitral regurgitation suggest primary mitral valve disease. This is further stressed by the presence of normal or increased left ventricular wall motion.

In contrast, mitral regurgitation secondary to myocardial disease is associated with diffuse or segmental left ventricular wall motion abnormalities. Such abnormalities are best assessed by two-dimensional rather than M-mode echocardiography because of the ability of two-dimensional echocardiography to display the entire left ventricle. In ischemic mitral regurgitation, segmental wall motion abnormalities may involve the left ventricle walls adjacent to one or both papillary muscles.

In non-ischemic myocardial failure with associated mitral regurgitation, the heart often appears dilated and diffusely hypokinetic with a low ejection fraction in the two-dimensional echocardiogram.

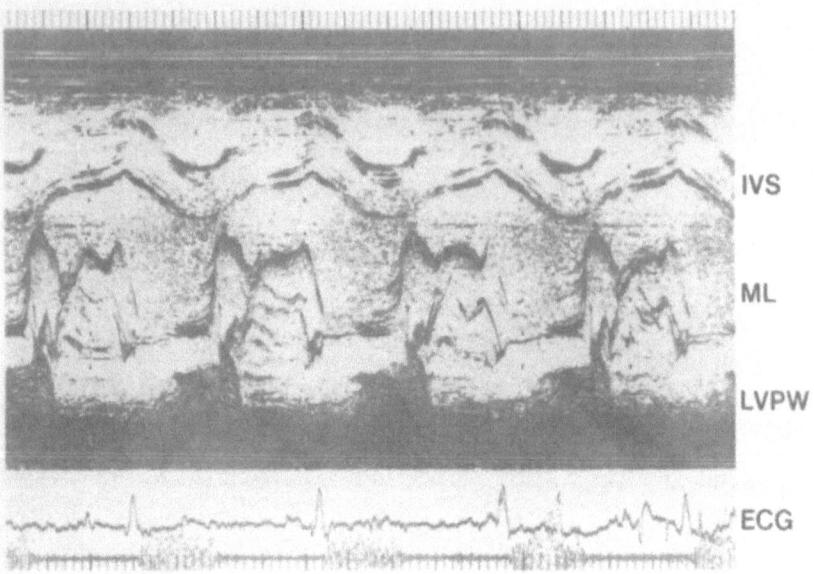

Figure 4. Abnormal diastolic fluttering of the posterior mitral leaflet due to partial rupture of the chordae tendineae. IVS : interventricular septum, ML : mitral leaflets, LVPW : left ventricular posterior wall.

The mitral valve echo appears to take a mid-ventricular position and the anterior as well as posterior leaflets are easily visualized on a Time Motion recording. An interrupted closure of the anterior mitral valve leaflet in the M-mode echocardiogram is compatible with increased diastolic pressure. The distance from maximum opening excursion of the anterior mitral leaflet to the ventricular septum is increased and the separation of the mitral valve leaflets reduced, both reflecting reduction in ventricular performance.

The differentiation between primary mitral valve disease and the various forms of mitral regurgitation secondary to myocardial processes is clinically important because of the different responses to medical and surgical treatment. If a patient with mitral regurgitation has echocardiographic evidence of primary disease of the mitral valve or ischemic mitral regurgitation with near normal left ventricular wall motion, we consider left heart catheterization, angiography, and send him to surgery for mitral valve replacement, if the indication is given clinically . The decision to proceed to catheterization and surgery is however, primarily based on clinical and not on echocardiographic parameters. If, on the other hand, the echocardiogram suggests mitral regurgitation secondary to dilated cardiomyopathy, an operative intervention would be less likely to benefit the patient and therefore this patient needs no left-heart catheterization. Aggressive medical therapy is in this case the therapy of choice.

Apart from these diseases, M-mode echocardiography may be of help as a diagnostic procedure in patients with suspected aortic regurgitation and hypertrophic obstructive cardiomyopathy. The latter especially may be difficult to differentiate clinically from other forms of mitral regurgitation.

Thus, the combined use of M-mode and 2-D echocardiography may be of great value in determining the diagnosis or etiology of suspected mitral valve disease as well as in the management of these patients.

REFERENCES

1. Cope GD, Kisslo JA, Johnson ML, Behar VS: A reassessment of the echocardiogram in mitral stenosis. Circul 52:664, 1975.
2. Henry WL, Griffith JM, Michaelis LL, Mc Intosh CL, Morrow AG, Epstein SE: Measurement of mitral valve orifice area in patients with mitral valve disease by real-time, two-dimensional echocardiography. Circul 51:827, 1975.
3. Wann LS, Weyman AE, Feigenbaum H, Dillon JC, Johnston KW, Eggleton RC: Determination of mitral valve area by cross-sectional echocardiography. Ann Intern Med 88:337, 1978.
4. Marlin RP, Rankowski H, Kleinman JH, Beaver W, London E, Popp RL: Reliability and reproducibility of two-dimensional echocardiographic measurement of the stenotic mitral valve orifice area. Amer J Cardiol 43:560, 1979.

14. TWO-DIMENSIONAL ECHOCARDIOGRAPHY OF THE AORTA AND AORTIC VALVE – IS QUANTITATION POSSIBLE?

R. Prasquier and P. Vervin

I. AORTIC STENOSIS

In Western-style countries adult valvular aortic stenosis has undergone recent unique changes, some of which are pertinent to echocardiographic examination:

1. It has become the most frequent surgical valvular disease.
2. Rheumatic aetiology has drastically decreased.

Accordingly calcific dystrophic aortic stenosis is presently the most common form of the disease; it can occur on bicuspid valves or as an ageing process on tricuspid valves. The latter, known as "senile" aortic stenosis has been largely neglected in the past. The present awareness of its potential severity, associated to the gratifying results of surgery at a very old age [1], to the high prevalence of auscultatory abnormalities in elderly patients, to the difficulties of clinical assessment, and to the wide availability of echocardiographic equipments is turning aortic valve stenosis into a geriatric problem. Along with frequently associated left ventricular failure and/or ischemic heart disease which reduce usefulness of phonomecanographic classical tests, this means for the echocardiographer difficulties in obtaining adequate tracings and pictures and for the clinician need for a non invasive test, sensitive enough to avoid unnecessary catheterization to large numbers of patients without critical lesions.

This serves to emphasize clinical potential usefulness for a non invasive independent quantitative anatomical assessment of aortic valvular area. Is two-dimensional echocardiography ready to play this role?

1.1. M-mode echocardiography

M-mode echocardiographic assessment of valvular aortic stenosis has already been reviewed [2] and will only be briefly summarized. Limitations are well recognized either in young patients where the single beam usually misses the flow restricting orifice of the domed leaflets, or in patients with calcific stenosis, where the calcific masses may prevent delineation of aortic leaflet motion: when

Roelandt, J. (ed.) The practice of M-mode and two-dimensional echocardiography
© *1983, Martinus Nijhoff Publishers. The Hague / Boston / London*
ISBN 978-94-009-6792-2.

leaflet opening is visible, beat-to-beat variations in systolic separation may prevent a representative quantitative measurement.

Measurements of left ventricular thickness are extremely important in the management of congenital stenosis: their value in elderly patients is more limited, because of associated hypertension, changes in thickness with age and possible occurrence of severe aortic stenosis with only moderate left ventricular hypertrophy.

Formulas based upon a constant stress hypothesis, either with end systolic LV wall thickness measurements [3], or more easily with end diastolic measurements [4], might derive clinically useful estimates of left ventricular systolic pressures in young patients without cardiac decompensation and aortic regurgitation. They have no predictive value in patients with heart failure and/or LV dilatation.

1.2. Anatomical basis for 2-D echocardiographic findings

Normal aortic valve is characterized by three equally sized cusps or leaflets attached to the aortic root at the level of commissures. Total cusp area being much greater than aortic root area, the normal closure line of the leaflets lies below the tip of the leaflet, leaving above a free overlapping portion, the lunula [5].

With commissural fusion, whether acquired (rheumatic heart disease) or congenital (without usually any commisural remnant), cusps may remain mobile for a long time, as long as there is no calcium deposit. A central orifice is situated at the distal tip of the valvular apparatus and preserved cusp mobility leads to the phenomenon of doming.

Dystrophic calcification of the aortic surface of the leaflet may occur on normal tricuspid valves, or at a younger age on bicuspid or rheumatical valves. Although it starts deep in the body of the leaflet, decreasing trivially (aortic sclerosis) or significantly its mobility, the lunula tends to fenestrate and disappear so that the tip of the leaflets, here again, becomes the closure line. Calcium deposits may extend from one cusp to another, leading to acquired ("false") bicuspid or unicommissural valves with grossly distorted eccentric orifices. In acquired as well as congenital bicuspidy, symphysis of right and left coronary cusps is much more frequent than symphysis of right and posterior leaflet, whereas symphysis of left and posterior leaflet is exceptional [6].

1.3. Cross-sectional echocardiographic assessment of valvular stenosis

The normal appearance of aortic valve in 2-D echocardiography is well known: in the long axis view during diastole, a single echo is seen in the middle of the aorta, whereas in systole two leaflets open briskly, adjacent to the aortic wall. It is unusual to see the complete leaflet motion throughout the cardiac cycle.

208

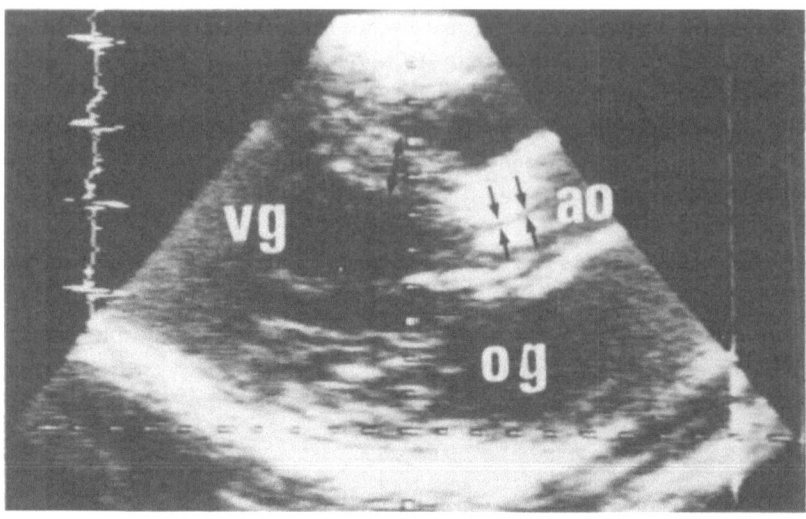

Figure 1. Extremely restricted MACS (multiple arrows) in a heavily calcified aortic valve (VG : left ventricule, OG : left atrium).

In the short axis parasternal view during diastole the closure lines of the three leaflets form a "Y" pattern; the commissures are more or less at 1, 5 and 9 o'clock of the aortic circle. Therefore left coronary cusp is more anterior, posterior non-coronary cusp is somewhat on the right and left coronary cusp is somewhat posterior. In systole, during the full opening of the leaflets cusp body is usually poorly visible but a definite triangular orifice area is clearly seen when there is aortic root dilatation or reduced left ventricular output. Some degree of lateral angulation is frequently necessary to delineate the left coronary cusp, so that the three leaflets may not be visible in one single section.

Long axis cusp separation
The most widely used 2-D index is, as in M-mode echocardiography, maximal aortic cusp separation (MACS) in the long axis view, measured at the inner aspects of the leaflets during systolic opening.

Careful medial to lateral sweep of the aorta is necessary to bring out the maximal aortic leaflet separation; whenever different degrees of leaflet separation can be recorded, the largest one is selected while the suspicion of an eccentric orifice is raised.

MACS is relatively easy to measure in young patients with flexible valves exhibiting systolic doming where a beam width artifact at the top of the leaflets frequently helps to define the flow restricting orifice [7].

Adequate long axis recordings of leaflet separation are not always obtainable in adult patients with calcific aortic stenosis; our failure rate (25%) is somewhat higher than what is usually reported [8, 9], and tends to increase with the age of the patients. Dense calcifications at the valvular level account for these difficulties. The aortic leaflets are recognized by their independent motion, perpendicular to the aortic wall, whereas non orificial calcium deposits, whether on the body of the cusp or on the adjacent aorta move in the direction of ventricular flow. However, a rigid valve may not move at all and lateral resolution limitations and/or large side lobes from highly reflectant calcium deposits may fill up the valvular orifice. Technical features of the echographic equipment and examination are therefore critical: the lowest possible gain settings should be used in order to reduce any blooming effect without, at the same time, leading to leaflet drop-out. Gain sensitivity, lateral resolution and side lobes differ from one equipment to another: a crispier valvular definition may usually presently be expected from good quality mechanical scanners.

The value of two-dimensional measurement of MACS as an index of aortic stenosis severity in the adult was assessed in relatively few published series [8, 9, 10].

Morard and col. [10] studied 24 patients (23 – 71 years) with a 30° mechanical scanner. Stenosis was categorized according to peak systolic ventriculo aortic gradient (PSG), as severe (PSG > 75mmHg), moderate (PSG 50 to 75mmHg) and mild (PSG < 50mmHg). Reanalysis of their data leads to the following conclusions: a – MACS was an accurate index of the presence or absence of aortic stenosis since there was no overlap between normal subjects (MACS 17 to 31mm) and affected patients (MACS 4.5 to 14.5mm). b – MACS mean group value was significantly lower with increasing degree of PSG (6mm vs 9mm vs 11.6 vs 22mm in normals). c – Although there was MACS overlap (severe 4.5 to 9mm, moderate 6.5 to 11.3mm, mild 9,2 to 14.5mm), specific cut-off points were found at 6mm (severe stenosis) and 12mm (mild stenosis). Besides, MACS < 9mm was found only among patients with PSG > 50mmHg, in 10/16 (63%) of the overall group of these patients. Although insensitive, it was therefore a specific index of potentially surgical aortic stenosis.

In a phased array echocardiographic study of 85 catheterized patients (14 – 78 years, mean 58) *De Maria and col* [8] could find no useful correlation (r = 0.4) between MACS and respectively PSG, aortic valve area and aortic valve index. Data rearrangement according to PSG shows a complete overlap (PSG < 50mmHg: MACS 0 to 15mm: PSG 50 to 75mmHg: MACS 0 to 11mm; PSG > 75mmHg; MACS 0 to 10mm). But on the published scatter plot only 3/31 (9.7%) patients with PSG > 50mmHg had MACS > 9mm. Regarding valve areas calculated through the Gorlin's formula mean MACS group values were significantly lower in critical (area < 0.75mm²) than in non critical aortic stenosis (4.5mm vs 10mm) and in normal subjects (19mm). Here, contrarily to the previous study MACS < 9mm was a sensitive (41/46: 91%) index of critical aortic stenosis, but not a specific one, since it was observed in 9/26: 34% of patients with mild stenosis. There was again no overlap between aortic stenosis patients (0 to 15mm) and normal subjects (15 to 24mm).

Feigenbaum's *group* which had first shown the value of 2-D MACS in the assessment of aortic stenosis in children [11] and in adults [12], recently extended their findings [9] in a series of 81 consecutive catheterized patients (28 – 74, mean 55 years) studied with a mechanical sector scanner. Data were compared to Gorlin's calculated aortic valve area with 3 groups (severe < 0.75cm², moderate 0.75 to 1cm², mild > 1 cm²). Mean MACS was also significantly different in each group (severe: 6.5 mm vs moderate 9.9mm vs mild 14.9mm), but the most impressive result of this study was the very good specificity of a MACS < 8mm: 29/30 pts (97%) had critical aortic stenosis. This cut-off point was however, rather insensitive since rearrangement of published data suggests that MACS was over 7mm in 21% of patients with critical stenosis, and only a cut-off point of 12mm was 100% sensitive. A MACS of 8 to 12mm was therefore in a "gray" zone. This range included unfortunately 44% of the study population.

The following factors may account for the apparently striking discrepancies between the comparable series from De Maria and Godley:

− 5/9 falsely critical (MACS < 9mm) De Maria's patients appeared on the scatter plot to have valve areas around 0.8cm² which might be considered as rather severe

− 3 falsely critical patients had marked decreased in LV stroke volume: this factor may be expected to decrease leaflet opening regardless the degree of stenosis

− choice of cut-off point of MACS < 8mm instead of 9mm would have decreased this index sensitivity for critical stenosis from 91% to 74%, very comparable to Godley's findings.

Taking into account the inadequacies of the Gorlin's formula for aortic valve area assessment [13], the axial echocardiographic resolution and the measurement error which may probably amount to ± 2mm, a more similar picture emerges from these two large independent studies.

Short axis measurement of aortic valve area
Whatever the value of long axis MACS in the qualitative assessment of valvular stenosis, it cannot be used as a quantitative index of severity. Direct planimetry of aortic valvular area on short axis echo sections is rarely achieved, reported success rate ranging from 13% [9] to 20% [8]. Besides the blooming effect of calcium deposits, specific difficulties arise from the overall systolic motion of the aortic valve apparatus in and out the tomographic plane [8] and the non planar shape of the aortic orifice in calcific stenosis. When the valve area can be entirely displayed on a single echo section, a reasonable similarity to Gorlin's formula's result is usually found: although this has never been systematically studied, a quantitative assessment of orifice size seems therefore possible in a minority of patients.

In many patients, although planimetry is not feasible, short axis aortic pictures bring useful qualitative information about orifice morphology and leaflet motion [8, 9].

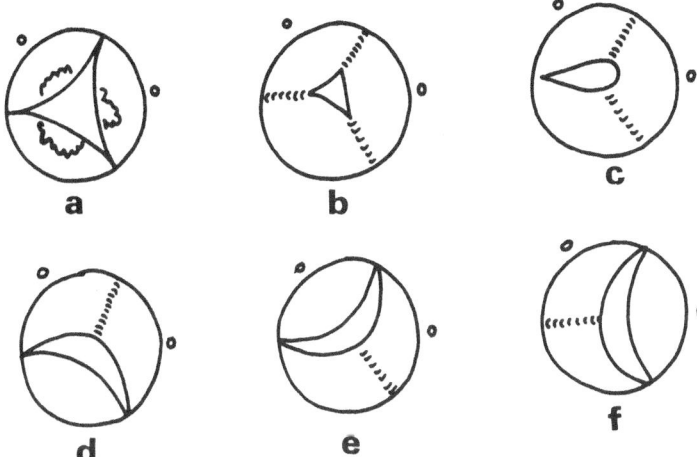

Figure 2. Schematic appearance of aortic orifices. a. Calcific aortic stenosis without commissural fusion. b. Rheumatic aortic stenosis with commissural fusion. c. Eccentric orifice with fusion of two commissures. d. Fusion of right coronary to left coronary cusp (usual case). e. Fusion of left coronary to posterior cusp. f. Fusion of right coronary to posterior cusp.

When the orifice keeps a relatively regular triangular or circular shape because of calcific deposits on a tricuspid valve without fusion of the leaflets (Figure 2a) or because of homogeneous commissural rheumatismal fusion (Figure 2b), long axis MACS is usually representative of overall valvular area. But irregularly shaped orifices explain most of the inadequacies of a single long axis measurement:

1. In many patients the orifice takes an elliptical or crescent shape because of leaflet fusion. Since this occurs more frequently between right and left coronary cusps (Figure 2d) the long axis measurement is close to the small diameter and degree of stenosis tends to be overestimated: whenever long axis leaflet separation is very restricted, the slit like actual aortic orifice (Figure 3) remains anyhow within the critical group but slightly larger long axis separations (over the 6mm range) could correspond to different degrees of stenosis. In the unusual case of bicuspidy involving the right and posterior coronary leaflet (Figure 2f) long axis leaflet separation would be expected to overestimate the size of an elliptical orifice.

2. Eccentric orifices (Figure 2c) which may result of fusion of two-commissures account for some of the major failures of long axis measurements. The following guidelines are useful:

— When there is only minimal motion on one leaflet and no motion on the others, stenosis is probably severe.

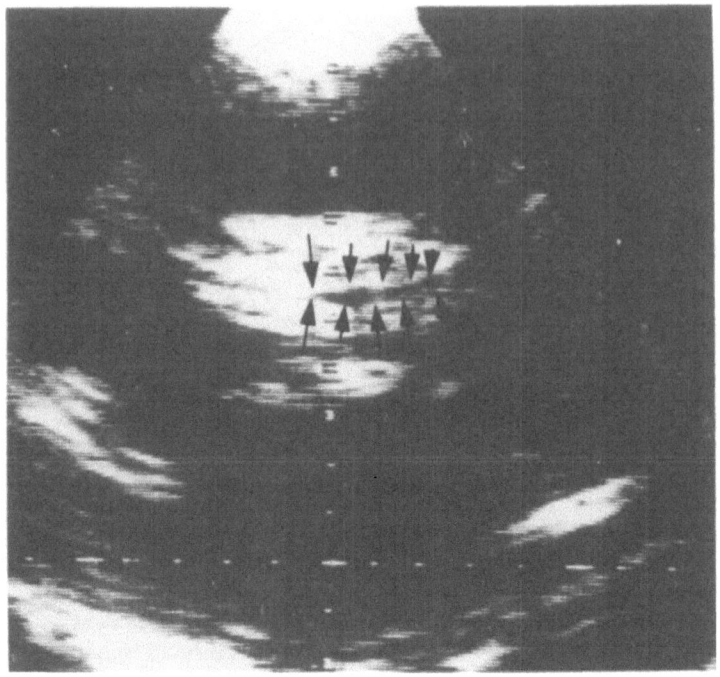

Figure 3. Short axis section of calcified slit-like orifice (arrows).

- When there is unrestricted motion of at least one leaflet, stenosis is likely to be mild.
- However when one leaflet appears to have kept moderate degree of mobility, while the others do not move at all, accurate echographic assessment of severity is unreliable without planimetry.

Short axis assessment of aortic stenosis has reportedly improved predictive accuracy of 2-D echocardiography from 46 to 86% [9]. These figures might not apply for every category of patients, of equipments and of echocardiographers.

1.4. Conclusions

The following conclusions regarding the use of 2-D echocardiography in the clinical management of patients with aortic valve stenosis are proposed:

1. Two dimensional echocardiography is the most sensitive and specific method for the diagnosis of aortic valve stenosis.

2. Planimetry of aortic orifice is feasible in a minority of patients; in these cases, it gives an acceptable quantitative assessment of the degree of stenosis.

3. A maximal long axis cusp separation of more than 11mm in systole rules out significant aortic stenosis.

4. In patients without left ventricular failure, a long axis MACS of less than 8mm is likely to correspond to severe stenosis, unless short axis shows a particularly eccentric orifice. In the 8 − 11mm range short axis qualitative analysis helps for a more accurate description of orifice size, but the final decision should take into account other non invasive indices: left ventricular wall thickness and endsystolic r/h ratio, corrected ejection time and Q waves to murmur's peak.

5. In patients with left ventricular failure and decreased stroke volume, echocardiographic indices tend to overestimate severity of valve stenosis, whereas phonomecanographic indices tend to underestimate it. Although it was suggested that short axis planimetry remains reliable [8], we see no reason why it should. Invasive testing is needed whenever ambiguity persists, although limits of the Gorlin's formula should not be dismissed and correlation between valve area and prognosis is far less than perfect [14]. Patients with poor left ventricular

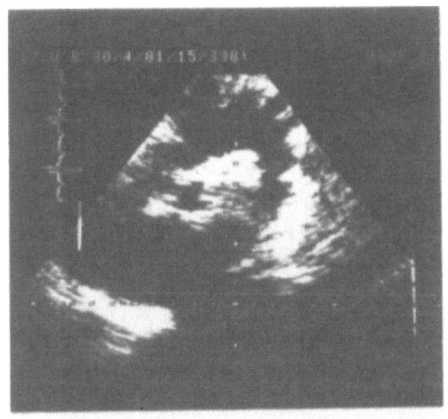

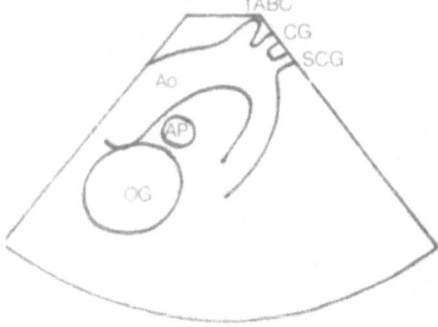

Figure 4. Suprasternal section of normal aortic arch (TABC : innomate artery, CG : left carotid artery, SCG : left subclavian artery, OG : left atrium, AP : pulmonary artery).

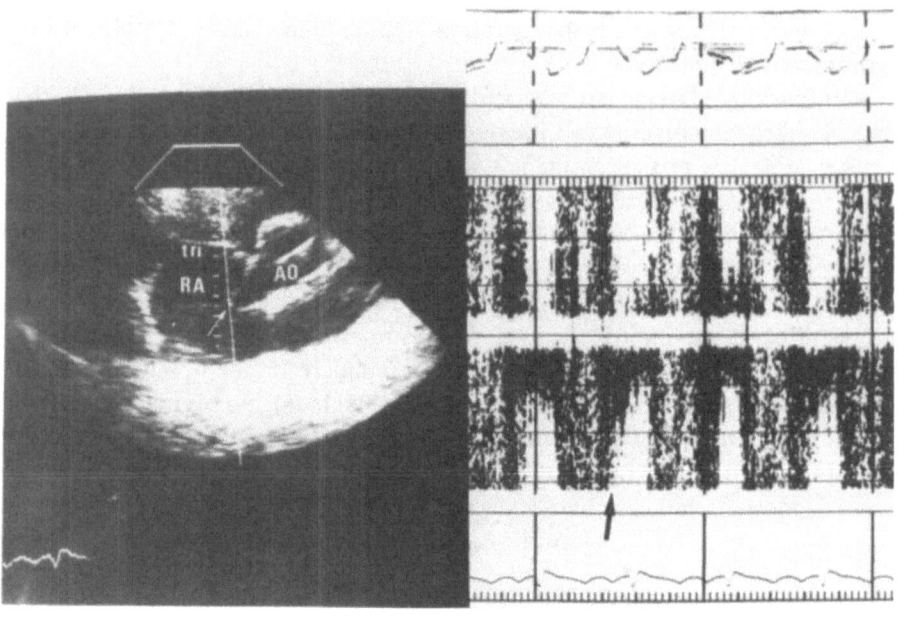

Figure 5. Sinus of Valsalva aneurysm (small arrow) ruptured into the right atrium (RA). Doppler recording at the point of rupture shows highly turbulent systolo diastolic regurgitant flow (large arrow). On the top, the M-mode recording of the tricuspid valve (TRI).

function and apparently only moderate degree of stenosis still represent in our experience a sizable, difficult to manage population.

6. Difficulties are maximal in very old patients, with usually poor echo recordings and very calcified valves. It must be stressed that neither hemodynamic nor echocardiographic available data do necessarily apply to this subset of patients, who are becoming frequent candidates for surgery.

II. EXAMINATION OF THE AORTA

Suprasternal notch cross sections allow an almost complete examination of the aorta in a sizable number of patients (Figure 4). Detection of aneurysmal enlargements of thoracic aorta [15], (Figure 5), of dissecting aneurysms [16] (Figure 6) and aortic coarctations is possible.

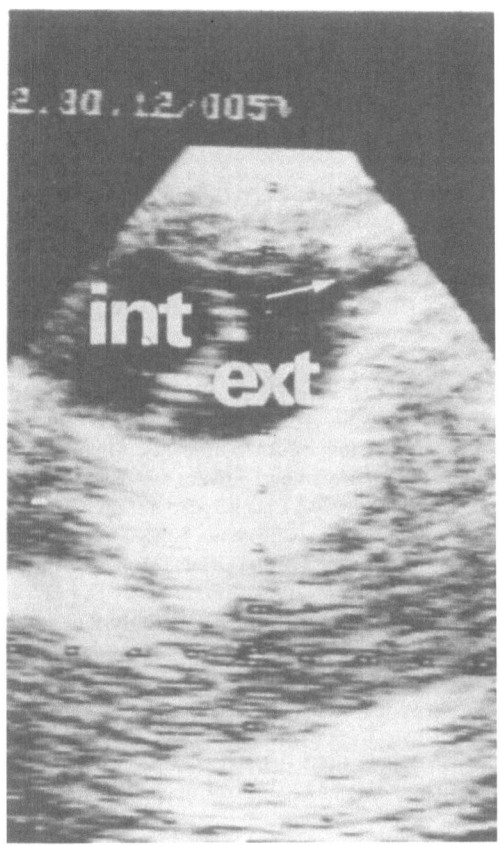

Figure 6. Dissection of the aortic arch: suprasternal view: an echo dense line separates aortic lumen from false channel. The arrow points to the left carotid artery.

Reliability of 2-D echocardiography in the assessment of aortic lesions will have to be tested in the future against other procedures of limited invasiveness such as computed axial tomography and digital angiography.

REFERENCES

1. Alam SE, Hutchinson J, Schwarz MJ: Replacing the aortic valve during the ninth decade of life. Geriatrics 31:100, 1977.
2. Leech GJ, Guiney TE, Davies MJ, Parker DJ: Echocardiography of the aortic valve, pp. 39 – 55, 4th Symposium on Echocardiology Rotterdam 1981 (M. Nijhoff Publ.).
3. Johnson GL, Myer RA, Schwartz DC, Korhagen J, Kaplan S: Echocardiographic evaluation of fixed left ventricular outlet obstruction in children. Pre and postoperative assessment of ventricular systolic pressures. Circulation 56:299, 1977.
4. Aziz KU, Van Grondelle A, Paul MH, Muster AJ: Echocardiographic assessment of the relation

between left ventricular wall and cavity dimensions and peak systolic pressure in children with aortic stenosis. Am J Cardiol 40:775, 1977.

5. Davies MJ: Pathology of cardiac valves 1979 Butterworths publ.

6. Cabrol C, Bensaid J, Doumeix JJ, Blanc G, Acar J, Morin B: Risques et résultats à moyen terme du remplacement valvulaire aortique pour sténose calcifiée chez 100 sujets de plus de 70 ans. Arch Mal Coeur 72:842, 1979.

7. Feigenbaum H: Echocardiography 3rd edition (L&Fibiger publ 1981).

8. De Maria AN, Bommer W, Joye J, Lee G, Bouteller J, Mason DT: Value and limitations of cross-sectional echocardiography of the aortic valve in the diagnosis and quantification of valvular aortic stenosis. Circulation 62:304, 1980.

9. Godley RW, Green D, Dillon J, Rogers EW, Feigenbaum H, Weyman AE: Reliability of two-dimensional echocardiography in assessing the severity of valvular aortic stenosis. Chest 79:657, 1981.

10. Morard JD, Bloch A, Mayor CH, Bopp P: L'échocardiographie bidimensionelle dans l'évaluation des sténosis mitrale et aortique. Arch Mal Coeur 72:165, 1979.

11. Weyman AE, Feigenbaum H, Hurwitz RA, Girod DA, Dillon JC: Cross-sectional echocardiography assessment of the severity of aortic stenosis in children. Circulation 55:773, 1977.

12. Weyman AE, Feigenbaum H, Dillon JC, Chang S: Cross-sectional echocardiography in assessing the severity of valvular aortic stenosis. Circulation 52:828, 1975.

13. Bird JJ, Murgo JP, Pasipoularides A, Phillip D, Rubal BJ: Left ventricular external work loss in valvular aortic stenosis: correlation with severity. Circulation 64:247, 1981.

14. Chizner MA, Pearle DL, DeLeon AC Jr: The natural history of aortic stenosis in adults. Am Heart J 99:419, 1980.

15. De Maria AN, Bommer W, Meumann A, Weinert L, Bogren H, Mason DT: Identification and localization of aneurysms of the ascending aorta by cross-sectional echocardiography. Circulation 59:755, 1979.

16. Roudaut R, Billes MA, Gateau P, Besse P, Dallocchio M: Two-dimensional echocardiography in the diagnosis of aortic dissection in 41 Patients. Circulation 64:314, 1981.

15. TWO-DIMENSIONAL ECHOCARDIOGRAPHY OF VENTRICULAR SEPTAL DEFECTS

G.R. Sutherland and S. Hunter

INTRODUCTION

The interventricular septum is that part of the ventricular mass which separates the two ventricular cavities. It is a highly complex three-dimensional structure formed from a number of morphologically distinct sub-units. It might be expected that such a septum should extend from the attachments of the atrioventricular valves (the septal portion of the atrioventricular junction) to the attachment of the arterial valves (the ventriculo-arterial junction). However, examination of the two septal surfaces of a dissected heart shows that the right and left sided extent of the ventricular septum do not entirely correspond. There are two reasons for this, (i) the septal leaflet of the tricuspid valve is attached to the atrioventricular junction at a more apical level than the septal leaflet of the mitral valve and (ii) the pulmonary valve is supported by a long muscular infundibulum which separates it from the tricuspid valve in contrast to the extensive left-sided area of aorto-mitral fibrous continuity. Thus at both the atrioventricular and arterial poles of septal musculature there are areas of ventricular myocardium which are not shared by both ventricles. The true extent of the interventricular septum is therefore bounded by projections of the tricuspid and aortic valve attachments to the opposing surfaces of the right and left ventricles.

The interventricular septum thus defined can be divided into a membranous and a muscular component, the membranous component being tiny in comparison to the vast bulk of the muscular septum. The muscular septum can be further sub-divided into (i) inlet, (ii) outlet and (iii) trabecular sub-units. Ventricular septal defects may involve any one of the above septal components or may involve two or more adjacent septal sub-units.

Ventricular septal defects can be classified into one of 3 morphological types on the basis of the structures which form the rim of the defect (Figure 1). Each type may then be further sub-divided on the basis of which septal sub-unit is predominately involved (Table 1).

Type 1 — Perimembranous Defects — These defects all involve the membranous septum, (this structure is normally totally excavated by the defect), and are roofed in part by either the aortic root or its posterior fibrous extension, the

Roelandt, J. (ed.) The practice of M-mode and two-dimensional echocardiography
© *1983, Martinus Nijhoff Publishers. The Hague / Boston / London*
ISBN 978-94-009-6792-2.

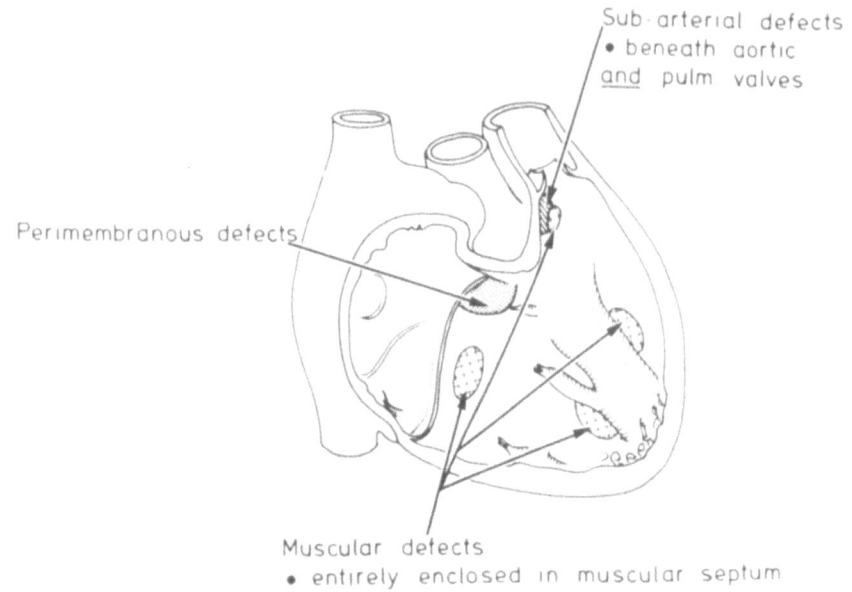

Figure 1. The 3 morphological types of VSD. Classification is on the basis of the structures which form the rim of the defect.

Table 1. Two-dimensional echocardiography of ventricular septal defects — classification of ventricular defects

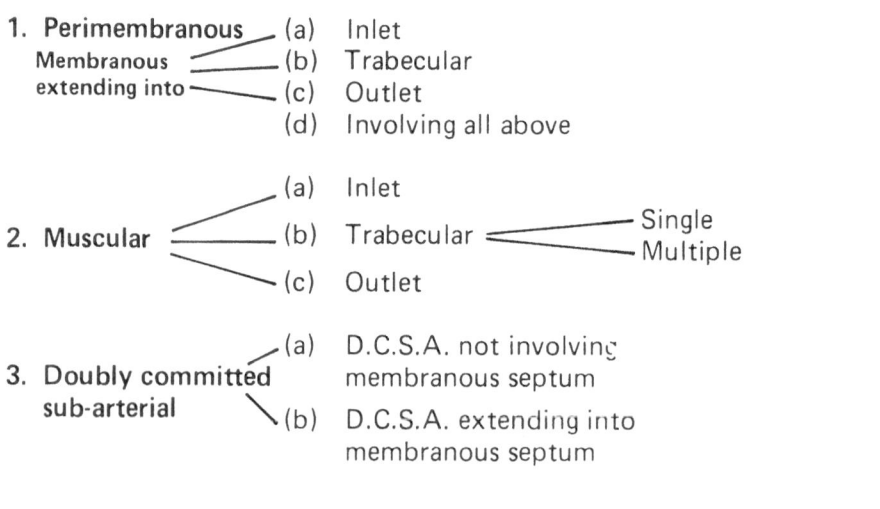

central fibrous body. However, these defects seldom confine themselves to the area of the membranous septum. Where the membranous defect extends posteriorly it involves the inlet muscular septum and is defined to be a perimembranous inlet defect. Where it extends anteriorly below the aortic root into the muscular outlet septum it is defined to be a perimembranous outlet defect. Where its major extension is inferiorly into the trabecular septum it is termed a perimembranous trabecular defect. Large perimembranous defects may extend equally into all three areas.

Type 2 – Muscular Defects – In contrast to perimembranous defects these defects are not roofed by the central fibrous body but have entirely muscular rims. They are sub-divided into muscular defects which involve the (i) inlet, (ii) trabecular or (iii) outlet components of the muscular septum. Defects in the trabecular portion are further sub-divided into two distinct morphological types – a. single trabecular defects and b. multiple trabecular defects of the swiss-cheese type.

A final type of defect completes this classification.

Type 3 – Doubly Committed Sub-Arterial Defects – These defects lie within the muscular outlet septum and are roofed by aortic and pulmonary valve rings, which lie at the same level and which are in fibrous continuity (Figure 1). This abnormal arrangement is caused by absence of a sub-pulmonary infundibulum and is usually associated with an abnormal side-by-side relationship of the great vessel roots. These defects may be sub-divided into two groups, (i) those which extend posteriorly to involve the membranous septum and (ii) those with an intact membranous septum.

The above morphological classification of ventricular septal defects is based on that proposed by Soto et al but has been significantly modified in the light of our subsequent correlative 2-D echocardiographic and morphological studies. It is a classification emminently suited to the ability of 2-D echocardiography to identify specific cardiac structures, as the main classification of defects in effected by identifying the structures which form the margins of a defect. Subdivision of defects is then carried out by defining their position within the ventricular septum. The initial classification of defects is relatively simple as membranous septum, central fibrous body and the fibrous aortic valve ring are all structures easily identified by two-dimensional echocardiography. However, further sub-division might in theory be difficult as apart from the small thin area of the membranous (Figure 2) the remainder of the ventricular septum appears as a thick homogeneous structure to the echocardiographer. Thus, a complete understanding of which septal sub-units form the composite septal echo in each of the standard 2-D echo planes must be available to allow accurate classification of any defect which is visualized.

2-D ECHOCARDIOGRAPHY OF
THE NORMAL INTERVENTRICULAR SEPTUM

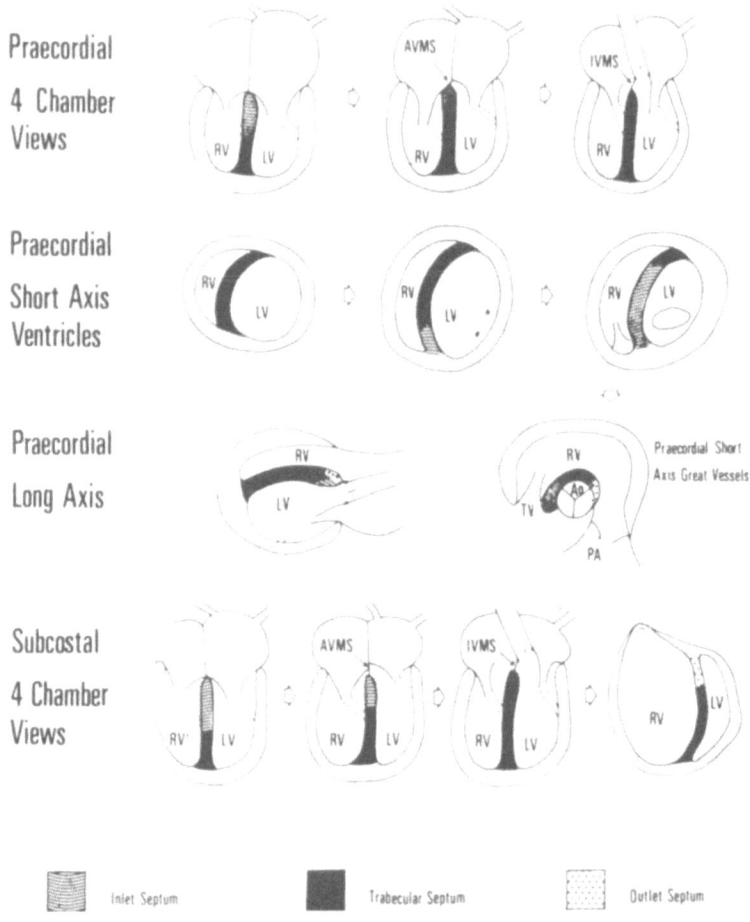

Figure 2. Two-dimensional Echo. Morphological correlation of the normal interventricular septum. RV : right ventricle, LV : left ventricle, Ao : aorta, PA : pulmonary artery, TV : tricuspid valve, IVMS : interventricular portion of membranous septum, AVMS : atrioventricular portion of membranous septum.

The normal interventricular septum – two-dimensional echocardiographic –
morphological correlations

The areas occupied by the individual septal sub-units in each of the standard
echocardiographic planes are shown in Figure 2. Note that the inlet portion of
the muscular septum is only profiled in a four chamber plane. The remainder of
the septal echo in this plane originates from the trabecular septum. At the
posterior aspect of the four chamber plane the septal atrioventricular valve
leaflet echoes insert almost at a common level to a central septal echo – dense
area which represents the atrioventricular muscular septum. As the echo beam is
swept anteriorly through the four chamber plane the atrioventricular valve septal
leaflets become further separated with the tricuspid leaflet septal attachment
placed more apically than the mitral septal leaflet. The thin structure which lies
between the atrioventricular valve septal leaflets and which now separates the left
ventricle from the right atrium is the atrioventricular membranous septum. Scanning anteriorly into the four chamber plus aortic root plane, the thin atrioventricular membranous septum is seen to become more echo dense as it fuses with
the posterior aspect of the aortic root to form the central fibrous body. It is
precisely at this point, (the junction of the four chamber and the four chamber
plus aortic root planes), that the interventricular portion of the membranous septum is initially recorded taking origin below the central fibrous body and aortic
root. Throughout the posterior aspect of the four chamber plus aortic root plane
the septal echo is formed by a thin superior membranous septal echo with the remainder being trabecular septal echoes.

From the praecordial transducer position it is usually impossible to scan
anteriorly from the four chamber plus aortic root plane. However, this is not the
case when using the subcostal approach. From this position the echo beam can be
swept forwards from the four chamber plus aortic root plane to record the subcostal right ventricular outflow tract plane. This is the only echocardiographic
approach which will consistently profile the small muscular outlet septum. This
therefore is a crucial echocardiographic plane to record in every patient suspected
of having a ventricular septal defect.

The septal sub-units which form the composite septal echo in both the short
and long axis planes are similarly illustrated in Figure 2. (Note that the muscular
outlet septum can theoretically be visualized in praecordial planes, but in practise
these planes have proved of little value in identifying muscular outlet defects).

Having thus correlated the morphology of the normal interventricular septum
with individual standard echocardiographic planes (Figure 3), it should be possible to accurately define which septal sub-unit is involved when a discrete area of
echo drop out is identified within the septal echo. By identifying the structures
which form the margins of such a defect, accurate classification on the basis of
the 2-D echo should be possible in every case.

The following echocardiographic descriptions of specific ventricular septal

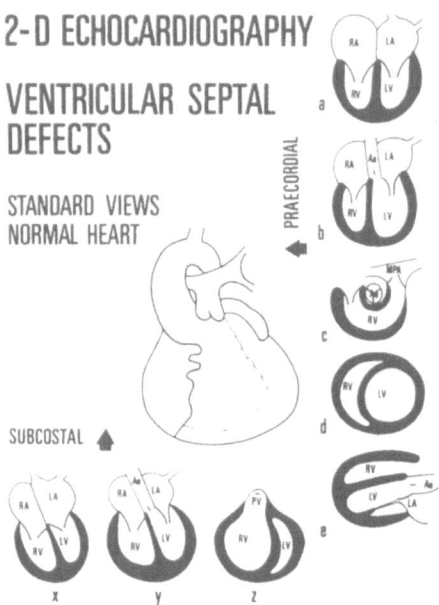

2-D ECHOCARDIOGRAPHY

VENTRICULAR SEPTAL
DEFECTS

STANDARD VIEWS
NORMAL HEART

Figure 3. The standard 2-D echo planes. Praecordial — a. Four chamber, b. Four chamber plus aortic root, c. Short axis great vessels, d. Short axis ventricles, e. Long axis. Subcostal — x. Four chamber, y. Four chamber plus aortic root, z. Right ventricular outflow.

defects are based on the results of a prospective study involving 280 infants and children. The 2-D echo findings were correlated with angiographic (280 pts), surgical (130 pts), and autopsy (31 pts) information. This correlative study confirmed that:

a. each type of ventricular septal defect could be correctly classified on the basis of a specific echocardiographic pattern, and
b. 2-D echocardiography was a highly effective technique for identifying the majority of haemodynamically important ventricular septal defects.

The two-dimensional features which differentiate ventricular septal defects

1. Perimembranous defects

These defects have as a common feature an area of echo drop out involving the membranous septum. This "drop out" will be best visualized at the junction of the four chamber and four chamber plus aortic root planes. At this point the defect is clearly seen to be roofed by the posterior portion of the aortic root and the central fibrous body.

Perimembranous inlet defects will extend posteriorly into the four chamber

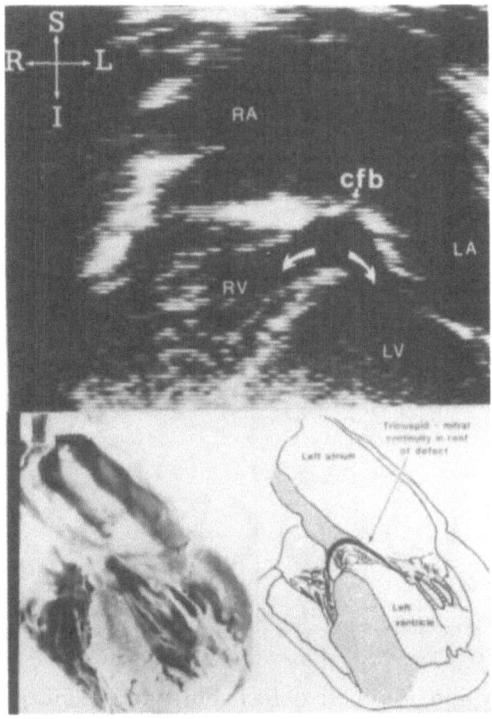

Figure 4a. A perimembranous inlet defect visualized in the four chamber plane.

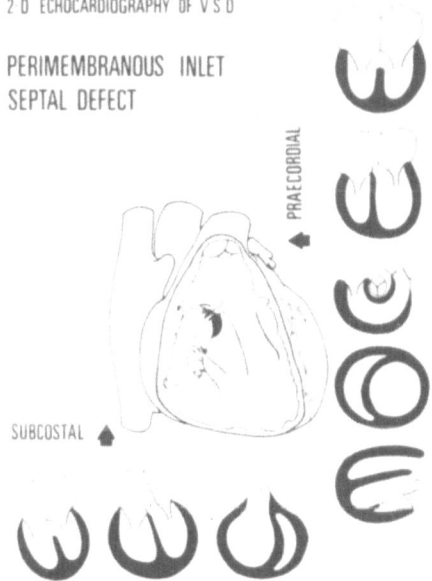

Figure 4b. The 2-D echo pattern diagnostic of a perimembranous inlet defect.

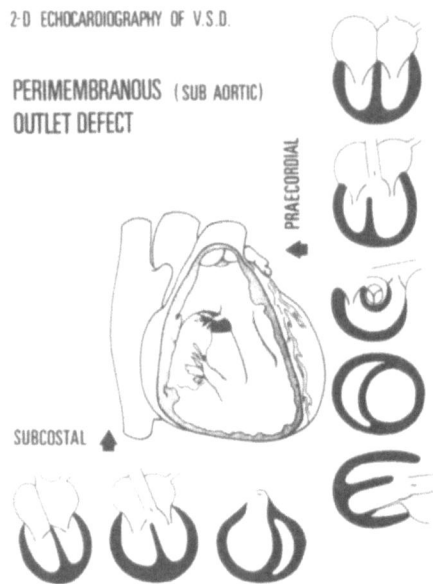

2-D ECHOCARDIOGRAPHY OF V.S.D.

PERIMEMBRANOUS (SUB AORTIC)
OUTLET DEFECT

PRAECORDIAL

SUBCOSTAL

Figure 5. The 2-D echo pattern diagnostic of a perimembranous outlet defect.

plane from this position. As these defects burrow posteriorly into the inlet septum they also excavate away the atrioventricular septum. They are thus roofed throughout their posterior extension by the atrioventricular valve septal leaflets as they implant at a common level into the atrioventricular junction (Figure 4a). The 2-D echo features diagnostic of a perimembranous inlet defect are illustrated in Figure 4b.

Defects which extend anteriorly from the membranous septal area to excavate into the muscular outlet septum below the aortic root are *perimembranous outlet defects*. The sub-aortic extension is visualized by scanning anteriorly through the four chamber plus aortic root plane. Large perimembranous outlet defects which extend anteriorly below the whole aortic root will also be visualized in the left ventricular long axis plane (Figure 5).

Defects which extend inferiorly to excavate away the superior portion of the trabecular septum are perimembranous trabecular defects. This inferior extension is best visualized in the four chamber plus aortic root planes. *Large perimembranous defects* will equally involve all three of the above neighbouring septal sub-units.

Muscular defects

Inlet muscular defects are only visualized in the four chamber planes. They are clearly seen on 2-D echo to lie within the inlet muscular septum and are separated from the atrioventricular junction by a muscle bar (Figure 6a). These defects do not involve either the atrioventricular or interventricular portions of the mem-

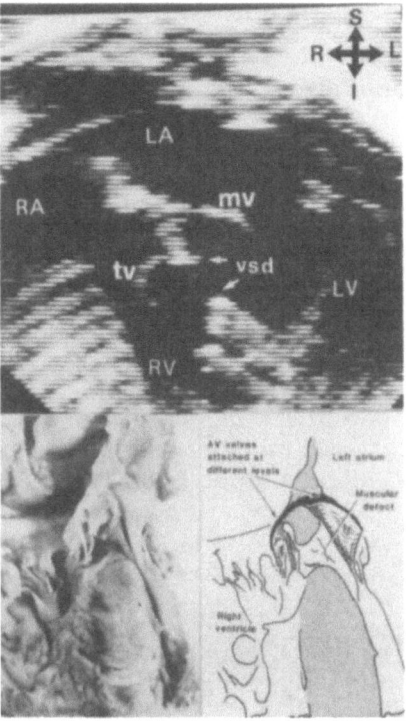

Figure 6a. A muscular inlet defect. (Note the intact atrioventricular septum).

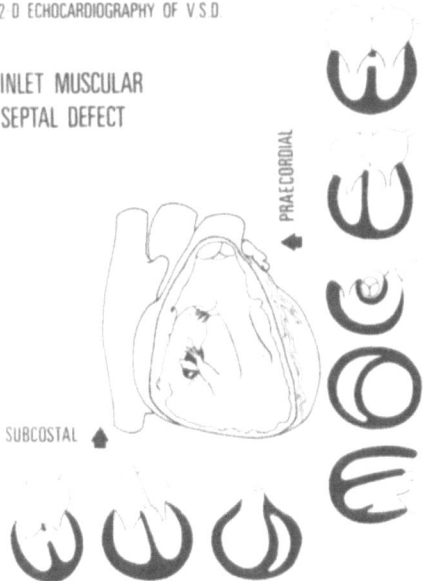

Figure 6b. The 2-D echo pattern diagnostic of a muscular inlet defect.

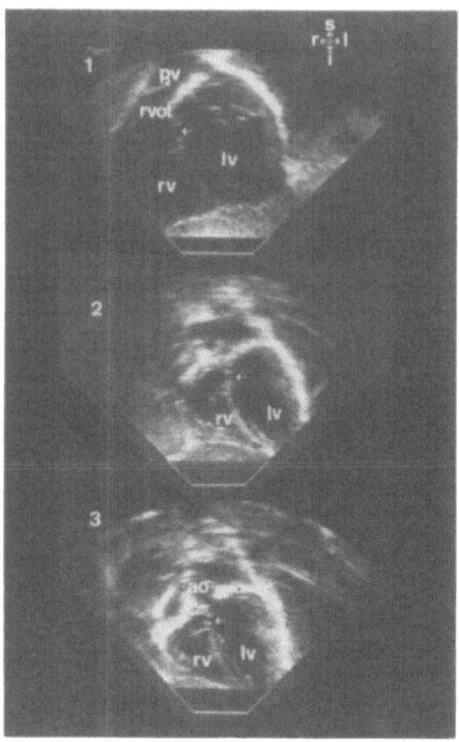

Figure 7a. A muscular outlet defect. This composite figure shows three still frames from a subcostal scan recorded by sweeping the echo beam posteriorly from the subcostal R.V.O.T. plane (1) to the four chamber plus aortic root plane (3). (Note the muscular outlet defect burrows posteriorly into the trabecular septum in plane (3)).

membranous septum. The above feature (Figure 6b) clearly distinguish these defects from perimembranous inlet defects.

Outlet muscular defects are only reliably visualized in the subcostal right ventricular outflow tract plane (Figure 7a), separated from the pulmonary valve by the long muscular infundibulum. In a significant number of patients this plane cannot be recorded and thus a muscular outlet defect cannot be excluded. These defects are clearly seen to be bounded by muscle and do not involve the membranous septum. The 2-D echo features diagnostic of this defect are illustrated in Figure 7b.

Single trabecular defects. Single trabecular defects are best visualised on short axis scanning. They are always clearly located within the trabecular (Figure 8) and never involve the membranous septum. Such defects are also frequently visualized on four chamber or long axis scanning. The multiple plane scanning technique used in this study should accurately locate them within the trabecular septum.

Multiple small trabecular defects (= the Swiss cheese defect) are not in our ex-

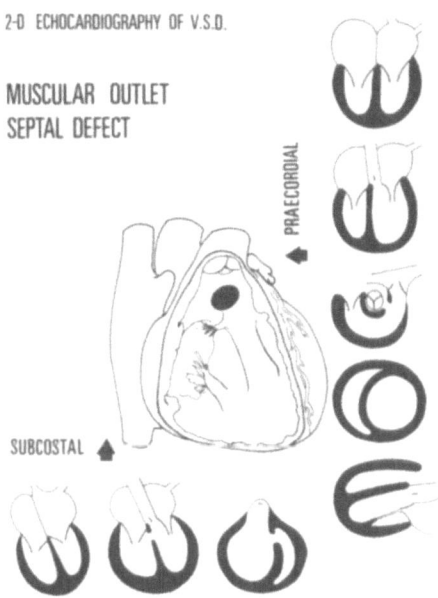

Figure 7b. The 2-D echo pattern diagnostic of a muscular outlet defect.

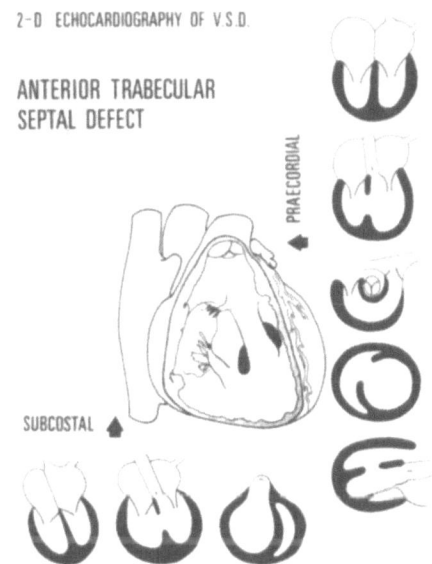

Figure 8. The 2-D echo pattern diagnostic of an anterior trabecular defect.

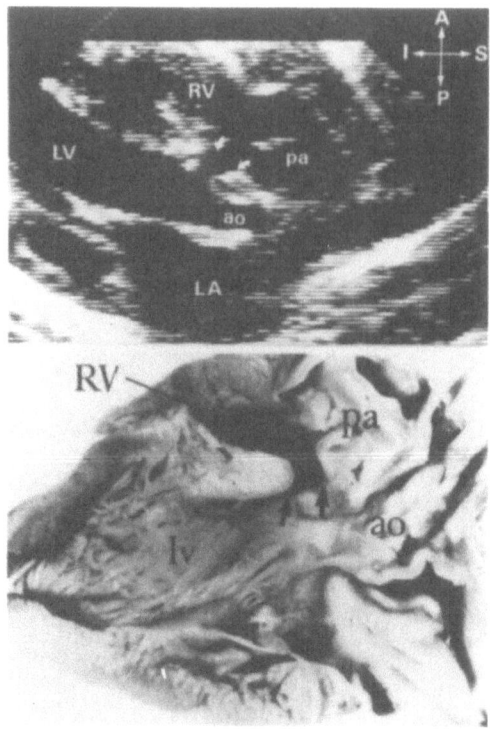

Figure 9a. Upper panel — a doubly committed subarterial defect. Note the conjoint aortic and pulmonary valves roofing the defect. Lower panel — the corresponding pathological specimen sectioned in a praecordial long axis plane.

Table 2. Two-dimensional echocardiography of ventricular septal defects

Types of defect			No. studied	No. correctly identified	% correctly identified
Perimembranous (extending mainly into)	(a) Inlet septum		43	43	100
	(b) Trabecular septum		19	16	84
	(c) Outlet septum		84	83	98
	(d) All of the above		39	39	100
Muscular	(a) Inlet		18	18	100
	(b) Single trabecular	Large	32	23	72
		Small	11	0	0
	(c) Multiple trabecular		4	0	0
	(d) Outlet		6	6	100
Doubly committed sub–arterial	(a) D.C.S.A. not involving membranous septum		15	15	100
	(b) D.C.S.A. extending into membranous septum area		9	9	100
	TOTAL		280	252	

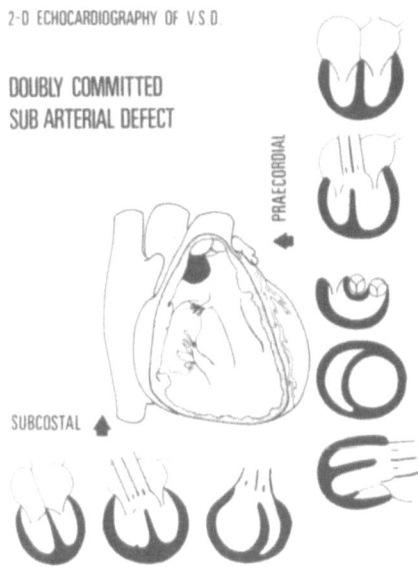

Figure 9b. The 2-D echo pattern diagnostic of a doubly committed subarterial defect.

perience visualised by 2-D echocardiography. This is because the multiple small defects burrow through the septum in an oblique fashion and thus fail to create a complete echocardiographic window across the width of the septum. In such cases the septum will appear intact in all views when scanned with the 2-D echo beam.

Doubly committed sub-arterial defects are roofed by conjoint aortic and pulmonary valve rings which lie at the same level. These features are well defined by 2-D echocardiography (Figure 9a). The echocardiographic pattern diagnostic of such a defect is illustrated in Figure 9b. These defects are best characterised by scanning through the four chamber plus aortic root planes.

DISCUSSION

Although the interventricular septum is formed from a number of morphologically distinct sub-units, it appears as a virtually homogeneous structure on two-dimensional echocardiography. The muscular septum varies little in width throughout the different echocardiographic planes. The only septal sub-unit which can be consistently differentiated is the thin interventricular portion of the membranous septum. Thus precise localisation of defects within the large mass of the muscular septum will only be possible if the echocardiographer appreciates which of the muscular septal sub-units form the composite thick septal structure visualised in each echocardiographic plane (Figure 2).

Where a ventricular septal defect is identified as an area of persistent septal "drop-out" in one or more of the echocardiographic planes recorded then an attempt should be made to determine three factors, 1. the cardiac structures which form the margins of the defect, 2. the septal sub-unit predominately involved and 3. any extension of the defect into neighbouring septal sub-units. By determining each of these 3 factors it should be possible to accurately classify each type of ventricular septal defect and determine its position within the septum.

As the resolution of two-dimensional systems has increased, it is now possible to accurately image the aortic root, the central fibrous body, (i.e. the area enclosed by the fibrous annuli of the tricuspid, mitral and aortic valves) the atrioventricular and interventricular portions of the membranous septum, the infundibular septum and the pulmonary valve. Thus, a classification of ventricular septal defects based on the structures forming their margins should be emminently suited to the imaging capabilities of two-dimensional echocardiography.

To determine if this method of classification was both practical and reliable we reviewed 280 patients with a ventricular septal defect. Using a multiplane scanning technique to construct an approximate three-dimensional model of the heart we identified a defect in 252 patients. In each case the structures forming the margins of a defect were readily identified thus allowing accurate classification into one of the three main groups (Figure 2). The further sub-division of these main groups, based on which septal sub-unit is predominately involved, was determined by the echocardiographic planes in which the defect was visualized, (e.g. a defect roofed in part by the central fibrous body but otherwise surrounded by muscle is a perimembranous defect. Where such a defect is only visualised in a four chamber plane which profiles the inlet septum, it is sub-classified as a perimembranous inlet defect). However, defects frequently extend across the boundaries of individual septal components and this information should be included in any description of a defect, (e.g. the majority of muscular outlet defects studied were not restricted to the right ventricular outflow plane but were traced postero-inferiorly into the four chamber plus aortic root plane where they burrowed into the trabecular septum. Such a defect should therefore be described as a muscular outlet defect which extends postero-inferiorly into the trabecular septum). In our experience, two-dimensional echocardiography accurately subdivided septal defects within each of the three main groups on the basis of which septal sub-unit was predominately involved, and in addition accurately identified any extension into an adjoining septal sub-unit.

Different defects were identified with different degrees of accuracy. (Table 2). Perimembranous inlet and outlet defects, doubly committed sub-arterial defects and inlet and outlet defects of the muscular septum were all identified with remarkable consistency, whereas defects of the trabecular septum were identified with varying degrees of success. Multiple small (swiss cheese) trabecular defects were not identified in this series. Single trabecular defects were inconsistently visualised with some correlation existing between defect size and defect recognition. When divided into two groups on the basis of intracardiac shunting (small defects with a Qp:Qs < 1.5:1 and large defects with a Qp:Qs > 1.5:1, Table 2) it was clear that small defects were not visualised at all compared with 72% recognition of large defects. However, some surprisingly large trabecular defects were not visualised.

The above findings show broad agreement with the results of previously published series [2, 3]. However, both these series have confined their investigation to the identification of septal defects in infants and have restricted their echocardiographic approach to the subcostal window. Although a subcostal approach will yield more information when compared to a praecordial aproach (the muscular outlet septum is only profiled from the subcostal window) it can be extremely difficult to record in older children and adolescents. In these cases a praecordial approach may be the only means of visualising a defect. However, information can be gained from the praecordial approach which is not readily obtainable from the subcostal window (e.g. the anterior extension of a perimembranous sub-aortic defect beneath the whole aortic root was only clearly visualised in a left ventricular long axis plane. Similarly, anterior trabecular defects were best visualised by praecordial short axis scanning, being frequently missed from the subcostal approach).

We would suggest that the composite approach adopted in this study in which the heart is visualised from both the subcostal and praecordial window and where a scanning technique is used to determine the extent of any defect will provide the maximum amount of information. It will accurately identify and classify the majority of ventricular septal defects in infants, children and adolescents, and thus offers considerable advantages over previously described echocardiographic techniques for studying the ventricular septum.

ACKNOWLEDGEMENTS

The authors wish to thank the editors of the British Heart Journal for their permission to reproduce Figures 4a, 4b, 5, 6a, 6b, 7b, 9a, 9b and Table 2.

REFERENCES

1. Soto B, Becker AE, Moulaert AJ, Lie JT, Anderson, RH: Classification of ventricular septal defects, Br Heart J 1980, 43:332–343, 1980.
2. Bierman FZ, Williams RG: Prospective identification of ventricular septal defects in infancy using subxiphoid two-dimension echocardiography. Circulation 1980, 62 No. 4, pp. 807–817, 1980.
3. Cheatham JP, Latson LA, Gutgesell HP: Ventricular septal defect in infancy: Detection with two-dimensional echocardiography. Am Heart J Jan. 1980 Vol. 47, pp. 85–89, 1980.

V. ASSESSMENT OF THE LEFT VENTRICLE BY M-MODE AND TWO-DIMENSIONAL ECHOCARDIOGRAPHY

Assessment of left ventricular function is essential in the evaluation and management of patients with cardiac disease. Echocardiography has unique advantages since it uses sound radiation which is harmless at the energy levels used so that it can be often repeated without untoward effects. M-mode measurements of the left ventricle have good accuracy and reproducibility. They can be used with advantage to assess left ventricular function in selected patients or when the patient serves as his own control (chapters 16 and 17). Computer-aided analysis is a versatile and attractive means to study left ventricular function but its clinical use is cumbersome. The method at present should still be considered as an investigational tool (chapter 17). Two-dimensional echocardiography offers many advantages over M-mode echocardiography for the assessment of left ventricular function since information in multiple tomographic views can be obtained. Area-length measurements in one or more representative views can be performed to obtain estimates of left ventricular volume by applying formulas largely tested in angiocardiography. However, since angiocardiography and echocardiography are basically different methods, good agreement between these two indirect methods should not be expected. Assessment of left ventricular ejection fraction is less dependent on geometric assumptions than volume assessment, and it is therefore not surprising that most studies have shown reasonable agreement between two-dimensional echocardiographic, angiocardiographic, and radionuclide determined ejection fraction although individual differences remain present (chapter 16 and 18). The major limitation of echocardiography remains the percentage of patients with unsatisfactory studies ranging between 10 to 40 percent depending on the type of patient being examined.

Roelandt, J. (ed.) The practice of M-mode and two-dimensional echocardiography
© *1983, Martinus Nijhoff Publishers. The Hague / Boston / London*
ISBN 978-94-009-6792-2.

16. QUANTIFICATION OF LEFT VENTRICULAR FUNCTION: HOW USEFUL IS IT FOR CLINICAL DECISION MAKING?

P. SCHWEIZER

The application of M-mode echocardiography has become well established in the morphological diagnosis of various cardiac diseases. More recently, the development of two-dimensional systems has enhanced this capability.

Now question arises, whether echocardiographic quantification of *global* and *regional* left ventricular function gives additional information about an individual patient's clinical condition and prognosis.

I. GLOBAL LEFT VENTRICULAR FUNCTION

M-mode echocardiography enables accurate measurement of distances because of the high axial resolution of the method being below 1 mm. Enddiastolic and endsystolic distances between the endocardium of the interventricular septum and the posterior left ventricular wall being recorded at the chordal level are reproducible and provide the main data for calculation of left ventricular performance. Several authors could demonstrate, that these "minor axes" of the left ventricle measured by ultrasound do significantly correlate with the dimensions and volumes obtained with cineangiography. [1 – 5].

However, in patients with dilated ventricles the used cubed diameter, which Feigenbaum first demonstrated to correlate with volume, induced a systematic overestimation [2, 4, 5]. This overestimation can be compensated partly by the introduction of linear regression equations [6, 7].

Echocardiographic indices of left ventricular function like fractional shortening are independent of artificial extrapolation to volume and permit also clinical useful estimation of ejections fraction [2]. Patients with normal ventricular function have values of fractional shortening greater than 25%.

The *limitations* encountered with the M-mode technique are due to the fact, that the echo samples only a small circumscript portion of the cardiac walls. In the presence of distorted geometry this portion is no longer representative for the total left ventricular cavity. [6, 8 – 10]. Especially in patients with coronary artery disease and patchy contraction abnormalities echo measurements may then be invalid. Those patients may appear to have normal function by M-mode and still have significant dysfunction by cineangiography.

Roelandt, J. (ed.) The practice of M-mode and two-dimensional echocardiography
© *1983, Martinus Nijhoff Publishers. The Hague / Boston / London*
ISBN 978-94-009-6792-2.

Therefore, to overcome this problem, the measurement of the so called mitral septal separation was recommended, a parameter being totally independent of left ventricular geometry [11, 12]. However, to our and others experience this parameter is a semiquantitative one, only demonstrating rough correlations to cineangiographic data [13, 14].

M-mode echocardiographic measurements are then useful, when they are made with knowledge of the limits of the technique. The method is especially helpful in the detection of various primary and secondary endstage myocardial diseases. In these cases the measurement of left ventricular diameter without artificial extrapolation to volume is a sufficient parameter of ventricular size [15]. Furthermore, in the evaluation of patients with suspected myocardial disease, M-mode echocardiography can demonstrate decreased indices of contractility before clinically apparent congestive heart failure has appeared. Serial determinations in the same patient allow therefore objective evaluation of the progression of the disease, especially of valvular heart disease [16 – 19]. In patients receiving cardiotoxic therapy M-mode echocardiography gives information about the reduction of left ventricular function (fractional shortening) before the clinical signs of heart failure appear [20]. However in patients with coronary artery disease and suspected regional contraction abnormalities all M-mode echocardiographic measurements must be interpreted cautiously [21].

Two-dimensional echocardiography offers more spatial orientation than the M-mode technique by displaying the global geometry of the left ventricle. Images can be obtained from multiple transducer positions including the apex impulse window [22, 23]. With the latter approach real-time non invasive ventriculograms similar to cineangiographic projections can be recorded.

The increase of dimensional data obtained with this technique should theoretically produce more accurate estimates of left ventricular volumes. In vitro studies have shown indeed a remarkable potential for accurate volume determination with the cross-sectional method [24 – 26].

But previously was reported, that in vivo volume determinations did not turn out as excellent as in vitro studies. The correlation between two-dimensional echocardiography and cineangiography obtained with single plane and/or biplane volume determinations ranged between acceptable (correlation coefficient r = 0.76 for enddiastolic volume) and excellent (r = 0.96) [23, 27 – 33].

Our own results, which we obtained with monoplane two-dimensional echocardiography (apical long axis view) and cineangiography (30° RAO-projection) are to be seen in Figure 1 and 2 [29].

A considerable underestimation of volumes could be observed in adult patients in correspondance with all other studies. More marked discrepancies between cineangiography and two-dimensional echocardiography were found in the case of larger ventricular volumes due to the established regression equations. This underestimation, exceeding in some cases 30%, held true regardless of whether monoplane or biplane methods were used or whether varying volume calcula-

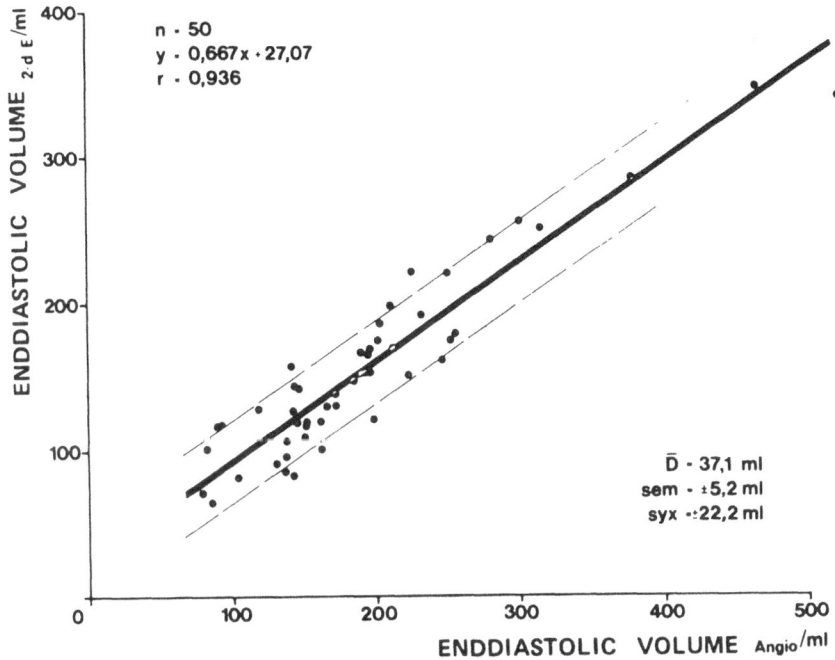

Figure 1. Correlation between the echocardiographically (2-d-E) and cineangiographically (Angio) determined enddiastolic volumes of the left ventricle in 50 patients. The 95% confidence limit is within the dashed lines.

tions were employed. The reasons for this underestimation, which needs correction formulas for compensation, are discussed elsewhere [29, 30].

In contrast to the significant underestimation of volumes by echocardiography the standard deviations obtained with correlation of ejection fraction were within tolerable limits (between 6 and 10%, mean value 7,6%). (see Figure 3) [23, 27 – 33].

These results make clear, that a point to point correlation between cineangiographic and two-dimensional echocardiographic measurements is not possible. However, when applied to an individual patient, the sensitivity of the echocardiographic method is sufficient enough to differentiate between normal and clearly pathological left ventricular function (sensitivity rates between 76 and 80%). According to our investigations in meanwhile 16 patients the intraobserver variability of measurements is within tolerable limits (day to day coeff. of var. 5,5 – 7%; EF: 1st day SD: 48,3 ± 6,5; 2nd day: 47,3 ± 8; 3rd day: 48,7 ± 8,5). Using the apical approach recordings can be obtained, even in critically ill patients, which are adequate for determination of volume and ejection fraction.

The methodological advantages to M-mode echocardiography especially for the evaluation of patients with coronary artery disease and suspected regional contraction abnormalities, are obvious. Quantitative evaluation of left ven-

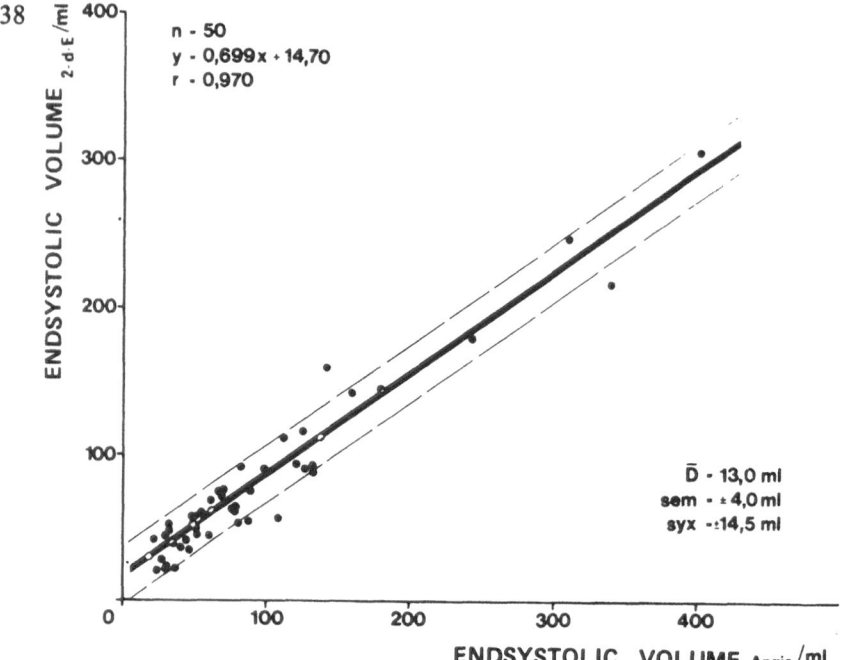

Figure 2. Correlation between the echocardiographically (2-d-E) and cineangiographically (Angio) determined endsystolic volumes of the left ventricle in 50 patients.

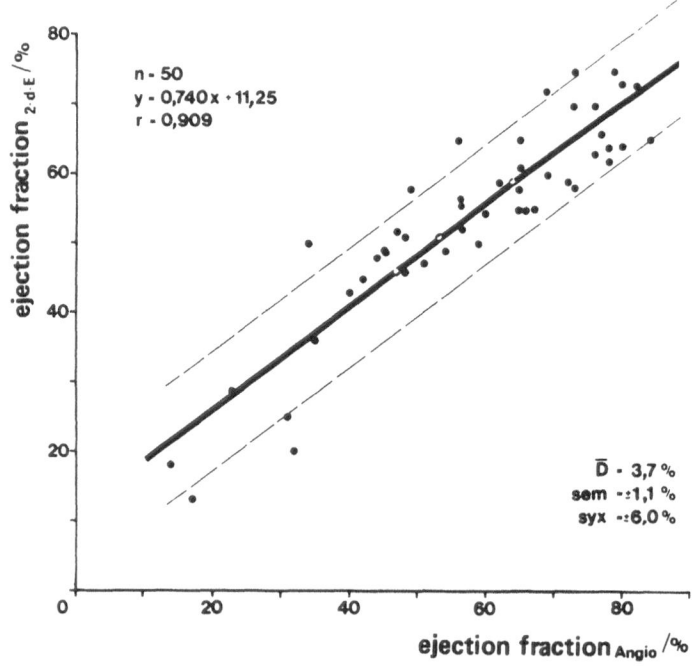

Figure 3. Correlation between the echocardiographically (2-d-E) and cineangiographically (Angio) determined endsystolic volumes of the left ventricle in 50 patients.

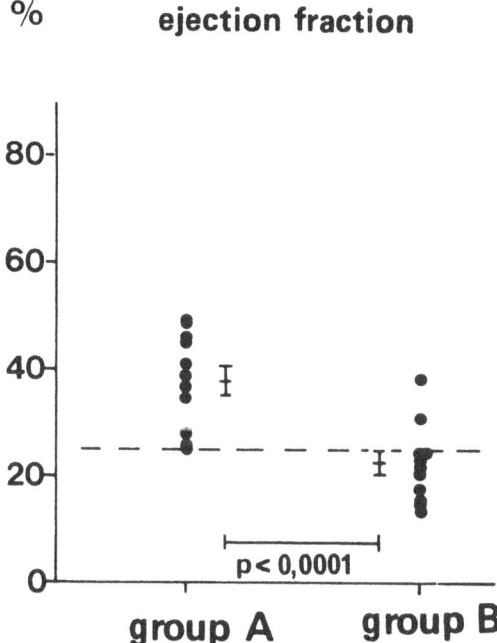

%   **ejection fraction**

Figure 4. Echocardiographically determined ejection fraction in patients with admission to the intensive care unit after resuscitation and different outcome (Group A and B).

tricular function proved to be valuable for the follow up of this patient group and helpful as a prognostic guide [34, 35]. For example the clinical course after resuscitation could be tested in 25 patients who were admitted to the intensive care unit. 11 of 25 patients could be discharged later on (Group A), whereas 14 of 25 patients died (Group B). The echocardiographically determined ejection fraction was significantly different between both groups ($38 \pm 3\%$ in group A and $23 \pm 2\%$ in group B) and could be used as a sensitive prognostic guide in those critically ill patients [35].

II. REGIONAL LEFT VENTRICULAR FUNCTION

The information gained with *M-mode echocardiography* is normally restricted to the basal portion of the left ventricle, which is least likely to be affected by ischemia. Only, when the contraction abnormalities are located in this basal near part they can probably be recorded with the single ultrasound beam. The successrate in the detection of abnormal wall motion in patients with acute myocardial infarction can be improved up to 84%, when, dependent of the investigator's skill, multiple areas of the left ventricle are scanned from multiple transducer positions [36, 37]. Only pathological findings should be used for diagnostic pur-

240

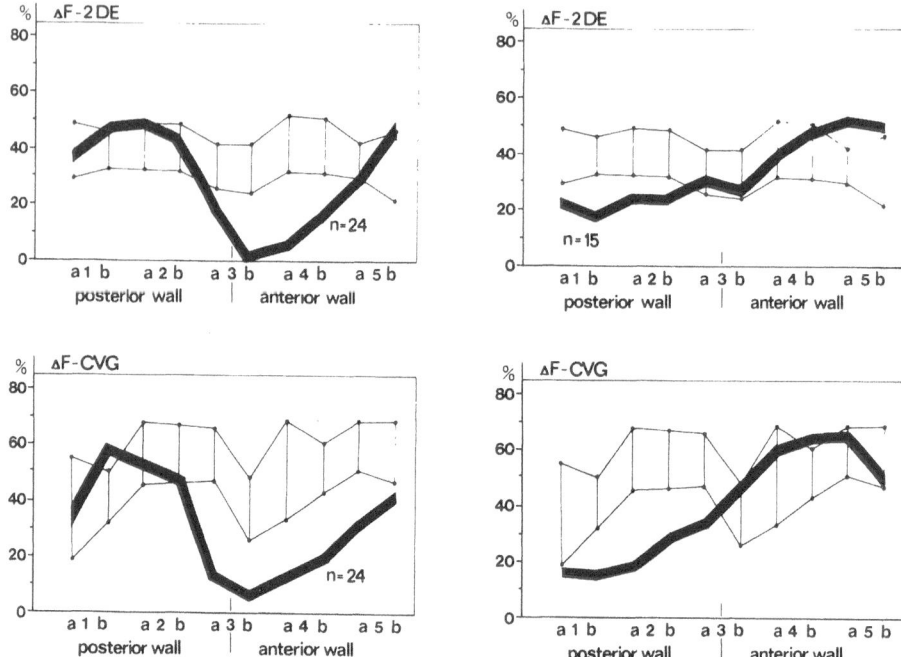

Figure 5. Plots of regional contraction in area segments ($\triangle$ F%) for the 24 patients with anterior wall infarction (left) and the 15 patients with inferior wall infarction (right). Correlation between two-dimensional echocardiography (2-d-E) and cineangiography (CVG). The normal contraction range represented by the tolerance limits (lower limits) and the mean values (upper limits) was established in 32 persons.

poses. No correct information can be given with the M-mode technique concerning the true extent of the pathological myocardial process [13, 37].

Two-dimensional echocardiography was at first used as a semiquantitative method for the delineation of wall motion abnormalities. Kisslo and coworkers prospectively analyzed the correlation between echocardiographically and cineangiographically detected wall motion abnormalities in 525 regions of the left ventricle from 105 patients [38]. Only 18 percent of these regions could not be visualized with multiple cross-sectional views and 87% of those imaged were correctly classified. These semiquantitative data in patients with chronic coronary artery disease were confirmed by other groups reporting sensitivity rates of 79 to 91% [39, 40]. Two-dimensional echocardiography further proved to be very sensitive in the qualitative and semiquantitative evaluation of akinetic zones in acute myocardial infarction [41, 42].

Newer efforts aim at quantitative echocardiographic wall motion analysis rather than the qualitative approaches. The practicability of those methods would be of special interest to estimation of changes secondary to therapeutic interventions, or, for example, to quantification of the extent of ischemia in acute myocardial infarction [43, 44].

Weiss and coworkers have recently shown in acute myocardial infarction in man, that the echocardiographic delineation of the contractile dysfunction was clearly correlated to the extent of pathologically proved myocardial damage [44]. These authors and several others quantified regional contraction at multiple short axis cross-sections from the cardiac basis to the apex. Visser and coworkers demonstrated, that the initial asynergic area obtained with two-dimensional echocardiography correlated well with the peak value of the isoenzyme of creatine kinase [45]. And Eaton and coworkers assessed the early topographic changes of acute myocardial infarction during the first two weeks by serial two-dimensional echocardiography. They could identify a group of patients with bad prognosis due to infarct expansion during the follow up period [46].

In a prospective study performed in 39 patients during the acute stage of transmural myocardial infarction we correlated echocardiographic and cineangiographic wall motion abnormalities [47]. Two chamber apical cross sections were compared with 30° – RAO-cineangiographic projections in a quantitative manner. An area-based method with the center of gravity of the end-systolic frame as inner fix point was used for quantification (10 segmental areas).

In correlation to cineangiography 138 of 190 segments were true abnormal with two-dimensional echocardiography (Sensitivity 73%). The specificity was 89% and the predictive accuracy of the echocardiographic method 85%.

The amount of pathological segments determined in each patient was in correlation to ejection fraction determined by echocardiography. A patient group with serious prognosis could be identified, having bad regional and global function with two-dimensional echocardiography. 4 patients of this group died during initial hospitalization (see Figure 6).

The echocardiographic assessment of diseased and residual myocardium in coronary artery disease appears, therefore, to be of prognostic interest. In patients with chronic ischemic heart disease and left ventricular aneurysms an index of residual myocardium was calculated from apical two- and four chamber views. This index proved to be of special prognostic value in the surgical or medical treatment [48].

In conclusion: M-mode measurement of left ventricular internal diameters and indices of function without extrapolation to volume are useful in the diagnosis and follow up of diseases envolving the entire myocardium. In patients with coronary artery disease and contraction abnormalities, quantitative M-mode echocardiographic diagnosis is limited or invalid because of the ''ice pick'' view of the technique. Two-dimensional echocardiography provides better spatial orientation and has the possibility to image the entire left ventricle. In patients with coronary artery disease the method is, therefore, superior to the M-mode technique. A point to point correlation of global and regional data to those ob-

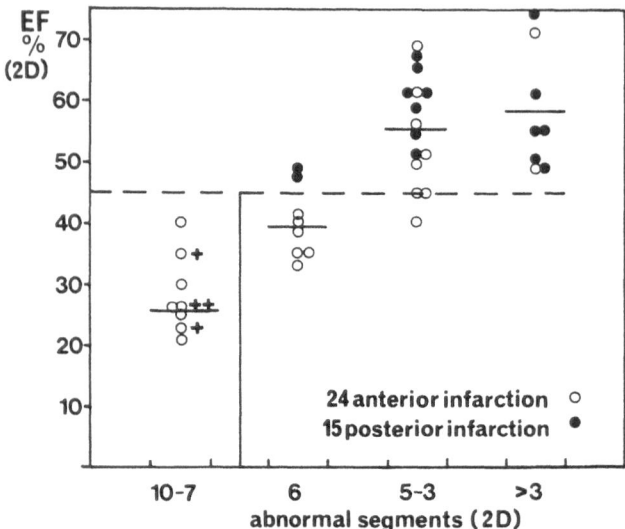

Figure 6. Regional and global left ventricular function in 39 patients with acute myocardial infarction. A high risk group with severe contraction abnormalities and reduced ejection fraction can be identified with echocardiography.

tained with invasive methods is impossible. However, quantitative evaluation with two-dimensional echocardiography is sensitive enough to give guidelines for management and prognosis of patients.

REFERENCES

1. Pombo JF, Troy BL, Russel RO: Left ventricular volumes and ejection fraction by echocardiography. Circulation 43:480, 1971.
2. Fortuin N, Hood WP, Sherman E, Craige E: Determination of left ventricular volumes by ultrasound. Circulation 44:575, 1971.
3. Murray JA, Johnston W, Reid JM: Echocardiographic determination of left ventricular dimensions, volumes and performance. Am J Cardiol 30:252, 1972.
4. Feigenbaum H, Wolfe SB, Popp RL: Correlation of ultrasound with angiography in measuring left ventricular diastolic volume. Am J Cardiol 23:111, 1969.
5. Feigenbaum H, Wolfe SB, Popp RL, Haine CL, Dodge HT: Ultrasound measurements of the left ventricle: a correlative study with angiocardiography. Arch int med 129:461, 1972.
6. Teichholz LE, Kreulen T, Herman MV, Gorlin R: Problems in echocardiographic volume determinations: echocardiographic – angiographic correlations in the presence or absence of asynergy. Amer J Cardiol 37:7, 1976.
7. Kronik G, Slany J, Mösslacher H: Comparative value of eight M-mode echocardiographic formulas for determining left ventricular stroke volume. Circulation 60:1308, 1979.
8. Linhart JW, Mintz GS, Segal BL, Kawai N, Kotler NW: Left ventricular volume measurement by echocardiography: Fact or fiction? Am J Cardiol 36:114, 1975.
9. Popp RL, Alderman EL, Brown OR, Harrison DC: Sources of error in calculation of left ventricular volumes by echocardiography. Amer J Cardiol 31:152, 1973.

10. Sweet RL, Moraski RE, Russel RO Jr: Relationship between echocardiography, cardiac output, and abnormally contracting segments in patients with ischemic heart disease. Circulation 52:634, 1975.

11. Massie BM, Schiller NB, Ratshin RA, Parmley WW: Mitral-septal separation: new echocardiographic index of left ventricular function. Amer J Cardiol 39:1008, 1977.

12. Child JS, Krivokapich J, Perloff JK: Effect of left ventricular size on mitral E point to ventricular septal separation in assessment of cardiac performance. Amer Heart J 101:797, 1981.

13. Erbel R, Schweizer P: Diagnostischer Stellenwert der Echokardiographie bei der koronaren Herzerkrankung – 1. M-mode Echokardiographie. Z Kardiol 69:391, 1980.

14. Kronik G, Mösslacher H, Korninger C, Ahmadi R: Echokardiographische Beurteilung der Myokardfunktion nach Vorderwandinfarkt. Ultraschall 1:182, 1980.

15. Mason SJ, Fortuin NJ: The use of echocardiography for quantitative evaluation of left ventricular function. Progr Cardiov Dis 21:119, 1978.

16. McDonald IG: Echocardiographic assessment of left ventricular function in aortic valve disease. Circulation 53:860, 1976.

17. Rosenblatt A, Clark R, Burgess J, Cohn K: Echocardiographic assessment of the level of cardiac compensation in valvular heart disease. Circulation 54:509, 1976.

18. Henry WL, Bonow RO, Ware JH, Kent KM, Redwood RD, McIntosh CL, Morrow AG, Epstein SE: Observations on the optimum time for operative intervention for aortic regurgitation – I. Evaluation of the results of aortic valve replacement in symptomatic patients. Circulation 6:471, 1980.

19. Henry WL, Bonow RO, Rosing DR, Epstein SE: Observations on the optimum time for operative intervention for aortic regurgitation – II. Serial echocardiographic evaluation of asymptomatic patients. Circulation 61:484, 1980.

20. Stein E, Hanrath P, Bleifeld W, Kupper W, Mathey D: Abnormales Kontraktions- und Füllverhalten des linken Ventrikels bei Tumorpatienten unter Adriamycin-Therapie. Dtsch med Wschr 103:1408, 1978.

21. Kerber RE, Marcus ML: Evaluation of regional myocardial function in ischemic heart disease by echocardiography. Progr Cardiov Diss 20:441, 1978.

22. Silverman NH, Schiller NB: Apex cardiography: A two-dimensional technique for evaluating congenital heart disease. Circulation 57:503, 1978.

23. Schiller NB, Acquatella H, Ports TA, Drew D, Goerke J, Ringertz H, Silverman NH, Brundage B, Botvinick EH, Boswell R, Carlsson E, Parmley WW: Left ventricular volume from paired biplane two-dimensional echocardiography. Circulation 60:547, 1979.

24. Eaton LW, Maughan WL, Shoukas AA, Weiss JL: Accurate volume determination in the isolated ejecting canine left ventricle by two-dimensional echocardiography. Circulation 60:320, 1979.

25. Helak JW, Reichek N: Quantitation of human left ventricular mass and volume by two-dimensional echocardiography: in vitro anatomic validation. Circulation 63:1398, 1981.

26. Bommer W, Chun T, Kwan OL, Neumann A, Mason DT: Biplane apex echocardiography versus biplane echocardiography in the assessment of left ventricular volume and function: validation by direct measurement. Amer J Cardiol 45:471, 1981.

27. Carr KW, Engler RL, Forsythe JR, Johnson AD, Gosink B: Measurement of left ventricular ejection fraction by mechanical cross-sectional echocardiography. Circulation 59:1196, 1979.

28. Folland ED, Parisi AF, Moynihan BS, Jones DR, Feldman CL, Jow DE: Assessment of left ventricular volumes and ejection fraction by real-time two-dimensional echocardiography. Circulation 60:760, 1979.

29. Schweizer P, Erbel R, Meyer J, Grenner H, Krebs W, Effert S: Möglichkeiten der Bestimmung von Volumina und Austreibungsfraktion der linken Kammer mit dem zwei-dimensionalen Ultraschallverfahren Herz 5:291, 1980.

30. Erbel R, Schweizer P, Krebs W, Pyhel N, Meyer J, Effert S: Monoplane und biplane zwei-

dimensionale echokardiographische Volumenbestimmung des linken Ventrikels. II. Untersuchungen bei koronarer Herzerkrankung. Z Kardiol 70:436, 1981.

31. Jenni R, Vieli A, Hess O, Anliker M, Krayenbuehl HP: Estimation of left ventricular volume from apical orthogonal two-dimensional echocardiograms. Europ Heart J 2:217, 1981.

32. Starling MR, Crawford MH, Sorensen SG, Levi B, Richards KL, O'Rourke RA: Comparative accuracy of apical biplane cross-sectional echocardiography and gated equilibrium radionuclide angiography for estimating left ventricular size and performance. Circulation 63:1075, 1981.

33. Touche T, Prasquier R, Merillon JP, Barthelemy M, Hanoun HC, Vervin P, Gourgon R: Mesure des volumes ventriculaires gauches par echographie bidimensionelle a partir d'une coupe apicale. Arch Mal Coeur 73:691, 1980.

34. Erbel R, Schweizer P, Bardos P, Meyer J, Minale S, Messmer BJ, Effert S: Long-term control of left ventricular function after aortocoronary bypass surgery by two-dimensional echocardiography. In: H Rijsterborgh ed.: Echocardiology, p. 25, Martinus Nijhoff, The Hague, 1981.

35. Erbel R Schweizer P, Lambertz H, Merx W, Meyer J, Effert S, Schoenmackers J: Prognostische Bedeutung der nicht invasiv bestimmten Ejektionsfraktion des linken Ventrikels bei reanimierten Patienten – Eine zwei-dimensionale echokardiographische Studie. Intensiv med 18:102, 1981.

36. Corya BC: Echocardiography in ischemic heart disease. Am J Med 63:10, 1977.

37. Feigenbaum H, Corya BC, Dillon JC, Weyman AE, Rasmussen S, Black MJ, Chary S: Role of echocardiography in patients with coronary artery disease. Am J Cardiol 37:775, 1976.

38. Kisslo JA, Robertson W, Gilbert BW, Ramm O, Behar VS: A comparison of real time two-dimensional echocardiography and cineangiography in detecting left ventricular asynergy. Circulation 55:134, 1977.

39. Grube E, Richter R, Otten H, Janson R, Lackner K, Simon H, Jörgens H: Darstellung linksventriulärer Kontraktionsanomalien mit Hilfe der zwei-dimensionalen Sektor-Echokardiographie. Dtsch med Wschr 104:703, 1979.

40. Kronik G, Hutterer B, Schmoliner B, Mösslacher H, Ehrenböck R: Sensitivität und Spezifität der zwei-dimensionalen Echokardiographie bei der Diagnose von Herzinfarktnarben. Klin Wsch 59:187, 1981.

41. Prasquier R, Barthelemy M, Vervin P, Hanoun CH, Touche T, Aumount MC, Gourgon R: Echocardiographie bidimensionelle dans l'infarctus aigu du myocarde. Arch Mal Coeur 72:1069, 1979.

42. Heger JJ, Weyman AE, Wann LS, Rogers EW, Dillon JC, Feigenbaum H: Cross-sectional echocardiographic analysis of the extent of left ventricular asynergy in acute myocardial infarction. Circulation 61:1113, 1980.

43. Parisi AF, Moynihan PF, Edward BS, Folland D, Feldman CL: Quantitative detection of regional left ventricular contraction abnormalities by two-dimensional echocardiography. II. Accuracy in coronary artery disease. Circulation 63:761, 1981.

44. Weiss JL, Bulkley BH, Hutchins GM, Mason SJ: Two-dimensional echocardiographic recognition of myocardial injury in man: comparison with postmortem studies. Circulation 63:401, 1981.

45. Visser CA, Lie KI, Kan G, Meltzer R, Durrer D: Detection and quantification of acute, isolated myocardial infarction by two-dimensional echocardiography. Am J Cardiol 47:1020, 1981.

46. Eaton LW, Weiss JL, Bulkley BH, Garrison JB, Weisfeldt ML: Regional cardiac dilatation after acute myocardial infarction. Recognition by two-dimensional echocardiography. New Engl J Med 300:57, 1979.

47. Schweizer P, Erbel R, Merx W, Krebs W, Erckelenz F v, Lambertz H, Effert S: Wall motion abnormalities in acute myocardial infarction. Correlation between two-dimensional echocardiography and cineangiography. Europ Heart J 2 (Abstr):108, 1981.

48. Barrett MJ, Charuzi Y, Corday E: Ventricular aneurysm: Cross-sectional echocardiographic approach. Am J Cardiol 46:1133, 1980.

17. COMPUTER-AIDED ANALYSIS OF M-MODE ECHOCARDIOGRAMS: PRACTICAL AND CLINICAL RELEVANCE OF RESULTS

P. HANRATH

M-mode echocardiography has rapidly become an established diagnostic technique in cardiology. Because of its non-invasive nature, high resolution and rapid sampling rate (1000 pulses/s) this method of examination has proven particularly valuable in determining cardiac chamber size, patterns of valve motion, structural abnormalities, velocity and amplitude of left ventricular wall motion. The growing interest in echocardiography since the early 50's has stimulated a desire to obtain increased diagnostic information from the heart using reflected ultrasound. This has led to the development of improved techniques of performing M-mode examinations and approaches to interpret the derived data. Computer-aided analysis of M-mode echocardiography was one of these approaches in order to improve the diagnostic information of M-mode echocardiograms in a quantitative manner.

TECHNIQUE OF COMPUTER ANALYSIS

A variety of techniques has been proposed for computer analysis of echocardiographic information [1 – 13]. Several groups tried to use the computer to identify certain echo structures with the aim of fully automatic analysis [1 – 3]. Other systems employed gated systems that look onto specific echoes. Both techniques have problems. Many echoes are close together and difficult to differentiate from each other. For example, the posterior left ventricular endocardium is frequently in proximity to structures of the mitral valve apparatus and the motion of the echoes can be very similar. In many cases it would be almost impossible to gate solely on the endocardium and eliminate the mitral valve echoes. It might also be extremely difficult to program a computer in order to distinguish endocardial echoes from those of chordal structures.

The most widely spread form of computer analysis of M-mode echocardiograms is therefore based on a semiautomatic system in which the physician or a technician identifies echoes and traces them using a digitizing pen [5 – 12]. Although this technique requires some time for manual tracing of the echoes, the mathematical calculations are performed by the computer.

This digitizing procedure is however very cumbersome if large series of heart

Roelandt, J. (ed.) The practice of M-mode and two-dimensional echocardiography
© *1983, Martinus Nijhoff Publishers. The Hague / Boston / London*
ISBN 978-94-009-6792-2.

beats have to be analysed. Therefore, van Zwieten and coworkers developed a system for automatic digitizing of pretraced M-mode echocardiograms with the aid of a TV camera [13].

LIMITATIONS OF COMPUTER ANALYSIS OF M-MODE ECHOCARDIOGRAMS IN CLINICAL PRACTICE

Apart from the calculation of wall thickness and cavity dimensions at endsystole and enddiastole, computer analysis of the M-mode echocardiogram has the advantage of permitting a continuous measurement of these parameters throughout the cardiac cycle with the simultaneous calculation of their instantaneous rate of change. The peak rates of wall and dimension changes measured from the echocardiogram during systole and diastole have shown a good correlation with similar measurements made from left ventricular cineangiograms [5]. However, comparing the peak rates of left ventricular dimension change with parameters derived from conventional echocardiographic measurements (mean circumferential fiber shortening velocity, LV fractional shortening), Kugler et al. [10] were not able to show that the computer-derived parameters were superior to the conventional indices in differentiating among patients with different kinds of heart disease and normal subjects.

A comparison of echocardiographic data analysed with a digitizing technique by different working groups so far yielded quite remarkable discrepancies, particularly in LV peak systolic shortening rate and peak filling rate. Kugler et al. [10] analysed peak shortening rates from 62 normal children that were significantly lower than those reported by Upton and Gibson [16] or by Sutton et al. [15] in a similar group of children.

The reason for these differences are related to technical as well as methodological problems. To perform a computer analysis, the XY coordinates of the echocardiographic boundaries of the septum and LV posterior wall have to be digitized. Hand-motion artefacts from the person digitizing the echo trace may result in distortion. Depending on whether or not and which technique of signal averaging or curve smoothing is used, the data may differ markedly. This becomes even more evident, if several consecutive cycles are analysed in one patient or if the same cycle is repeatedly analysed. Data concerning the reproducibility and the beat-to-beat variability of peak values derived by the digitizing technique vary between 3 and 20%, resp. 6 and 11% [6, 8, 10, 14, 15].

In literature several publications exist stressing the importance of the measurement of wall thickening or thinning velocities [16]. However, in my opinion, a note of caution is needed concerning these measurements. Although the boundaries of the left ventricular posterior wall are easily delineated in a good-quality echocardiogram, those of the right ventricular wall and the interventricular septum are more difficult. In a study performed by Sutton et al. the diastolic thickness of the right ventricular anterior wall averaged 2.4 ± 0.3 mm[17]. Although values of such small dimension can be obtained with a digitizing system, instantaneous velocities calculated from these values may not be reliable, and may represent tracing artefacts more than true wall excursion.

Other measurements done on a computer system are measurements of specific systolic or diastolic time intervals derived from the simultaneous recording of the M-mode echocardiogram along with the phono- or apexcardiogram [15, 17]. The combined recording of these parameters made it possible to determine isovolumic contraction and relaxation times which, however, have not proven to be very useful for decision-making in clinical practice.

Because of the ease with which computers can perform mathematical manipulations, it happened that some of the systems which are now on the market perform unjustified calculations based on one-dimensional measurements, e.g. the calculation of left ventricular volumes. If the physician is not familiar with the limitations of left ventricular volume calculation derived from M-mode recordings, he may not recognize the inaccuracies involved in such calculations and this may lead to serious patient mismanagement.

If further attention is paid to the fact that the M-mode technique only allows to analyse the basal portion of the left ventricle which in patients without coronary artery disease may not represent global left ventricular function, the value of computer-aided analysis of M-mode echocardiography in clinical practice and for clinical decision-making is doubtful.

In conclusion, computer analysis of M-mode echocardiograms allows calculations of echocardiographic parameters not easily made with conventional methods. There is no doubt that the introduction of this technique more than seven years ago revealed important basic information concerning left ventricular systolic and diastolic mechanical and myocardial performance in different kinds of heart disease. Yet this kind of analysis of M-mode data has not proven be a practical tool in clinical cardiology. This is most likely due to the fact that the computer-derived variables such as peak rates of cavity dimension change or wall thickness change have not proven superior to conventional echocardiographic indices in differentiating patients with different heart diseases. Therefore, this technique will at present primarily remain an important research tool and not a method for the routine evaluation of M-mode echocardiograms.

REFERENCES

1. Hirsch M, Sanders WJ, Popp RL: Computer processing of ultrasonic data from the cardiovascular system. Comput Biomed Res 6:336, 1973.
2. Kunahara M, Eicho S, Kitagawa H, Minato K, Mihi N: Computer analysis of ultrasonic echocardiogram. Proc. U.S.-Japan Seminar on image analysis, 1978.
3. Ledley FU, Wilson JB: Computer analysis of ultrasound cardiograms. Comput Biol Med 4:27, 1974.

4. Griffith JM, Henry WL: Video scanner-analog computer system for semiautomatic analysis of routine echocardiograms. Amer J Cardiol 32:961, 1973.
5. Gibson BG, Brown DJ: Measurement of peak rates of left ventricular wall movement in man. Comparison with angiography. Brit Heart J 37:677, 1974.
6. Brower RW, Dorp WG van, Vogel JA, Roelandt JR: Am improved method for the quantitative analysis of M-mode echocardiograms. Europ J Cardiol 3:171, 1975.
7. Saffer SL, Nixon JV, Mischelevich DJ: A simple method for computer-aided analysis of echocardiograms. Amer J Cardiol 38:34, 1976.
8. Decoodt PR, Mathey DG, Swan HJC: Automated analysis of the left ventricular dimension time curve from echocardiographic recordings. Computers and Biomed Res 9:549, 1976.
9. Krebs W, Hanrath P, Bleifeld W, Effert S: Rechnergestützte Auswertung von M-mode Echokardiogrammen. Herz/Kreislauf 9:519, 1977.
10. Kugler JD, Gutgesell HP, Nihill MR: Instantaneous rates of left ventricular wall motion in infants and children. Ped Cardiol 1:16, 1980/80.
11. Friedman MJ, Sahn JJ: Computer-assisted analysis of M-mode echocardiogram: Is it a goldmine? Ped Cardiol 1:47, 1979/80.
12. Menke JA, Behren PA von, Baolum M, Bada HS, Khama NN: The use of a microcomputer in the evaluation of echocardiograms. Catheterization and Cardiovascular Diagnosis 6:649, 1980.
13. Zwieten G, Bastiaans OL von, Honhoop J, Vogel JA: Video tracings of M-mode echocardiograms in Ch. Lancée (ed.) Echocardiology, Martinus Nijhoff Publishers, The Hague, 469, 1979.
14. Decoodt PR, Mathey DG, Swan HJC: Assessment of left ventricular filling by echocardiography in normal subjects and subjects with coronary artery disease and with asymmetric septal hypertrophy. Acta Cardiol 24, II, 1979.
15. Hanrath P, Mathey DG, Kremer P, Sonntag F, Bleifeld W: Effect of Verapamil on left ventricular isovolumic relaxation time and regional left ventricular filling in hypertrophic cardiomyopathy. Amer J Cardiol 45:1258, 1980.
16. Upton MT, Gibson DG: The study of left ventricular function from digitized echocardiograms. Progr Cardiovasc Dis 20:359, 1978.
17. Sutton StJ, Hagler DJ, Tajik AJ, Giuliani ER, Seward IB, Ritter DG, Ritman EL: Cardiac function in the normal newborn: Additional information by computer analysis of the M-mode echocardiograms. Circul 57:1198, 1978.

18. A CRITICAL LOOK AT QUANTITATION OF THE LEFT VENTRICLE FROM M-MODE AND TWO-DIMENSIONAL ECHOCARDIOGRAPHY

R. JENNI, O.M. HESS, J.D. CARROLL, AND H.P. KRAYENBUEHL

The clinical application of ultrasound to the examination of the heart has presently found a wide application: the one- and two-dimensional echocardiography are diagnostic tools of utmost importance for diagnosis of cardiac disease and assessment of left ventricular function. Left ventricular internal diameter, left ventricular shortening of the minor axis, left ventricular volume and systolic ejection fraction are echocardiographic parameters for assessing left ventricular function. There have been several papers [1 – 3] comparing these parameters to angiocardiography for validation of the echocardiographic method in determining left ventricular function. There are several problems in measuring left ventricular function by one- or two-dimensional echocardiography such as underestimation of the true internal diameter, rotational movements of the heart or geometric factors for evaluation of left ventricular volume and ejection fraction. The purpose of the present study is to evaluate the accuracy of one- and two-dimensional echocardiography for quantitative assessment of left ventricular size and function, and to discuss probable factors causing misinterpretation or under- or overestimation of left ventricular myocardial function.

1. ONE-DIMENSIONAL ECHOCARDIOGRAPHY

The one-dimensional echocardiography is still an important method for assessing left ventricular myocardial function because spatial resolution and sampling rates are higher than that of two-dimensional echocardiography allowing accurate determination of left ventricular internal diameter and wall thickness of the interventricular septum and posterior wall. Computerized evaluation of systolic shortening and diastolic filling parameters [4, 5] have been used to determine time-dependent changes in left ventricular function.

Standard measurements: Routinely, the left ventricular internal diameter (D) is obtained from the standard interspace, where the head of the ultrasonic transducer is in a right angle to the chest wall and the interventricular septum and the posterior wall are recorded simultaneously just below the mitral valve apparatus. The following standard parameters are determined in our laboratory:

Roelandt, J. (ed.) The practice of M-mode and two-dimensional echocardiography
© *1983, Martinus Nijhoff Publishers. The Hague / Boston / London*
ISBN 978-94-009-6792-2.

Left ventricular end-diastolic (D_D) and end-systolic (D_S) internal diameter, systolic shortening of the internal diameter (%Sh) and the mean circumferential fiber shortening velocity (V_{CF}). In Table 1 the normal values for D_D, %Sh and V_{CF} are given.

Problems in echocardiographic dimension measurements

1. Resolution problems
Poor lateral resolution, dropout of echoes and overlapping of echoes might affect the quality of the evaluated echocardiogram, and might be, therefore, a major problem to determine the "true" endocardial surface of the posterior left ventricular wall [9]. These technical problems might be important for determination of left ventricular function using one-dimensional echocardiography, and this might be a source of misinterpretation of "true" left ventricular internal diameter.

2. Ventricular geometry
Left ventricular geometry might become very important for assessing the longest or "true" left ventricular internal diameter (Figure 1). The more spherical the left ventricle becomes, the more the error in assessing left ventricular size from only the midchamber diameter increases, whereas this error is relatively small in an elliptical left ventricle. This shape change of the left ventricle might become important from end-diastole to end-systole because it is well known that the long/short axis ratio is much higher during systole than diastole.

3. Rotational movements of the heart
The rotation of the heart from diastole to systole might cause misinterpretation of the internal diameter because the ultrasonic beam is not directed at the same site during diastole and systole (Figure 2). This means that the calculated systolic shortening of the left ventricular internal diameter is based on two different ventricular sites. Furthermore McDonald [10] showed that the heart moves anterior-

Table 1. Normal values (given are mean values and range) for left ventricular end-diastolic internal diameter (D_D), systolic shortening of the internal diameter (Sh) and mean circumferential fiber shortening velocity (V_{CF}).

	D_D (cm)	Sh (%)	V_{CF} (circ/sec)
Mc Donald et al. [6]	4.4(3.8 − 5.0)	35.5(30 − 44)	1.22(0.91 − 1.50)
Feigenbaum [7]	4.7(3.5 − 5.7)	− −	1.30(1.01 − 1.94)
Felner and Schlant [8]	5.0(4.2 − 6.0)	32.9(28 − 37)	1.26(0.95 − 1.60)
Our data*	5.1(4.4 − 6.5)	36.8(29 − 46)	1.25(0.98 − 1.62)

* 35 patients (15 women and 20 men) with a mean age of 33 years and an average heart rate of 71 beats/min.

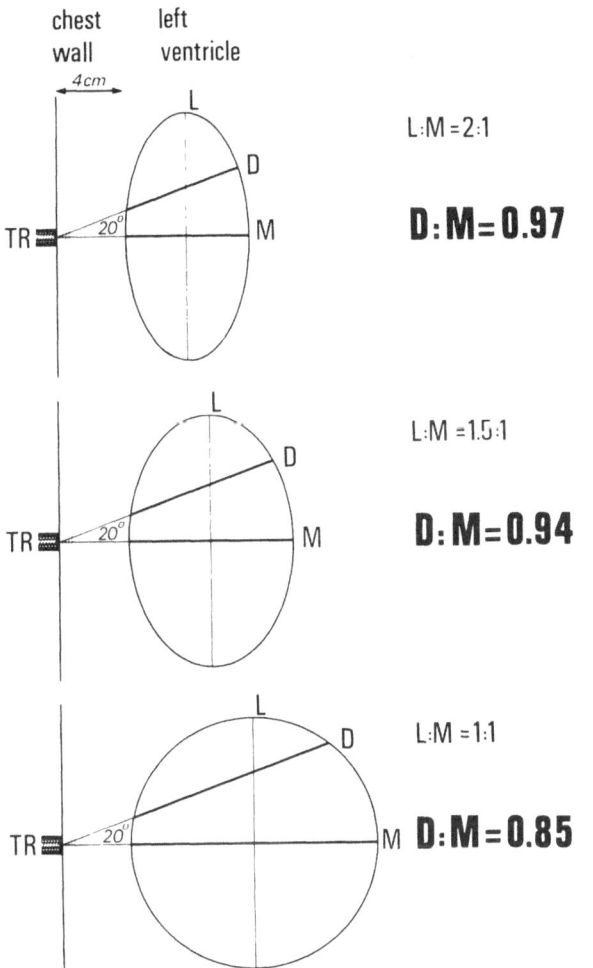

Figure 1. Importance of the left ventricular geometry on the assessment of the true internal diameter. This figure illustrates the possible error in not measuring the longest internal transverse diameter by echocardiography. TR : Transducer, L : Left ventricular long axis, M : Left ventricular short axis, D : Echocardiographic ventricular diameter (Reproduced from 12).

ly during systolic contraction. This might be the reason why the anterior movements of the posterior wall are usually more pronounced than the posterior movements of the interventricular septum.

4. Validation of the method

Simultaneous measurements of the left ventricular internal transverse diameter by one-dimensional echocardiography and angiocardiography in the dog showed a reasonable good correlation between the echocardiographic and angiocardiographic shortening of the left ventricular internal diameter, whereas the ab-

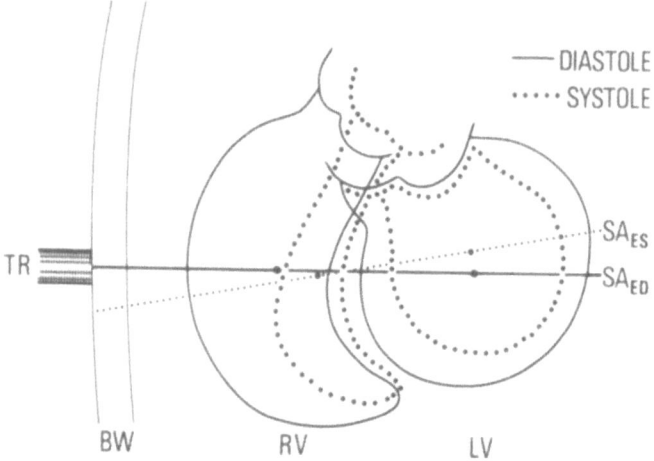

Figure 2. Importance of the rotational movements of the heart for the correct assessment of left ventricular internal diameter. This figure illustrates that the echocardiographic technique is not measuring at the same site during diastole and systole. TR : Transducer, BW : Chest wall, RV : Right ventricle, LV : Left ventricle, SA_{ed} : End-diastolic axis of the center of gravity of the RV and LV, SA_{es} : End-systolic axis of the center of gravity of the RV and LV (Reproduced from 12).

solute values for the internal diameter showed significant variations between the two methods [11]. Comparisons of the echo- and angiocardiographic internal diameter and systolic shortening of the internal diameter in patients showed reasonable good correlations between both methods [1, 2].

2. TWO-DIMENSIONAL ECHOCARDIOGRAPHY

In contrast to the M-mode echocardiography the development of two-dimensional (2-D) echocardiography has permitted tomographic visualization of the entire left ventricle in different views. The American Society of Echocardiography [13] has recently published recommendations about a uniform nomenclature and a standardization of the various cross-sectional images.

Technique

2-D ultrasonic cardiac images are usually obtained by mechanical or electronic steering of one or more transducer crystals back and forth through an arc or sector.

For M-mode echocardiography the ultrasound instrument is pulsed at a rate of 1000 pulses per second. The 2-D echocardiography uses the same B-mode information as the one-dimensional echo, but the sound beam is automatically moved through the body to create an imaging plane. This 2-D echocardiographic images are essentially tomographic sections of the heart. Most 2-D echocardiographic instruments provide 30 frames per second, that means that very rapidly moving structures will be better recognized by M-mode because of its higher sampling rate. The phased array 2-D echo can simultaneously display the 2-D image and a M-mode echocardiogram at a certain area of the 2-D image. The sampling rate of this single line is higher than the frame rate of the whole image. With mechanical sector scanners the transducer must be stopped to create a M-mode record and it is not possible to produce simultaneously a M-mode and a 2-D image.

For quantitative evaluation the various 2-D echocardiographic views are usually recorded on video tape for playback, slow motion and stop action. Stop action and single-frame images suffer from image degradation compared to dynamic motion display. In stop action and single-frame images the endocardial borders are often not visualized properly and it is difficult to draw the left ventricular boundaries. If portions of the endocardium cannot be visualized in the stopped frame, slow motion or frame by frame analysis is helpful in defining the internal left ventricular boundaries.

Left ventricular volumes

Assessment of left ventricular function can be done by 2-D echocardiograms. Recent attempts have been made to determine the left ventricular volume and ejection fraction from various tomographic 2-D images [14 – 19]. Whereas the echocardiographic ejection fraction compared favourably with that estimated from mono [16] and biplane [14, 15, 17, 18] cine-angiograms, the left ventricular volumes were smaller than those obtained from cine-angiography.

Standard determination of left ventricular volume by cine-angiography is based of the area-length method [20] or Simpson's rule [21]. The area-length method uses the left ventricular angiographic area of the right and left anterior oblique projection and the longest left ventricular axis in either one of the two projections. The Simpson's rule is based on a multiple slices theory. Comparison of these calculated angiographic volumes with casts [22] showed reasonable good correlations between both techniques. Therefore, angiography was used as reference method for validation of echocardiographic volume determination.

However, the comparison of the angio- and echocardiographic data is limited by the fact that the raw data, namely the echocardiographic cross-sectional images and the angiographic silhouettes, generally do not provide the same information. In contrast to the echo images, which yield information from a given plane and not more, the angiographic silhouette represents the maximal outer borders of the left ventricle perpendicular to the X-ray beam. It is obvious that the areas of biplane echocardiographic ellipsoids tend to be smaller than the corresponding angiographic silhouettes and hence lead to an underestimation of the true left ventricular volume.

Table 2. Left ventricular volumetry by 2-D-echocardiography

Author	Views	Method	EDV r	Δ%	ESV Δ%	r	EF r	Δ%	Angio
1. Carr [14]	parasternal long axis, parasternal short axis, apical two-ch, apical 4-ch	AL	0.93	(−30%)			0.93	(−2%)	14xbiplane 8xRAO
2. Schiller [15]	apical 2-ch, parasternal short axis	modified Simpson	0.80	(−30%)	(−33%)	0.90	0.87	(+10%)	biplane
3. Folland [16]	apical 4-ch, 2 x parasternal short axis	modified Simpson	0.84				0.78		monoplane 30° RAO
4. Silverman [17]	apical 4-ch, apical long axis	AL	0.94	(−2%)	(+25%)	0.91			biplane
5. Jenni [18]	apical 4-ch, RAO equivalent	AL	0.98	(−8%)	(−2%)	0.97	0.87	(−3%)	biplane
6. Edelman [19]	apical 4-ch, apical 2-ch	modified Simpson	0.90	(−35%)			0.91	(+1.1%)	biplane

Abbreviations: AL : Area-length, EDV : end-diastolic volume, ESV : end-systolic volume, EF : ejection fraction, RAO : right anterior oblique projection, ch : chamber, r : correlation coefficient, Δ% : % difference of the mean value between angio- and echocardiography.

Left ventricular end-diastolic and end-systolic volumes (Table 2) were significantly underestimated in all studies. The correlation coefficient are between r = 0.80 and 0.98 for end-diastolic volume and 0.78 − 0.97 for end-systolic volumes. The underestimation for the mean value between angio and echocardiography for end-diastolic volumes varies between − 30% and − 2% and for end-systolic volumes between − 33% and + 25%. It is interesting that in both studies with two apical orthogonal views, i.e. the classical four chamber view and the "RAO-equivalent" view [18] or the apical long axis view [17], the underestimation of left ventricular volume was minimized, because only in the "RAO-equivalent" and apical long axis view the left ventricular outflow tract was included.

Ejection fraction

Left ventricular ejection fraction (Table 2) calculated from different 2-D echocardiographic views, correlated well with those from cine-angiograms (r = 0.78 − 0.93) including patients with localized wall motion abnormalities.

Left ventricular axis measurements

Table 3 shows the comparison between the angiographic (RAO long and short axis and LAO short axis) and the echocardiographic axes ("RAO equivalent" long and short axis, four chamber view short axis from our own study [18]). In the "RAO equivalent" view, the long axis is underestimated by 7 at end-diastole and 14% at end-systole (p < 0.001). This underestimation is due to the transducer not being placed at the true apex of the heart and, therefore, causing a foreshortening of the left ventricle [23]. Also the comparison of the area of the "RAO-equivalent" view to the area of the angio RAO-projection yielded a significant underestimation at end-diastole. At end-systole there was no significant difference between the two areas.

Conclusions

We conclude that ejection fraction can be accurately estimated using various 2-D echocardiographic views. Left ventricular volumes were underestimated with this noninvasive procedure, but if two orthogonal apical views, in which the left ventricular outflow tract is included, were used, suitable raw data for noninvasive left volumetry are available.

Two-dimensional echocardiography can be performed serially without risk for the patients, this analysis has potential utility in longterm studies of left ventricular function.

Table 3. Comparison between echocardiographic and angiographic axes and areas (mean values ± 1 s.d. of 42 patients)

Angiography								Echocardiography							
RAO						LAO		'RAO equivalent' view						Four chamber view	
Long axis (cm)		Short axis (cm)		Area (cm²)		Short axis (cm)		Long axis (cm)		Short axis (cm)		Area (cm²)		Short axis (cm)	
ED	ES	ED	ES	ED	ES	ED	ES	ED	ES	ED	ES	ED	ES	ED	ES
10.8	9.2	6.2	4.1	54.9[b]	31.4†	6.1†	4.4†	10.0	7.9	6.0	4.4	51.2[b]	30.4†	5.9†	4.4†
±1.3[a]	±1.5[a]	±1.2[c]	±1.3[b]	±16.4	±16.9	±1.2	±1.1	±1.7[a]	±1.6[a]	±1.3[c]	±1.3[b]	±18.6	±13.3	±1.1	±1.2

Abbreviations: ED : end-diastolic axis, ES : end-systolic axis, RAO : right anterior oblique, LAO : left anterior oblique, †NS : not significant.
[a] $P < 0.001$.
[b] $P < 0.005$.
[c] $P < 0.05$.

256

REFERENCES

1. Cooper RH, O'Rourke RA, Karliner JS, Peterson KL, Leopold GR: Comparison of ultrasound and cineangiographic measurements of the mean rate of circumferential fiber shortening in man. Circulation 46:914, 1972.
2. Fortuin NJ, Hood WP Jr, Craige E: Evaluation of left ventricular function by echocardiography. Circulation 46:26, 1972.
3. Gibson DG, Brown DJ: Measurement of peak rates of left ventricular wall movement in man. Comparison of echocardiography with angiography. Brit Heart J 37:677, 1975.
4. Gibson DG, Brown DJ: Measurements of instantaneous left ventricular dimension and filling rate in man, using echocardiography. Brit Heart J 35:1141, 1973.
5. Hanrath P, Mathey DG, Kremer P, Sonntag F, Bleifeld W: Effect of verapamil on left ventricular isovolumic relaxation time and regional left ventricular filling in hypertrophic cardiomyopathy. Am J Cardiol 45:1258, 1980.
6. McDonald IG, Feigenbaum H, Chang S: Analysis of left ventricular wall motion by reflected ultrasound. Circulation 46:14, 1972.
7. Feigenbaum H: Echocardiography, 2. Aufl. Lea & Febiger, Philadelphia, 1976.
8. Felner JM, Schlant RC: Echocardiography. A teaching atlas. Grune & Stratton, New York, 1976.
9. Roelandt J, Dorp WG van, Bom N, Laird JD, Hugenholtz PG: Resolution problems in echocardiology: a source of interpretation errors. Am J Cardiol 37:256, 1976.
10. McDonald IG: The shape and movements of the human left ventricle during systole. Am J Cardiol 26:221, 1970.
11. Brunner HH, Turina M, Turina J, Krayenbühl HP: Simultane Bestimmung der linksventrikulären Dimensionen beim Hund mittels Kineangiokardiographie und Echokardiographie. Schweiz Med Wschr 106:1553, 1976.
12. Krayenbühl HP, Turina J, Hess O, Ettori F: Die Echokardiographie in der Beurteilung der Ventrikelfunktion. Schweiz Med Wschr 107:1317, 1977.
13. Henry WL, De Maria A, Gramiak R et al: Report of the American Society of Echocardiography Committee on nomenclature and standards in two-dimensional echocardiography. Circulation 62:212, 1980.
14. Carr KW, Engler RL, Forsythe JR, Johnson AD, Gosink B: Measurement of left ventricular ejection fraction by mechanical cross-sectional echocardiography. Circulation 59:1196, 1979.
15. Schiller NB, Acquatella H, Ports TA et al: Left ventricular volume from paired biplane two-dimensional echocardiography. Circulation 60:547, 1979.
16. Folland ED, Parisi AF, Moynihan PF, Jones DR, Feldman CL, Tow DE: Assessment of left ventricular ejection fraction and volumes by real-time, two-dimensional echocardiography. A comparison of cine-angiographic and radionuclide techniques. Circulation 60:760, 1979.
17. Silverman NH, Ports TA, Snider AR et al: Determination of left ventricular volume in children: echocardiographic and angiographic comparisons. Circulation 62:547, 1980.
18. Jenni R, Vieli A, Hess O, Anliker M, Krayenbühl HP: Estimation of left ventricular volume from apical orthogonal 2-D echocardiograms. Europ Heart J 2:217, 1981.
19. Edelman SK, Rowe DW, Pechacek LW, Garcia E: Cardiovascular Diseases. Bulletin of the Texas Heart Institute 8:344, 1981.
20. Dodge HT, Sandler H, Baxley WA, Hawley RR: Usefulness and limitations of radiographic methods for determining left ventricular volume. Am J Cardiol 18:10, 1966.
21. Chapman GB, Bakter O, Reynolds J, Bonte FJ: Use of biplane cinefluorography for measurements of ventricular volume. Circulation 18:1105, 1958.
22. Bentivolglio LG, Griffith LD, Cuesta AJ, Geczy M, Radiographic evaluation of formulas for left ventricular volume using canine casts. J Appl Physiol 33:365, 1972.
23. Erbel R, Schweizer P, Meyer J, Grenner H, Krebs W, Effert S: Left ventricular volume and ejection fraction determination by cross-sectional echocardiography in patients with coronary artery disease: A prospective study. Clin Cardiol 3:377, 1980.

VI. APPLICATION OF M-MODE AND TWO-DIMENSIONAL ECHOCARDIOGRAPHY IN CORONARY ARTERY DISEASE

Two-dimensional echocardiography has become an useful adjunct in the clinical management of patients with coronary artery disease although it is of little value for the assessment of patients with uncomplicated obstructive coronary artery disease. It is a sensitive technique, however, for the early detection and localization of myocardial infarction as is outlined in chapter 19. A concept of regional analysis and a standardized nomenclature is presented which is of considerable help for the analysis of patients with coronary artery disease where regional wall motion abnormalities are common. Echocardiography is extremely useful method for the detection of complications of coronary artery disease. In many instances it provides a definitive diagnosis as well as comprehensive picture of global left ventricular function as is presented in chapter 20. The finding of very poor left ventricular function with a two-dimensional echocardiogram could obviate catheterization risks and costs in these patients. The unique capabilities of the echocardiographic method for serial follow-up studies and testing the effects of interventions in patients with coronary artery disease are nicely illustrated by the data presented in chapter 25.

Roelandt, J. (ed.) The practice of M-mode and two-dimensional echocardiography
© *1983, Martinus Nijhoff Publishers. The Hague / Boston / London*
ISBN 978-94-009-6792-2.

19. THE VALUE OF ECHOCARDIOGRAPHY IN THE CORONARY CARE UNIT: LEFT VENTRICULAR WALL MOTION STUDIES IN THE ASSESSMENT OF THE PATIENT WITH ACUTE MYOCARDIAL INFARCTION

R. PRASQUIER AND T. TOUCHE

Several reports [1, 2] have shown the potential value of echocardiography during acute myocardial infarction (MI), but it is only since the advent of two-dimensional (2-D) recordings that this technique has become an important clinical adjunct for patients in the coronary care unit. With the beam directed by the 2-D picture, M-mode recordings should always be simultaneously performed, because of better resolution and temporal discrimination; this report will however focus upon 2-D echocardiography in acute MI, emphasizing both methodological requirements and clinical utility.

I. METHODS

1. Echocardiographic examination

The echocardiographer should attempt to record as many different ventricular sections as possible and relate all these sections one to another in order to build a three dimensional mental image of the left ventricle. Reports are more reliable when written immediately after the examination. For reproducibility and comparison purposes, it is necessary to single out in each view, the particular section which covers the largest ventricular area.

Parasternal short axis sections are the most difficult to adequately visualize, but prolonged attempts are rewarding. Misinterpretations of the left atrial wall at systole as an akinetic ventricular posterior wall and false anterior distensions on oblique sections may be read with careless technique. Short axis sections are extremely important, because they show the entire ventricular circumference and lend themselves more easily to quantitative analysis. Besides, many small posterior infarctions (Figure 1) are seen only in these views.

The apical views are frequently the easiest to record in coronary patients. The 4 cavities views allow for the best description of septal and lateral involvement; different degrees of transducer rotation between the 4 cavities and the 2 cavities views with the corresponding meridian sections offer an almost entire overview of left ventricular involvement. The apex is a strategic portion, always involved in anterior infarctions; since it lies under the point of maximal impulse, it should

Roelandt, J. (ed.) The practice of M-mode and two-dimensional echocardiography
© *1983, Martinus Nijhoff Publishers. The Hague / Boston / London*
ISBN 978-94-009-6792-2.

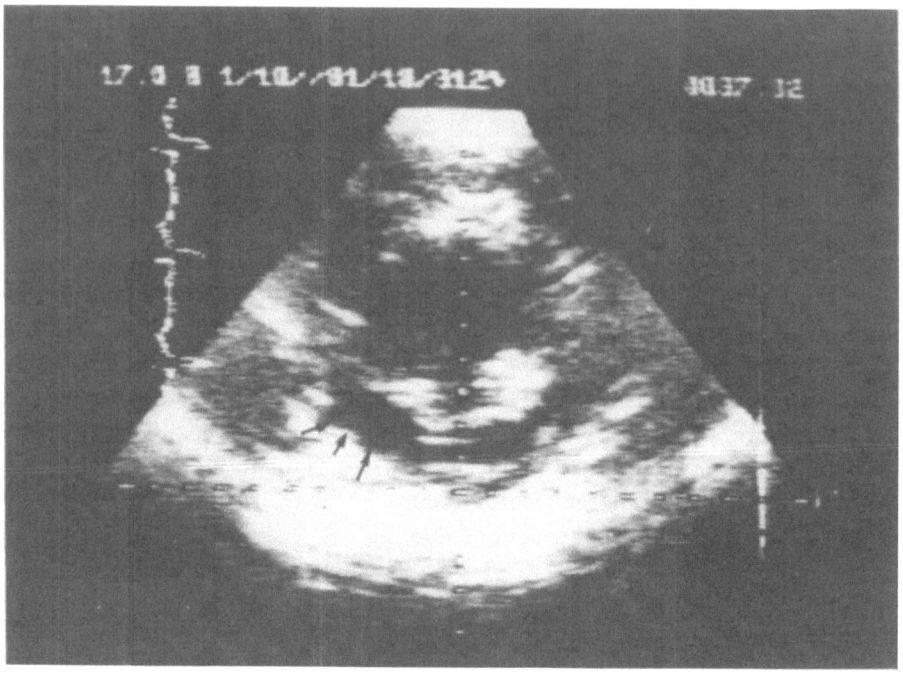

Figure 1. Short axis section of a small posterior MI. The arrows point towards the inferobasal akinetic segment.

be specifically looked for through slightly inferior positioning and lateral transducer angulation.

Subcostal views are most necessary in patients with emphysema, or in patients with posterior infarction in order to assess right ventricular wall motion abnormalities and/or tricuspid regurgitation.

2. Echocardiographic abnormalities during myocardial infarction

2.1. Changes in echo structure

Dense echoes on a thinned myocardial wall [3] are specific but not sensitive indices of infarcted tissue. Echographic structure identification of myocardial injury [4] might become a useful clinical tool in the future.

2.2. Changes in wall motion

These include different assessment criteria, loosely lumped together under the names of hypo, a- and dyskinesis.

2.2.1. Wall motion relative to an intracavitary reference point or axis. This commonly used index requires adequate endocardial visualization. Computer aided endocardial outline contouring aids in the definition of a fixed reference system and permits easier measurements of chordal shortening or regional area shrinkage [5]. In our hands poor interobserver reproducibility, mainly due to inadequate still frame endocardial visualization did not yield acceptable results for individual assessment. This problem was recently thoroughly reviewed [6].

Qualitative analysis may lead to a wall motion index, normal segments being for instance scored 0, hypokinetic 1, akinetic 2, dyskinetic 3 [7]. Hypokinesis should be assessed with great caution because of 1. poor reproducibility, 2. wide range of normal wall motion and 3. unsettled signification, since no difference in contraction pattern was found on quantitative echographic studies conducted in normal and coronary patients without prior MI [8].

2.2.2. Wall thickening. Wall thickening is a more specific index of myocardial ischemia or infarction than wall motion. M-mode systolic myocardial thinning was described as a characteristic feature of acute MI [9]. 2-D measurements of systolic thickening require perfect quality endocardial and epicardial outlines and are prone to even greater relative errors than endocardial displacement measurements. Visual assessment of absence of thickening is however the best clue to the presence of infarction. It is the only useful index, when conduction abnormalities (complete LBBB) are associated to the MI.

2.2.3. Relative displacement of adjacent wall segments. The simplest way of assessing wall motion is to see the differences in motion between a normal and an abnormal adjacent segment, well defined breakpoint being often visible in systole. Distinction should be made in dyskinetic segments between passive bulging because of preserved adjacent segment motion and active systolic expansion.

A frequent geometrical distortion is the lack of intracavitary narrowing at the papillary level, a clue to wall expansion. Aneurysm is defined by the persistance of an internal breakpoint during diastole.

Recognition of these abnormal displacements is an index of rather gross dysynergy: it is most helpful in apical views where endocardial outlines are inadequate because of tangential beam orientation.

3. Assessment of anatomical extent

There is a wide variability in the number, the names, the anatomical description of the involved segments. For instance, the segment between the two papillary muscles is called inferior, posterior or lateral. Other ambiguities include the amount of involvement required to call a segment abnormal, the different sizes of the segments, and the difficulties to relate to anatomical contours when internal geometry is distorted.

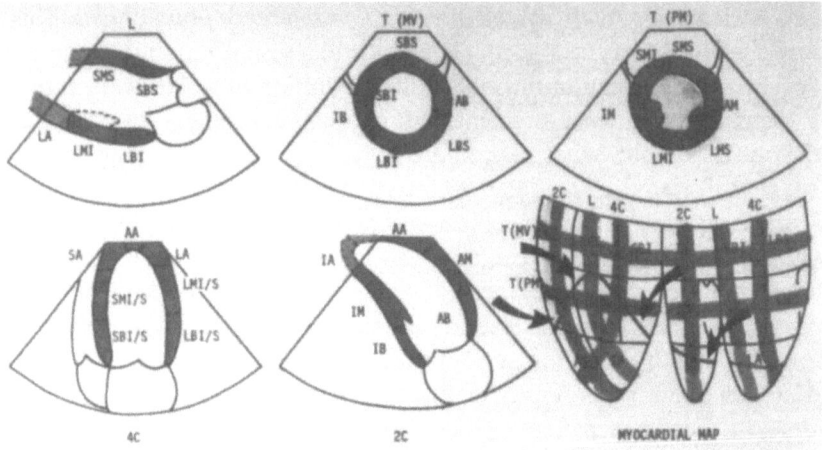

Figure 2. Display of segmental abnormalities. Wall motion abnormalities are traced on the corresponding lines on the myocardial map. (2C apical 2 cavities, 4C apical 4 cavities, L long axis, TMV short axis at mitral level, TPM short axis at papillary level). Limits of the infarcted area are then joined together (arrows) yielding a visual display of an anterior infarction (S : septum, A : anterior, L : lateral, I : inferior, A : apical, M : mid ventricular, B : basal, S : superior, I : inferior).

This is why we favour a method based upon anatomical internal landmarks. Our present segmental analysis (Figure 2) is based upon the division of the left ventricle into 4 walls (anterior, lateral, inferior and septal) and 3 levels: apical, midventricular at papillary level, and basal, with further subdivision in two halves (superior and inferior) of the mid ventricular and basal portions of the septum and lateral wall. This leads to 16 segments of internal similar size. The boundaries of abnormal motion are then precisely redrawn on the different views, and these drawings are retraced on a pre set myocardial map, allowing for a three-dimensional visual display of asynergy.

Similar use of anatomical descriptors has been recently proposed by Tajik and col [10]. This approach has in our experience improved anatomical accuracy, observer reproducibility and use by the clinician of the echographic data.

II. RESULTS

1. Diagnostic value of wall motion studies

1.1. Sensitivity

We performed two similar prospective blind studies, each one with a different phased array equipment, on a total number of 95 patients with acute MI and no prior infarction, consecutively admitted to the coronary care unit [11]. Echocarcardiograms were performed from the first to the fourth day after the acute event, and were read as asynergic only if akinesis or dyskinesis existed. Among 44 patients with anterior transmural MI, 40 had adequate complete recordings of the anterior portions of the left ventricle (91%): all of them (40/40) had some degree of segmental asynergy. Among 44 patients with posterior transmural MI, 35 had adequate complete recordings of the posterior portions of the left ventricle (79%): 34/35 (97%) had some degree of posterior asynergy. Among 7 patients with subendocardial infarctions, all of whom had adequate recordings, only 5 (71%) had segmental asynergy.

Similar results have been obtained by other investigators [7, 12]. A normal recording of an adequate quality (i.e. more than 50% visualization of segmental endocardium) virtually rules out transmural infarction; adequate recordings of posterior wall were more difficult to achieve although our success rate has presently somewhat improved (85%).

Subendocardial infarction may exist with an apparently normal echocardiogram; recent canine heart studies have similarly demonstrated that abrupt decrease in systolic thickening is seen only when the infarction involves at least 20% of transmural thickness [13].

1.2. Specificity

Specificity of segmental asynergy is extremely high for the diagnosis of MI. Although acute ischemic events may lead to transitory akinesis [14, 15], this is not found in patients with chronic ischemic heart disease without infarction [8]. Occasional asynergic areas may be observed in patients without apparent coronary disease (often with aortic regurgitation) but much more frequently when trying to overread segments with inadequately recorded endocardial outlines.

1.3. Early diagnosis

The value of 2-D echocardiography is enhanced by its ability to diagnose with a similar accuracy a myocardial infarction within the first hours of the event [16] at a time when enzyme and EKG changes are still non diagnostic. This would be particularly helpful if early aggressive management (thrombolysis) were contemplated.

Radionuclide angiography is significantly less sensitive than 2-D echocardiography for the diagnosis of acute posterior MI, and comparable for anterior myocardial infarction [17].

2. Topographical extension of the infarction

2.1. Anatomy of the infarction

The apicoseptal segment was always involved in anterior infarctions, and the inferobasal segment in posterior infarctions. In a retrospective study of 100 old

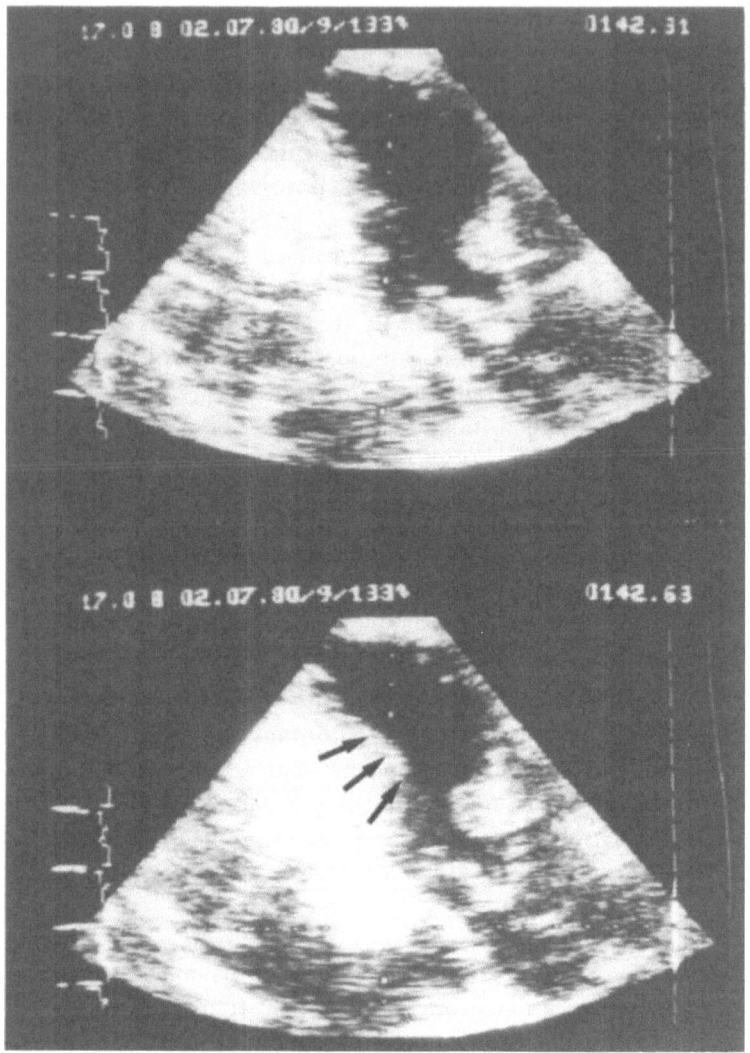

Figure 3. Patient in pulmonary edema and extensive Q waves (2, 3, F, V_{1-5}). Good residual motion of inferior wall (arrows) and in other sections of basal septum and lateral wall. Uneventful clinical improvement.

MI's, we could find only 3 lateral infarctions without asynergy of either of these 2 segments. Different degrees of extension of asynergy along myocardial walls around these two "key-segments" can be seen, but no clear-cut correlation with EKG topography could be found.

2.2. Prognostic value

2.2.1. Extent of infarction.

There is some relation between the extent of 2-D echographic asynergy and the outcome of the infarction. This was described through wall motion scores [7, 17] or ejection fraction measurements.

Limited asynergy, in the absence of mechanical complication, always means favorable outcome for the acute stage; it is most useful in patients with small infarctions as a confirmatory tool, and in Killip class II patients [18] (Figure 3).

The anatomical studies of Weiss and col [19] showed a good correlation between wall motion abnormalities and post mortem extent of infarcted myocardium, with some degree of echographic overestimation. This could be due to vicinity tethering effect on normal myocardium or to adjacent small foci of necrosis.

2.2.2. Serial changes

Difficulties in interpretation of serial studies have already been emphasized. In our experience, contrarily to some other studies [17], a definite improvement in the extent of asynergy is an unusual finding beyond the first day of infarction, most patients having similar serial wall motion studies during the acute phase.

Expansion of the infarcted area [20] (Figure 4) was found in 15% of our anterior infarction patients. It may exist as early as the first day in patients in cardiogenic shock, but peaks usually at the end of the first week. It carries a more severe but not uniformly fatal prognosis.

III. ASSOCIATED FINDINGS

1. RV infarction

RV infarction occurs only in posterior MI with involvement of the lower septum. Although frequently mentioned, it still remains to be thoroughly echographically described. We found RV enlargement or segmental asynergy in a small minority (3/44: 7%) of posterior MI's, all of whom had suggestive clinical features. Systematic use of subcostal views might increase the sensitivity of the method.

RV infarction can readily be echographically recognized from compressive pericarditis, which may occur during MI with a similar clinical and hemodynamic picture.

2. Thrombi

Apical thrombi can be detected during acute, and usually extensive myocardial infarctions, although embolic episodes are extremely unusual. Progressive frequent disappearance was found in a recent study [21].

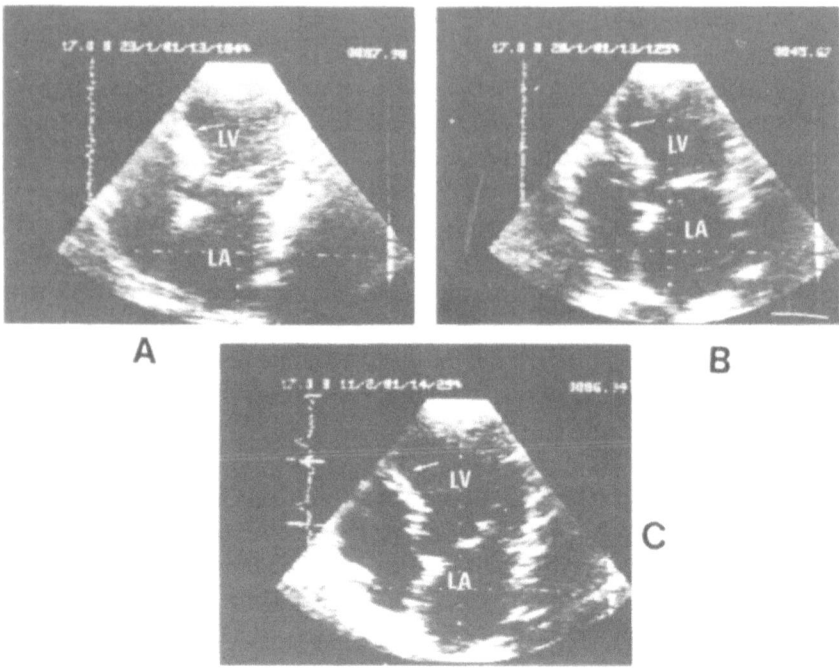

Figure 4. (upper panel) – Anterior MI with progressive expansion (arrows) A, B, C : 3rd, 8th, 21st day after MI.

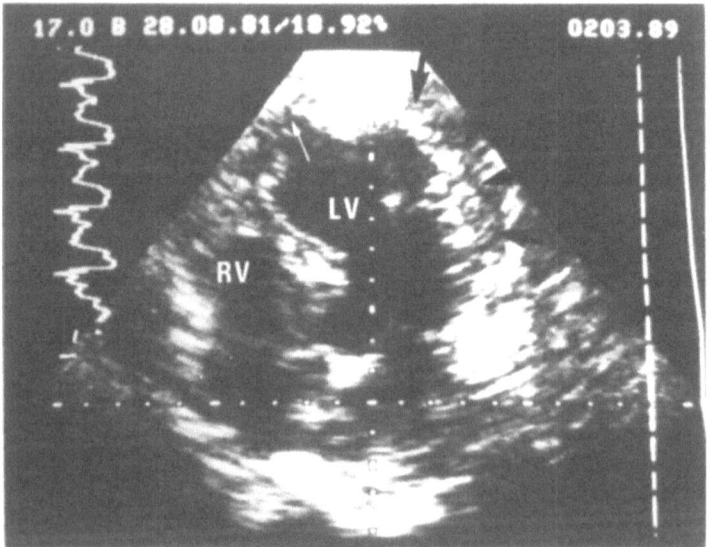

Figure 5. (lower panel) – Free wall rupture (white arrow) during acute anterior MI. Black arrows in partially filled with clots pericardial cavity. Successful emergency surgical repair.

3. Mechanical complications

This subject being dealt with elsewhere in this book, it will only be emphasized that this is a major field of contribution of 2-D echocardiography in acute coronary care, where it should be performed on an emergency basis, whenever suspicion arises. This allows for early recognition of rupture of papillary muscle, septum or free wall (Figure 5).

In conclusion, two-dimensional echocardiography is nowadays the simplest and most powerful diagnostic tool in acute coronary care, besides EKG recordings. Some of the present difficulties, related to inadequate handling of large amounts of tomographic data will hopefully be solved in the future, for more accurate quantitative description of myocardial infarction.

REFERENCES

1. Corya BC, Rasmussen S, Knoebel SB, Feigenbaum H: Echocardiography in acute myocardial infarction. Am J Cardiol 36:1, 1975.
2. Nieminen H, Heikkila J: Echoventriculography in acute myocardial infarction. Br Heart J 38:271, 1976.
3. Rasmussen S, Corya BC, Feigenbaum H, Knoebel SB: Detection of myocardial scar tissue by M-mode echocardiography. Circulation 57:237, 1978.
4. Bauwens D, O'Donnell M, Miller JG, Mimbs JW: Detection of acute myocardial ischemia in vivo with qualitative ultrasonic backscatter. Circulation 60 Suppl II:152, 1979.
5. Parisi AF, Moynihan PF, Folland ED, Strauss WE, Sharma GVRK, Sasahara AA: Echocardiography in acute and remot myocardial infarction. Am J Cardiol 46:1205, 1980.
6. Bastiaans OL, Meltzer RS, McGhie J, Verbeek PW, Roelandt J: Quantification from two-dimensional echocardiographic images. In: Rijsterborgh ed. Echocardiology. Martinus Nijhoff, The Hague, 131, 1981.
7. Heger J, Weyman A, Wann S, Rogers E, Dillon J, Feigenbaum H: Cross-sectional echocardiographic analysis of the extent of left ventricular asynergy in acute myocardial infarction. Circulation 61:1113, 1980.
8. Moynihan PF, Parisi AF, Feldman CL: Quantitative detection of regional left ventricular contraction abnormalities by two-dimensional echocardiography. Circulation 63:752, 1981.
9. Corya BC, Rasmussen S, Feigenbaum H, Knoebel SB, Black MJ: Systolic thickening and thinning of the septum and posterior wall in patients with coronary artery diseases. Circulation 55:109, 1977.
10. Edwards WD, Tajik AJ, Seward JB: Standardized nomenclature and anatomic basis for regional tomographic analysis of the heart. Mayo Clin Proc 56:479, 1981.
11. Prasquier R, Barthelemy M, Vervin P, Hanoun CH, Touche T, Aumount MC, Gourgon R: Echocardiographie bidimensionnelle dans l'infarctus aigu du myocarde. Arch Mal Coeur 72:1069, 1979.
12. Nixon JV, Narahara KA, Smitherman TC: Estimation of myocardial involvement in patients with acute myocardial infarction by two-dimensional echocardiography. Circulation 62:1248, 1980.
13. Lieberman AN, Weiss JL, Jugdutt BI, Becker LC, Bulkley BH, Garrison JB, Hutchins GM, Kallman CA, Weisfeldt ML: Two-dimensional echocardiography and infarct size: relationship of regional wall motion and thickening to the extent of myocardial infarction in the dog. Circulation 63:739, 1981.

14. Distante A, Michelassi C, Rovai D, Benassi A, Landini L, L'Abbate A: Computerized analysis of continuous echocardiographic recordings: study of trends in myocardial ischemia. Computers in cardiology IEEE Computers 1980.
15. Wann LS, Ferris JV, Childress RH, Dillon JC, Weyman AE, Feigenbaum H: Exercise cross-sectional echocardiography in ischemic heart disease. Circulation 60:1300, 1979.
16. Monaghan MJ, Daly K, Jackson G, Jewitt DE: Early detection of acute myocardial ischemia and infarction by cross-sectional echocardiography. In: Rijsterborgh ed. Echocardiology 93, Martinus Nijhoff Publishers, 1981.
17. Reet RE van, Quinones MA, Waggoner AD, Nelson JG, Winters WL Jr, Miller RR: Assessment of global function and regional wall motion in acute myocardial infarction by two-dimensional echocardiography. Circulation 64:95, 1981. (Abstr.)
18. Abrams DS, Starling MR, Crawford MN, O'Rourke RA: Value of non invasive techniques for predicting complications in patients with acute class II myocardial infarctions. Circulation 64:29, 1981. (Abstr.)
19. Weiss JL, Bulkley BH, Hutchins GM, Mason SJ: Two-dimensional echocardiography recognition of myocardial injury in man. Comparison with postmortem studies. Circulation 63:401, 1981.
20. Eaton LW, Weiss JL, Bulkley BH, Garrison JB, Weisfeldt ML: Regional cardiac dilatation after acute myocardial infarction. Recognition by two-dimensional echocardiography. N Engl J Med 300:57, 1979.
21. McEntee CW, Reet RE van, Winters WL, Nelson JG, Waggoner AD, Miller RR, Quinones MA: Incidence and natural history of mural thrombi in acute myocardial infarction by two-dimensional echocardiography. Circulation 64:93, 1981. (Abstr.)

20. ECHOCARDIOGRAPHIC DIAGNOSIS OF COMPLICATIONS OF MYOCARDIAL INFARCTION

R.S. MELTZER AND J. ROELANDT

1. INTRODUCTION

The complications of acute myocardial infarction where echocardiography can play an important role are listed in Table 1. Echocardiography is especially important in assessing anatomic complications such as aneurysms, thrombus, papillary muscle rupture, and ventricular septal defect. The technique is applicable at the bedside and this is important since there is reluctance to subject patients with acute infarction to catheterization. Some of the complications listed in Table 1 have surgical implications, and it is thus frequently useful to have a rapid and safe noninvasive method of confirming or making the diagnosis.

Table 1. Complications of MI where echo may be useful

I. Acute
    1. Poor pump function
    2. Rupture
       a. Free wall
       b. Interventricular septum
    3. Mitral regurgitation
       a. Papillary muscle dysfunction
       b. Flail mitral leaflet
    4. Right ventricular infarction

II. Chronic
    1. Aneurysm
       a. Subacute regional LV dilatation
       b. True aneurysm
       c. False or pseudo-aneurysm
    2. Left ventricular thrombus
    3. Pericardial effusion

Roelandt, J. (ed.) The practice of M-mode and two-dimensional echocardiography
© *1983, Martinus Nijhoff Publishers. The Hague / Boston / London*
ISBN 978-94-009-6792-2.

2. ACUTE COMPLICATIONS OF INFARCTION

Both M-mode and two-dimensional echocardiography are sensitive methods for assessing left ventricular function [1 – 3]. Furthermore, two-dimensional echocardiography can assess local myocardial contactility and the state of the entire left ventricle in most patients [4, 5], while allows examination of the cardiac base alone. Two-dimensional echocardiography has an advantage over M-mode echo in that it can assess lateral wall motion of the left ventricular walls and the apex of the LV where most often the pathology occurs in coronary disease.

2.1. Pump failure

Hypotension in the setting of acute infarction has multiple etiologies. If it is not caused by a dysrhythmia it may be due to hypovolemia, tamponade, mechanical problems such as VSD or mitral regurgitation, or primary myocardial failure. These entities may be differentiated echocardiographically, and myocardial failure from regional aneurysmal dilatation may also be distinguished from more global dysfunction due to "ischemic cardiomyopathy". We have several times been called to the coronary care unit to evaluate a patient in cardiogenic shock who was thought to have primary myocardial dysfunction but echocardiographically had a normal size left ventricle and hyperactive motion of at least a part of the left ventricle. These patients have either ventricular septal defects or mitral regurgitation, with soft or nonexistent murmurs due to low output, frequently masked by the noise from the multiple "apparati" of a modern CCU-balloon pump, respirators, etc. Patients with hypotension due to VSD's or mitral regurgitation from papillary muscle rupture always have hyperkinetic hearts. These are easy to differentiate from the grossly dilated hypocontractile heart of a patient with primary pump failure due to myocardial infarction. Cardiac tamponade is a rare complication of infarction, sometimes due to free wall rupture, rarely to catheter perforation, and occasionally related to the same disease process that caused the infarction – aortic root dissection, uremia, collagenvascular diseases. In these cases pericardial effusion is present, though specific echocardiographic diagnosis of tamponade is difficult and tamponade remains a clinical diagnosis [6 – 9].

2.2. Acute mitral regurgitation

Acute mitral regurgitation may complicate myocardial infarction via two different mechanisms with similar causes. That is, the papillary muscle may be dysfunctional, especially in inferior infarctions, and cause mitral regurgitation mainly late in systole due to its lack of contraction [10]. The same area may also rupture and cause flail mitral leaflet. The first condition may also progress the second. The echocardiographic hallmark of flail mitral leaflet is classically a systolic echo in the left atrium which disappears during diastole, and frequently a picture of accentuated holosystolic prolapse in the M-mode tracing at the mitral level.

The diagnosis is by no means always so simple, however, and flail mitral leaflet can closely simulate a left atrial myxoma or mitral mass. Two-dimensional echocardiography can more reliably differentiate these conditions than can M-mode. This difference is usually apparent from the clinical setting, however. Papillary muscle dysfunction is recognized on M-mode echocardiography by a largely intact mitral apparatus. Recent abstracts have suggested that papillary muscle dysfunction can be recognized on two-dimensional echocardiography by abnormal mitral leaflet coaptation, but we have serious reservations about the reliability of this sign. Further confirmation will be required before papillary muscle dysfunction becomes an echocardiographic diagnosis.

Though two-dimensional echocardiography can frequently detect associated conditions in mitral regurgitation and thereby help elucidate its etiology and significance [11], we are currently witnessing early studies of another technique which promises to yield important and clinically useful information about mitral regurgitation in the future: pulsed Doppler echocardiography [12]. Doppler echocardiography can directly detect and perhaps eventually quantify the extent and severity of the mitral regurgitation [13, 14]. The problems with this approach are largely technical: it has been difficult to create a ''duplex'' instrument with coordinated and reliable two-dimensional images and an operator-directed volume smaple for pulsed Doppler signals.

Also, the physical limitations of the pulsed Doppler method are such that the higher velocity jets of either mitral or aortic regurgitation cannot be quantified in real-time at the depths necessary in adult echocardiographic work.

Parenthetically, this may not be the case in infants, where a shorter transducer-to-target distance in allows more frequent sampling of the Doppler signal. Laboratories testing a new clinical Doppler equipment are currently trying to map the extent of mitral regurgitation in time and space within the left atrium − and even pulmonary veins. Perhaps new developments such as color-coded Doppler echocardiography using digital multigate technique [15, 16], or the application of fast Fourrier transform chips to allow real-time Doppler signal quantification, will improve our ability to yield clinically useful information in mitral regurgitation in the future.

2.3. Ventricular rupture

Left ventricular frcc wall rupture is usually immediately fatal, though several case have been diagnosed ante-mortem in Rotterdam using the commerecially available MiniVisor (Organon Teknika) [17, 18].

Ruptures of the interventricular septum are a complication of myocardial infarction that may be survived and are important to diagnose, since they lead to an abrupt worsening of hemodynamics. Classically this diagnosis is made to the new presence of a holosystolic murmur, frequently heard better at the sternal border than axilla, and significant increases in oxygen saturation from the right atrium to pulmonary artery. Echocardiography can frequently visualize VSD's as "dropout" of echoes in the interventricular septum though this sign is unreliable due to its poor sensitivity and specificity. A much better echocardiographic sign of intracardiac shunting is the detection of contrast crossing the septal defect [19, 20]. Unlike the case for ASD's were the large majority of shunts can be detected peripheral venous injections, VSD's are often not detected by right-to-left shunting after peripheral vein injections. This is one of the reasons why our group [21, 22] and other [23] are interested in the possibilities of transmission of echocardiographic contrast through the lungs. We are currently pursuing a course of studying microbubble dynamics and their removal by the lungs [24, 25], with the goal of developing noninvasive and safe methods of transmission of ultrasonic contrast through the lungs. If this can be obtained, the echocardiographic diagnosis of VSD's using contrast echocardiography to image left-to-right shunts may be improved.

2.4. Right ventricular infarction

At present right ventricular infarction is usually diagnosed by hemodynamic or scintigraphic techniques. It can occsionally be suspected or diagnosed echocardiographically by finding a dilated hypocontactile right ventricle, sometimes associated with "paradoxical" interventricular septal motion in the absence of septal infarction. The right ventricle is best examined by two-dimensional echocardiography in the parasternal and apical four chamber views.

3. CHRONIC COMPLICATIONS OF MYOCARDIAL INFARCTION

3.1. Aneurysm

Though M-mode echocardiography can show local diskinesis and suggest the presence of a left ventricular aneurysm [26 – 28], it was only with the advent of two-dimensional echocardiography that noninvasive evaluation of patients for the presence of left ventricular aneurysms became a reality [29]. Echocardiography shares with angiography and radionuclide scintigraphy the disadvantage that localized dyskinesis does not always imply that a surgeon will find a discrete aneurysm at operation. Echocardiography does have an advantage over the other two techniques, however, in that it can not only image endocardial wall

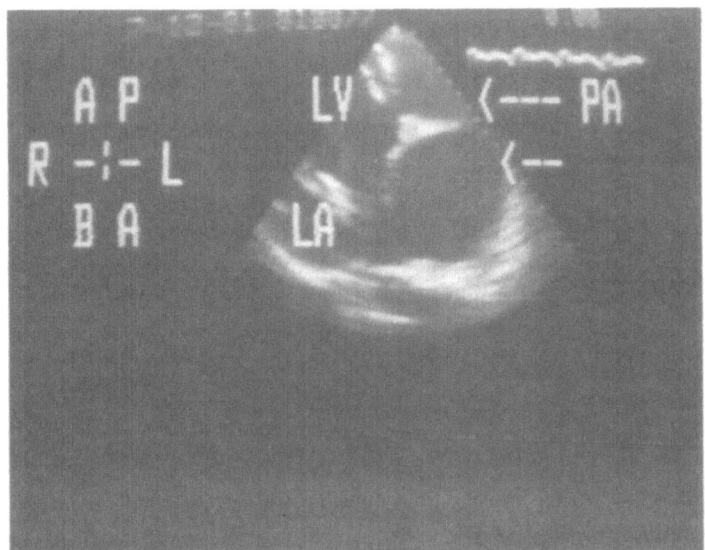

A

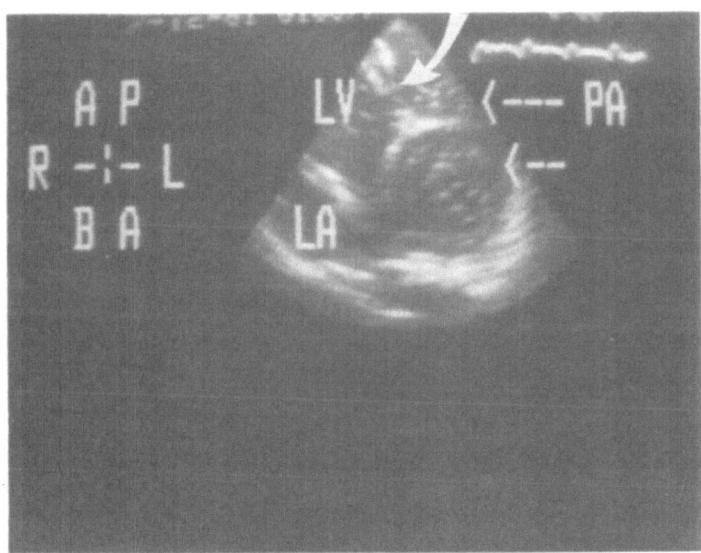

B

Figure 1. Pseudo-aneurysm. A: Apical four chamber view with transducer angled towards the patient's left side. A large, seemingly loculated echo-free area represents the pseudo-aneurysm (PA, arrows). B: After left ventricular injection of saline, contrast was seen to cross from the left ventricle (LV) through the small orifice (curved arrow) into the pseudo-aneurysm. Abbreviations: AP : apical, BA : basal, R : right, L : left, LA : left atrium.

motion but also can assess local left ventricular wall thickening. A true aneurysm has a thin wall which does not thicken during systole and often actually thins. Using quantitative techniques such as that of Eaton et al [30], it may even be possible to echocardiographically diagnose those patients at risk for aneurysm development due to semiacute infarct expansion.

Due to the non-invasive nature of this technique, all patients with persistent ST elevation on ECG after infarction, or other signs of possible aneurysm (difficult to control failure or ventricular dysrhythmias, prolonged apical impluse on physical examination) should have two-dimensional echocardiographic evaluation for the possibility of a ventricular aneurysm.

3.2. Pseudo-aneurysm

A pseudo-aneurysm is a more dangerous complication of myocardial infarction than a true left ventricular aneurysm, because its natural history is rupture and death and its detection frequently should be followed by an operation. One of the first uses of two-dimensional echocardiography reported from our institution was the detection of a left ventricular pseudo-aneurysm, in 1975 [31]. At that time two-dimensional echocardiographic equipment developed at the Thoraxcenter and available to us was considerably more primitive than the equipment now commercially available. The important signs by which a pseudo-aneurysm can be recognized include a smaller orifice size compared to maximal aneurysm dimention, sometimes the imaging of a discontinuity in the myocardial echo, and the lack of a clearcut myocardial echo surrounding the aneurysm (Figure 1).

Like true aneurysm, pseudo-aneurysm exhibit dyskinetic motion and frequently harbor mural thrombi [32].

3.3. Left ventricular thrombi

Left ventricular thrombi are a frequent complication of myocardial infarction coming to autopsy [33] (Figures 2 and 3) and about half of the chronic left ventricular aneurysms operated on at Stanford contain mural thrombi. The large majority of these thrombi are silent — that is, they never cause a clinically apparent embolus. Thus the natural history of left ventricular thrombus, and even its prevalence, is unknown. An important reason for this was the lack of a noninvasive screening test to diagnose left ventricular thrombi. Until the recent past the only test for left ventricular thrombi was cardiac catheterization with left ventricular angiography, and even this is not always reliable and may miss even giant left ventricular mural thrombi [34].

This situation has changed in the past few years due to the introduction of two-dimensional echocardiography and the realization that it is a good, though by no

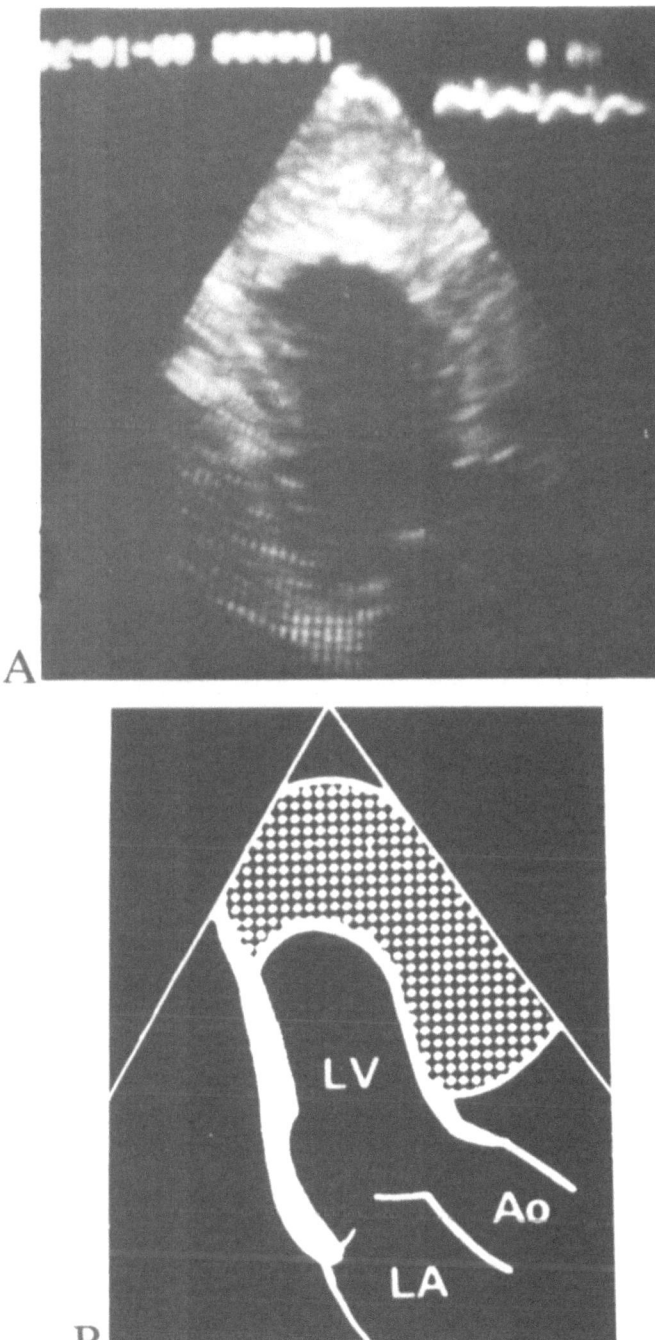

Figure 2. A: Stop-frame photograph from the two-dimensional echocardiogram of a patient with a giant apical left ventricular thrombus inside a thin-walled apical aneurysm. The patient had suffered an apical myocardial infarction 4 months previously. This thrombus was missed on left ventricular angiography. Apical four chamber view. B: diagrammatic representation, with stippled area representing thrombus. Abbreviations: LV : left ventricle, Ao : aorta, LA : left atrium.

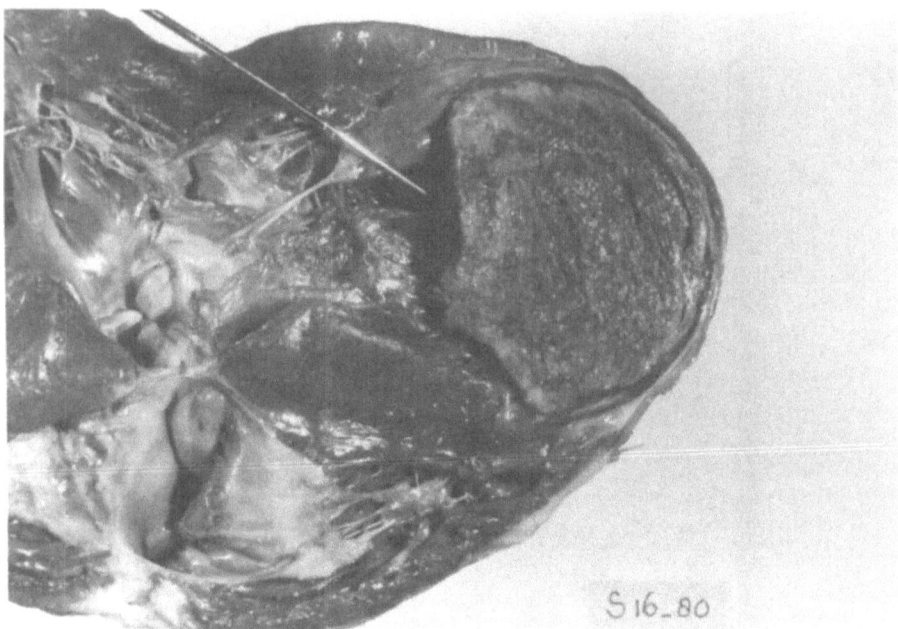

Figure 3. The heart of the patient whose echocardiogram is shown in Figure 2, at autopsy 1 week later (the patient died of a repeat infarction). The apical thrombus is being separated from the aneurysmal wall by a probe.

means perfect, diagnostic test for left ventricular thrombi [35 – 38]. Two-dimensional echocardiography has unique characteristics that enhance its ability to detect left ventricular thrombi compared to the other widely used cardiac imaging techniques: its tomographic form of image processing allows display of different soft tissue characteristics at all points in its output, whereas angiography and scintigraphy integrate all information throughout the body thickness in the formation of their images. However, both false positive and false negative two-dimensional echocardiograms for left ventricular thrombi have been reported, and the interpretation of some studies requires considerable experience. Some useful criteria for the diagnosis are listed in Table 2.

Now that a simple noninvasive technique is available for the diagnosis of left

Table 2. Criteria for the diagnosis of left ventricular thrombi

- Mass which moves with the heart (artifactual echoes may also do this)
- Attached to an aneurysmal or abnormally moving portion of myocardium
- Site usually in LV apex
- Can be imaged from different echocardiographic views
- Mass is adjacent to myocardium but separate myocardial echo is present
- Occasionally texture of mass is distinct from myocardium

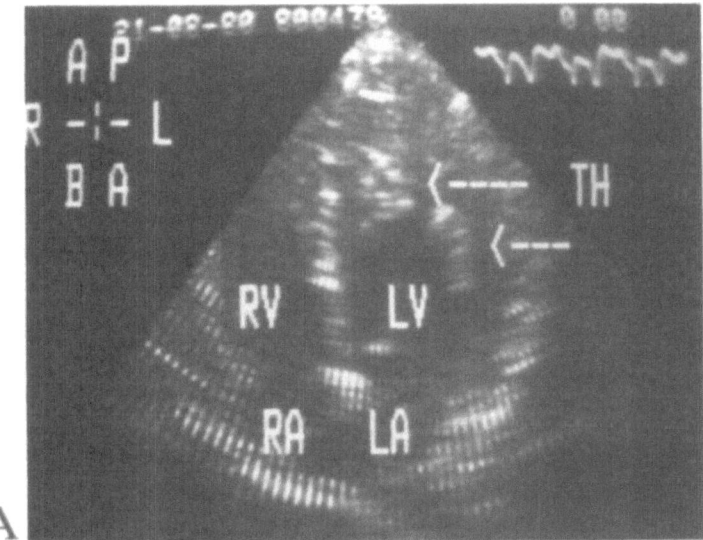

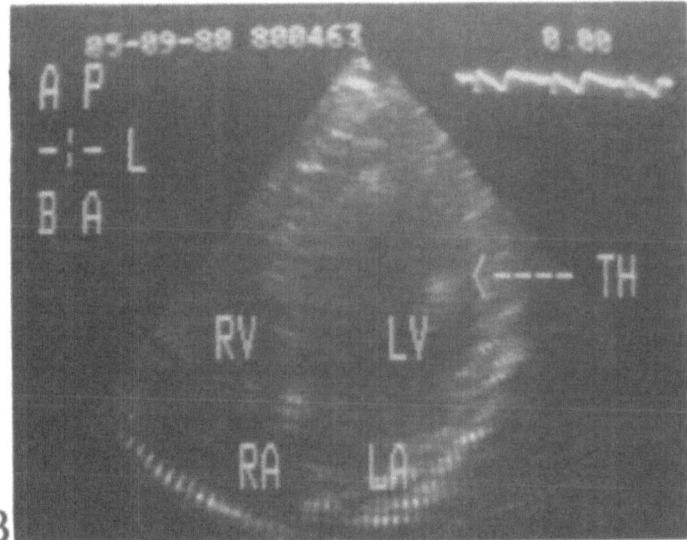

Figure 4. Serial follow-up of a left ventricular thrombus. The patient was a 31 year old male who presented with a cerebral embolus 2 weeks after a myocardial infarction. All panels are stopframe photographs from his two-dimensional echocardiogram, apical four chamber view. A: A large thrombus (TH) divided into several smaller pieces is seen in the left ventricle (LV). B: 2 weeks later the thrombus is smaller. C: 5 months after presentation the thrombus in the LV body is gone. In real-time it was apparent that the echoes in the LV apex were reverberations and did not move with the heart cycle, as the former thrombus did.

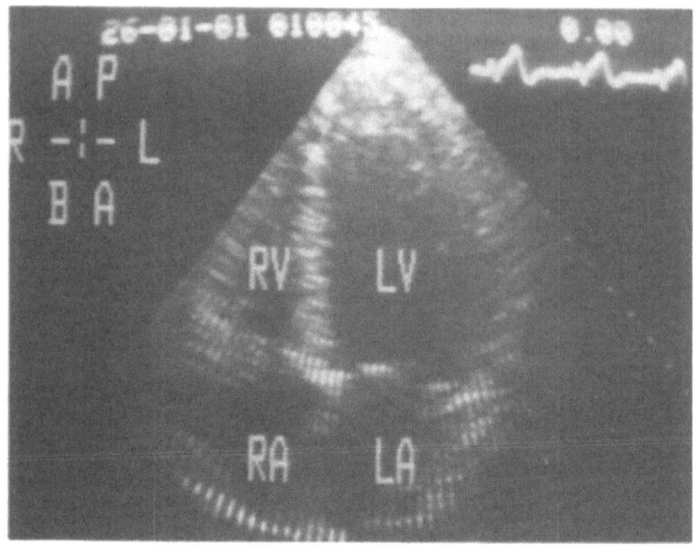

Figure 4C.

ventricular thrombi, the way is open for studies of the natural history and response to anticogulation of this previously silent condition (Figure 4).

3.4. Pericardial effusion

Dressler's syndrome is usually though not always associated with a pericardial effusion echocardiographically. The size of these effusions is usually small, and they can be detected using standard M-mode echocardiographic techniques [39, 40].

4. CONCLUSION

Many of the important complications of myocardial infarction can be readily detected by echocardiography. Since echocardiographic equipment is rapidly improving, we feel that an echocardiographic capability will be more and more helpful in the future. This applies both to the coronary care unit, where many surgically correctable complications of acute myocardial infarction can be identified [41], and to the out-patient treatment of coronary artery disease.

REFERENCES

1. Popp RL: Echocardiographic evaluation of left ventricular function. New Engl J Med 296:856, 1977.
2. Meltzer RS, Popp RL: Echocardiographic analysis of left ventricular function. Indian Heart J (in press).
3. Roelandt J: Practical echocardiology. Forest Grove, Oregon: Research Studies Press. Chapter 8: Assessment of left ventricular function, pp. 117–136, 1977.
4. Kisslo JA, Robertson D, Gilbert BW, Ramm O Von, Behar VS: A comparison of real-time, two-dimensional echocardiography and cineangiography in detecting left ventricular asysnergy. Circulation 55:134, 1977.
5. Bansal RC, Tajik AJ, Seward JB, Offord KP: Feasibility of detailed two-dimensional echocardiographic examination in adults: prospective study of 200 patients. Mayo Clin Proc 55:291, 1980.
6. Schiller NB, Botvinick EH: Right ventricular compression as a sign of cardiac tamponade. Circulation 56:774, 1977.
7. Settle HP, Adolph RJ, Fowler NO et al: Echocardiographic study of cardiac tamponade. Circulation 56:951, 1977.
8. Horowitz MS, Schultz CS, Stinson EB et al: Sensitivity and specificy of echocardiographic diagnosis of pericardial effusion. Circulation 50:239, 1972.
9. Hancock EW: Management of pericardial disease. Modern Concepts Cardiovasc Dis 48:1, 1979.
10. Roberts WC, Perloff JK: Mitral valvular disease. Ann Int Med 77:939, 1972.
11. Mintz GS, Kotler MN, Segal BL, Parry WR: Two-dimensional echocardiographic evaluation of patients with mitral insufficiency. Am J Cardiol 44:670, 1979.
12. Baker DW: The present role of Doppler techniques in cardiac diagnosis. Prog Cardiovasc Dis 21:517, 1977.
13. Kalmanson D, Veyrat C, Bouchareine F, Groote A de: Noninvasive recording of mitral valve flow velocity patterns using pulsed Doppler echocardiography. Brit Heart J 39:517, 1977.
14. Abbasi AS, Allen MW, DeCristofaro D, Ungar I: Detection and estimation of the degree of mitral regurgitation by rangegated pulsed Doppler echocardiography. Circulation 61:143, 1980.
15. Brandestini M, Howard A, Eyer M, Stevenson J, Weiler T: Visualization of intracardiac defects by M/Q mode echo: Doppler ultrasound. Circulation 59–60 (Suppl II):II–13, 1979.
16. Stevenson G, Brandestini M, Weiler T, Howard A, Eyer M: Digital multigate Doppler with color echo and Doppler display – diagnosis of atrial and ventricular septal defects. Circulation 59–60 (Suppl II):II–205, 1979.
17. Hagemeijer F, Verbaan CJ, Sonke PCG, Rooij CH de: Echocardiography and rupture of the heart. Brit Heart J 43:45, 1980.
18. Meltzer RS, Verheugt FW, Roelandt J: Left ventricular free wall rupture diagnosed by two-dimensional echocardiography. Circulation, in press (letter to the editor).
19. Meltzer RS, Schwartz J, French J, Popp RL: Ventricular septal defect noted by two-dimensional echocardiography. Chest 76:455, 1979.
20. Scanlan JG, Seward JB, Tajik AJ: Visualization of ventricular septal rupture utilizing wide-angle two-dimensional echocardiography. May Clin Proc 54:381, 1979.
21. Meltzer RS, Serruys PW, McGhie J, Verbaan N, Roelandt J: Pulmonary wedge injections yielding left sides echocardiographic contrast. Brit Heart J 44:390, 1980.
22. Meltzer RS, Sartorius OEH, Lancée CT, Serruys PW, Verdouw PD, Essed C, Roelandt J: Transmission of echocardiographic contrast through the lungs. Ultrasound in Med & Biol 7:377, 1981.
23. Reale A, Pizzuto F, Gioffre PA, Nigri A, Romeo F, Martuscelli E, Mangieri E, Scibilia G: Contrast echocardiography, transmission of echoes to the left heart across the pulmonary vascular bed. Eur Heart J 1:101, 1980.

24. Meltzer RS, Tickner EG, Sahines TP, Popp RL: The source of ultrasonic contrast effects. J Clin Ultrasound 8:121, 1980.

25. Meltzer RS, Tickner EG, Popp RL: Why do the lungs clear ultrasonic contrast? Ultrasound in Med & Biol 6:261, 1980.

26. Kreamer R, Kerber RE, Abboud FM: Ventricular aneurysm: use of echocardiography. J Clin Ultrasound 1:60, 1973.

27. Dillon J, Feigenbaum H, Weyman AE et al: M-mode echocardiography in the evaluation of patients for aneurysmectomy. Circulation 53:657, 1976.

28. Peterson JL, Johnston W, Hessel EA, Murray JA: Echocardiographic recognition of left ventricular aneurysm. Am Heart J 83:24, 1972.

29. Weyman AE, Peskoe SM, Williams ES et al: Detection of left ventricular aneurysm by cross-sectional echocardiography. Circulation 54:936, 1976.

30. Eaton LW, Weiss JL, Bilkley BH, Garrison JB, Weisfeldt ML: Regional cardiac dilatation after acute myocardial infarction. Recognition by two-dimensional echocardiography. New Engl J Med 300:57, 1979.

31. Roelandt J, Brand M van den, Vletter WB, Nauta J, Hugenholtz PG: Echocardiographic diagnosis of pseudoaneurysm of the left ventricle. Circulation 52:466, 1975.

32. Catherwood E, Mintz GS, Kotler MN, Parry WR, Segal BL: Two-dimensional echocardiographic recognition of left ventricular pseudo-aneurysm. Circulation 62:294, 1980.

33. Garvin CF: Mural thrombi in the heart. Am Heart J 21:713, 1941.

34. Meurs H van, Meltzer RS, Brand M van den, Essed CE, Michels HR, Roelandt J: Illustrative echocardiogram: superiority of echocardiography over angiography in diagnosing a left ventricular thrombus. Chest 80:321, 1981.

35. DeMaria AN, Bommer W, Neumann A, Grehl T, Weinart L, Denardo S, Amsterdam E, Mason DT: Left ventricular thrombi identified by cross-sectional echocardiography. Ann Int Med 90:14, 1979.

36. Ports TA, Cogan J, Schiller NB, Rappaport E: Echocardiography of left ventricular masses. Circulation 58:528, 1978.

37. Meltzer RS, Gothaner D, Rakowski H, Popp RL, Martin RP: Diagnosis of left ventricular thrombi by two-dimensional echocardiography. Brit Heart J 42:261, 1979.

38. Asinger RW, Mikell FL, Sharma B, Hodges M: Observations on detecting left ventricular thrombus with two-dimensional echocardiography: emphasis avoidance of false positive diagnosis. Am J Cardiol 47:145, 1981.

39. Teicholz LE: Echocardiographic evaluation of pericardial diseases. Prog Cardiovasc Dis 21:133, 1978.

40. Horowitz MS, Schultz CS, Stinson EB, Harrison DC, Popp RL: Sensitivity and specificity of echocardiographic diagnosis of the pericardial effusion. Circulation 50:239, 1974.

41. Mintz GS, Victor MF, Kotler MN, Parry WR, Segal BL: Two-dimensional echocardiographic identification of surgically correctable complications of acute myocardial infarction.

21. USEFULNESS OF ECHOCARDIOGRAPHY FOR THE ASSESSMENT OF INTERVENTIONS IN PATIENTS WITH ACUTE AND CHRONIC CORONARY ARTERY DISEASE (THROMBOLYSIS, VASODILATORY THERAPY ETC.)

P. Schweizer

One application of M-mode – and recently of two-dimensional echocardiography is to assess in sequential studies the progression or regression of a disease process, the effect of surgical therapy or the effect of pharmacological interventions.

Those studies are legitimate provided that the echocardiographic registrations and measurements are standardized and the spontaneous as well as the methodological variations are known.

With *M-mode echocardiography* there exist meanwhile clear guidelines for standardization of measurements [1]. Left ventricular dimensions should be picked up at the chordal level and the leading edge method should be preferred, that means, dimensions should always be measured from the onset of the echoes in the M-mode recordings [2, 3].

Despite standardization of measurements there exists interobserver and intrapatient variability when doing serial studies. Several factors, that do increase variability and which are often encountered when evaluating serial echocardiograms in a clinical setting, can be minimized (see Table 1).

The variability of measurements can for example be attributed to the different experience of technicians performing the echocardiograms. To improve reproducibility it is therefore advisable that all recordings are produced by one experienced echocardiographer with one ultrasonic system [4]. Errors can be further introduced into the measurement of the left ventricle by inconsistent placement of the transducer on the chest wall. The details of the intercostal space used

Table 1. Guidelines for serial echocardiographic evaluation

- Perform all recordings by one experienced echocardiographer (technician) and with only one ultrasonographic system
- Study the patient in a basal state and take variations, produced by changes in heart rate, into account
- Record at constant respiratory phase (held mid-exspiration)
- Hold spatial orientation between the transducer probe and the heart (thorax) constant
- Select only technically adequate tracings and use the suggested recommendations for standardization of measurements
- Be cautious with the interpretation of wall amplitude- and wall thickness changes

---

Roelandt, J. (ed.) The practice of M-mode and two-dimensional echocardiography
© *1983, Martinus Nijhoff Publishers. The Hague / Boston / London*
ISBN 978-94-009-6792-2.

and the degree of left lateral tilt of the patients upper body should therefore be documented in a patient who is being followed serially [2, 5]. Some workers propose an inclinometer or other external reference systems for reproduction of body- and transducer position [5 – 7].

The patient should be studied in a basal state and variations produced by changes in heart rate should be taken into account. In normal subjects progressive increases in heart rate result in proportional decreases in both end-diastolic and endsystolic left ventricular dimensions [8]. Recently it has been demonstrated, that echocardiographic left ventricular dimensions significantly decrease during quiet phasic inspiration. Measuring at a constant part of the respiratory cycle, as determined by a respirometer, will therefore further improve reproducibility [9].

One inherent technical problem is lateral resolution due to ultrasonic beam width leading to difficulty in identifying wall margins by echocardiography [3]. Echo "drop-outs" are due to an improper angle of beam incidence to the structure being studied. For these reasons only technically adequate tracings should be selected for quantification.

Axial ultrasonic resolution is about 1 mm, which means, that there is a potential error in the system of 10% when measuring a small 10 mm structure [10]. Besides improper delineation of the interventricular septum and the posterior left ventricular wall, this is one reason, why variability of measurements is greatest with wall thickness and wall amplitudes. Several studies have demonstrated bad reproducibility of wall thickness and wall amplitude measurement from day to day in the same individual. Caution should therefore be used in ascribing quantitative changes in wall thickness or wall amplitude to any intervention [10 – 13].

With rigid standardization of technique according to the cited guidelines, the largest measures, namely the left ventricular diameters, were the most reproducible. Reproducibility decreased with increasing time intervals, but even with weekly intervals time variability was within tolerable limits, the coefficient of variation being 5% or below [4, 6, 7, 14].

Pharmacological effects can therefore be deduced from changes in echocardiographic cavity dimensions and derived parameters of left ventricular function. The analysis can be facilitated and the parameters can be assessed more widely and more accurately using computer based digitizing techniques [15 – 17]. Measurements of instantaneous left ventricular dimension and its rate of change are then possible as well as the evaluation of combined hemodynamic-echocardiographic studies (see Figure 1).

Vasodilatory agents: To evaluate the short term effects of a potent new antianginal drug (molsidomin) simultaneous echocardiographic-hemodynamic studies were performed in 8 male patients with coronary artery disease [18]. Heart rate was controlled by atrial pacing before and 40 min. after an i.v.dose of 4 mg molsidomin was given. Measurements were performed during heart rate 80 and 100 beats per minute respectively.

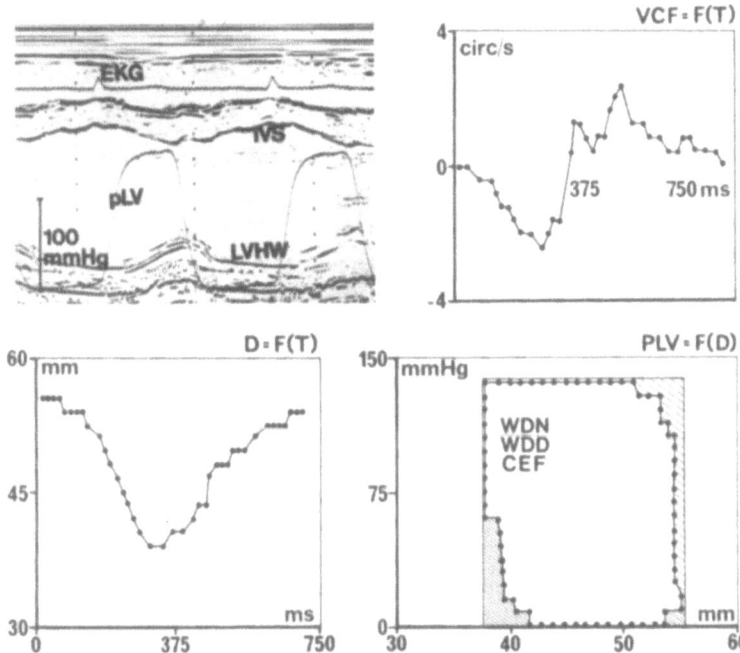

Figure 1. Computer-based pressure-dimension analysis. Upper left: recording showing simultaneous echocardiogram of left ventricular cavity (paper speed 100 mm/s) and left ventricular pressure (pLV, Millar-tip manometer). Bottom left: Corresponding computer output of instantaneous left ventricular dimension (D) as function of time F (T). Bottom right: Pressure (PLV) − dimension (D) loop. The surface area enclosed by the loop represents left ventricular dimension stroke work (WDN). Other derived parameters are left ventricular diastolic dimension work (WDD) and cycle efficiency (CEF) [16]. IVS : interventricular septum; LVHW : left ventricular posterior wall.

As can be seen from Figure 2, with both heart rates there was a significant fall of mean aortic pressure and left ventricular enddiastolic pressure whereas total peripheral resistance remained nearly constant. Therefore the vasodilatory effect of the drug is predominantly on the capacity vessels. The echocardiographie enddiastolic and endsystolic dimensions of the left ventricle both decreased significantly, from 51 ± 5 to 47 ± 4 mm and from 34 ± 4 to 32 ± 5 mm respectively.

The reduction of myocardial oxygen demand was documented by a shift of the left ventricular pressure-dimension loop downwards and to the left. The diastolic left ventricular dimension-pressure work significantly decreased and the incoordinate contraction of the left ventricle became more sufficient (see example in Figure 3).

These results are in correlation with similar combined hemodynamic-echocardiographic and -cineangiographic studies performed with isosorbide dinitrate, amylnitrite and molsidomin [19 − 21]. The findings are consistent with the concept of the antianginal action of the nitrates and similar drugs being

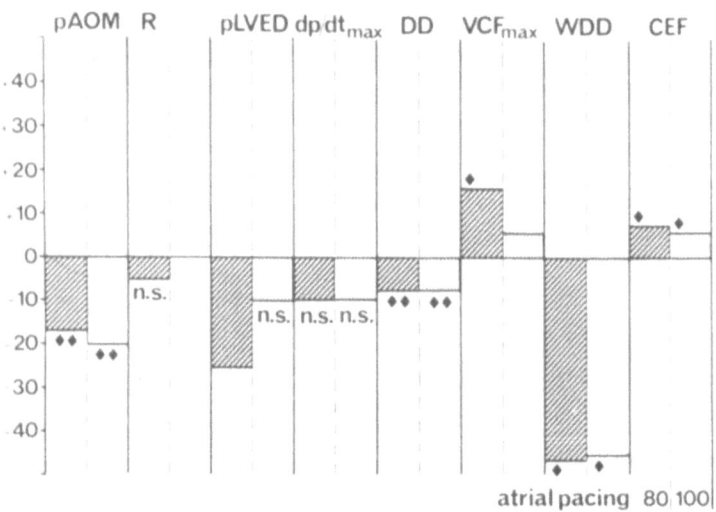

Figure 2. Graph of the percent changes in hemodynamic parameters (mean aortic pressure, total peripheral resistance, left ventricular enddiastolic pressure, dp/dt max), echocardiographic parameters (enddiastolic diameter, maximal velocity of circumferential fiber shortening) and parameters derived from pressure-dimension diagrams (diastolic pressure dimension work, cycle efficiency) obtained with 8 patients after 4 mg molsidomin ($\triangle$ p < 0.05; $\triangle\triangle$ p < 0.01).

related to extra-cardiac-induced lowering of myocardial oxygen consumption.

M-mode echocardiography is also a suitable method for the noninvasive assessment of the *long term effects* of vasodilatory agents. In a controlled double blind study 12 patients with coronary artery disease received orally 4 mg of molsidomin or placebo. Heart rate, arterial blood pressure, echocardiographic left ventricular dimensions and derived parameters of left ventricular function were obtained before and up to 360 minutes after drug application (see Figure 4).

In contrast to placebo the systolic blood pressure significantly decreased with molsidomin, reaching its maximal change (17%) after one hour. The diastolic arterial blood pressure slightly (7%) but significantly decreased as well. The pressures remained reduced for at least 4 hours. The echocardiographically determined enddiastolic and endsystolic diameters also significantly (p < 0.05) decreased within the first 30 minutes reaching their maximum of change after 2 hours. The diameters remained reduced for up to 4 hours. In comparison with the placebo measurements heart rate did not change during the follow up and the parameters of contractility (max VCF) also remained constant.

A similar prolonged effect on left ventricular dimensions determined with echocardiography has been observed with isosorbide dinitrate and with

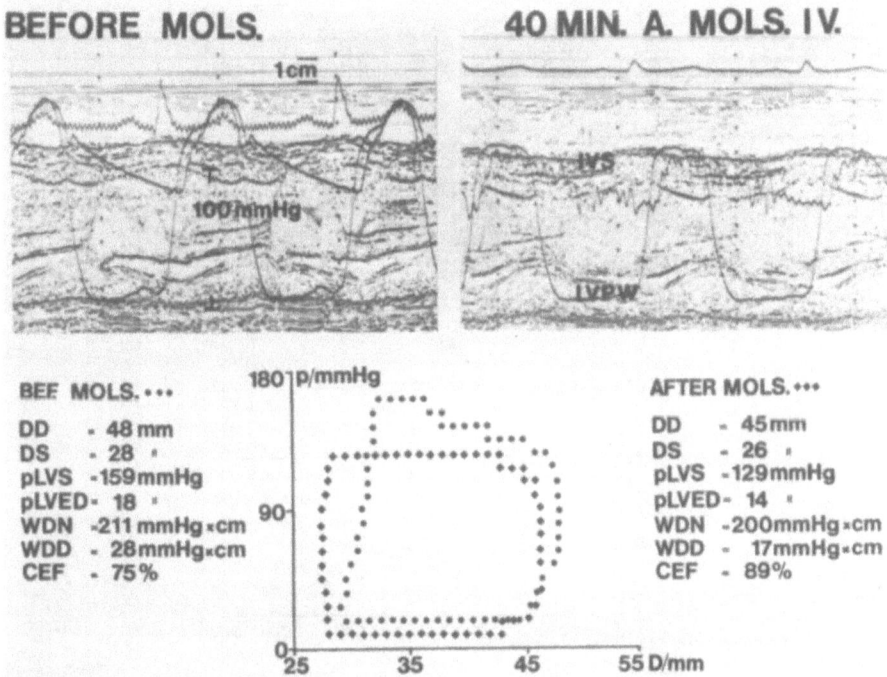

Figure 3. Representative example of a pressure-dimension analysis in a patient with coronary artery disease, obtained from simultaneous echocardiographic-hemodynamic registrations before and 40 min. after 4 mg of molsidomin. The shift of the pressure-dimension loop downward and to the left is accompanied with a decrease of diastolic pressure-dimension work (WDD) and a more sufficient and coordinate left ventricular contraction.

nitroglycerin ointment [22]. These echocardiographic studies confirm several earlier reports that vasodilators (isosorbide dinitrate) given orally or sublingually produce beneficial hemodynamic effects, that may last for several hours [23 – 27].

Effects on left ventricular cavity size and function determined with M-mode echocardiography, partly in combination with other noninvasive methods, have been systematically investigated before and after the administration of inotropic agents and of several beta blockers [28 – 31].

In respect to the evaluation of pharmacological interventions M-mode echocardiography has methodological inherent limits since this procedure can only delineate a small, circumscript portion of the left ventricle. In the presence of an asymmetric contraction pattern the regional parameters which are obtained are not by all means representative for global left ventricular function.

M-mode echocardiography does remain valid in intrapatient studies, as has been demonstrated, since each subject serves as his own control. But the noninvasive study of the total left ventricle would be more attractive especially in patients with acute or chronic coronary artery disease.

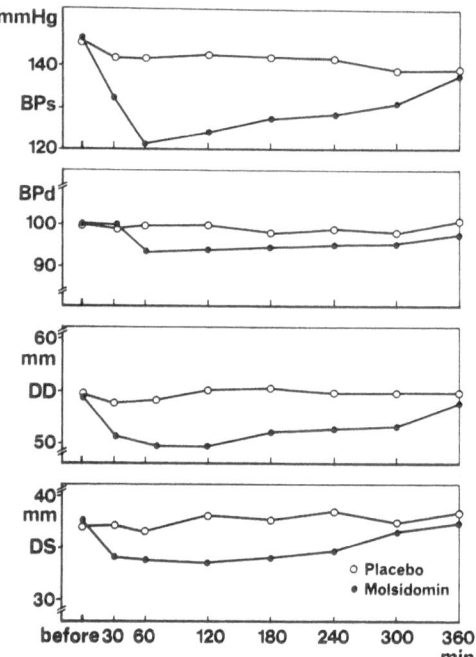

Figure 4. Graph demonstrating the significant (p < 0.05) changes of systolic and diastolic blood pressure (BP), enddiastolic (DD) and endsystolic (DS) diameters after the administration of 4 mg of molsidomin in correlation to placebo. The reduction of blood pressures and the reduction of echocardiographically determined diameters are measurable for at least four hours.

Two-dimensional echocardiography principally enables visualization of all parts of the left ventricle including the anterior wall and the apical-near segments. The sectional images registered from the region of the apical impulse are anatomically similar to the usual cineangiographic projections and therefore well adaptable to volume determinations.

Cross-sectional echocardiography is a relatively new method and there exists only limited experience with its application to interventional studies. From a practical standpoint the suggested guidelines for serial echocardiographic evaluation (see Table 1) are also applicable to this method. But until now very few reports have paid attention to intrapatient and interobserver variability of two-dimensional echocardiographic volume measurements and of quantitation of wall motion abnormalities [32 – 36].

With animal experiments it could be demonstrated, that two-dimensional echocardiography provides reproducible images for quantitative measurements of left ventricular function, both in control states and during acute myocardial ischaemia [37]. Furthermore, a modification in infarct size due to different pharmacological interventions could be observed. The extent of motion abnormalities measured at different cross-sectional levels significantly increased after the application of phenylephrine [38]. In contrast, a pronounced improvement in contraction was noted after infusion of nitroglycerin or nitroprusside [38, 39].

According to those optimistic experimental studies two-dimensional echocardiography was applied to a clinical follow up study. 48 consecutive patients with acute transmural myocardial infarction – 28 anterior and 14 inferior wall infarctions – were evaluated before and from the first up to the third day after intracoronary streptokinase therapy. A further control registration followed within 3 – 4 weeks after the acute event.

Investigations were performed according to the strict guidelines for serial echocardiographic evaluation, mentioned above (see Table 1). The long axis view of the left ventricle was registered from the apex impulse window using a wide angle sector scanner. The slicesummation method was applied to the determination of left ventricular volumes and ejection fraction. The length of the enddiastolic segment in which abnormal contraction occurred during systole was measured and its percentage part of the total length of the enddiastolic left ventricular outline was calculated. (%AKS). This method of measuring segmental wall motion abnormality being previously introduced by Beeder et al demonstrated good interobserver and intrapatient reproducibility [40].

In group A, consisting of 16 patients, fibrinolytic treatment was successful within four hours from the beginning of chest pain. In group B intracoronary thrombolysis was unsuccessful or the reopening of the occluded coronary vessel occurred later than 4 hours after the beginning of clinical symptoms.

It can be seen from Table 2, that patient group A showed a significant reduction of the percentage part of akinetic myocardial contraction and a significant increase in ejection fraction, beginning with the second day after therapy. In group B the global and regional left ventricular function remained nearly constant during the follow up period.

These preliminary results demonstrating a positive effect of early streptokinase therapy must be validated with corresponding invasive investigations in future. But they support earlier reports of Eaton and coworkers who also demonstrated the usefulness of two-dimensional echocardiography for following up of patients with acute myocardial infarction [41].

Table 2. 2-D-echocardiographic control of global and regional left ventricular function before and after streptokinase therapy

		before	1st day	2nd day	3rd day	3 – 4 weeks	
A	EF:	47 ± 8	52 ± 9	52 ± 7*	54 ± 8*	53 ± 8*	%
	AKS:	22 ± 9	19 ± 13	15 ± 13*	13 ± 11*	13 ± 12*	%
B	EF:	43 ± 10	44 ± 10	45 + 9	44 ± 9	44 ± 10	%
	AKS:	29 ± 12	27 ± 11	27 ± 8	27 ± 8	27 ± 9	%

* p < 0.05.

In conclusion, M-mode echocardiography is meanwhile an established method, whose advantages and disadvantages for the assessment of interventions are well known. Two-dimensional echocardiography for follow up studies, which are necessarily based on quantitative evaluation of left ventricular function, is still at the beginning. Intrapatient and interobserver variability are objects of controversies. The cited experimental and clinical studies give promise to optimism.

REFERENCES

1. Sahn DJ, De Maria A, Kisslo J, Weyman A: Recommendations regarding quantitation in M-mode echocardiography: results of a survey of echocardiographic measurements. Circulation 58:1072, 1978.
2. Popp RL, Filly K, Brown OR, Harrison DC: Effect of transducer placement on echocardiographic measurement of left ventricular dimensions. Am J Cardiol 35:537, 1975.
3. Roelandt J, Dorp WG van, Bom N, Leird JD, Hugenholtz PG: Resolution problems in echocardiography: a source of interpretation errors. Am J Cardiol 37:256, 1976.
4. Lapido GOA, Dunn FG, Pringle TH, Bastian B, Lawrie TDV: Serial measurements of left ventricular dimensions by echocardiography. Assessment of week-to-week, inter- and intraobserver variability in normal subjects and in patients with valvular heart disease. Br Heart J 44:284, 1980.
5. Stafadouros MA, Canedo MI: Reproducibility of echocardiographic estimates of left ventricular dimensions. Br Heart J 39:390, 1977.
6. Martin MA, Fieller NJR: Echocardiography in cardiovascular drug assessment. Br Heart J 41:536, 1979.
7. Wong M, Shah PM, Taylor RD: Reproducibility of left ventricular internal dimensions with M-mode echocardiography: effects of heart size, body position and transducer angulation. Am J Cardiol 47:1068, 1981.
8. De Maria AN, Neumann A, Schubart PJ, Lee G, Mason DT: Systematic correlation of cardiac chamber size and ventricular performance determined with echocardiography and alterations in heart rate in normal persons. Am J Cardiol 43:1, 1979.
9. Brenner IR, Waugh RA: Effect of phasic respiration on left ventricular dimensions and performance in a normal population. Circulation 57:122, 1978.
10. Monoson PA, O'Rourke RA, Crawford MH, White DH: Measurements of left ventricular wall thickness and systolic thickening by M-mode echocardiography: interobserver and intrapatient variability. J Clin Ultrasound 6:215, 1978.
11. Pietro AD, Voelker G, Ray BJ, Parisi AF: Reproducibility of echocardiography. A study evaluating the variability of serial echocardiographic measurements. Chest 79:29, 1981.
12. Corya B: Significance of serial echocardiographic measurements. Chest 79:1, 1981.
13. Vignola PA, Bloch A, Kaplan AD, Walker HJ, Chiotellis PN, Meyers GS: Interobserver variability in echocardiography. J Clin Ultrasound 5:238, 1977.
14. Clark RD, Korcuska K, Cohn K: Serial echocardiographic evaluation of left ventricular function in valvular disease, including reproducibility guidelines for serial studies. Circulation 62:564, 1980.
15. Gibson DG, Brown DJ: Measurement of instantaneous left ventricular dimension and filling rate in man using echocardiography. Br Heart J 35:1141, 1973.
16. Gibson DG, Brown DJ: Assessment of left ventricular systolic function in man from simultaneous echocardiographic and pressure measurements. Br Heart J 38:8, 1976.
17. Krebs W, Hanrath P, Bleifeld W, Effert S: Rechnergestützte Auswertung von M-mode Echokardiogrammen. Herz/Kreislauf 9:519, 1977.

18. Schweizer P, Meyer J, Merx W, Erbel R, Krebs W: The hemodynamic effects of molsidomin. VIIIth World Congress of Cardiology Tokyo 1978, I, 1238.

19. Meyer J, Sprauer R, Krebs W, Erbel R, Schweizer P, Effert S: Wirkung von Molsidomin auf die Belastung des linken Ventrikels bei koronarer Herzkrankheit. Dtsch med Wschr 105:1210, 1980.

20. Miller RR, Palomo AR, Brandon TA, Hartley CJ, Quinones MA: Combined vasodilator and inotropic therapy of heart failure: Experimental and clinical concepts. Am Heart J 102:500, 1981.

21. Meyer J, Hagemann K, Krebs W, Merx W, Schweizer P, Erbel R, Effert S: Computeranalyse der Druck-Volumen-Beziehung vor und nach Gabe von Isosorbiddinitrat. 2. Nitrat-Symposion Berlin. ed. W. Rudolph, A Schrey, Urban & Schwarzenberg, München, Wien, Baltimore 1980, p. 135.

22. Hardarson T, Henning H, O'Rourke R: Prolonged salutary effects of isosorbide dinitrate and nitroglycerin ointment on regional left ventricular function. Am J Cardiol 40:90, 1977.

23. Williams DO, Bommer W, Miller RR, Amsterdam EA, Mason DT: Hemodynamic assessment of oral peripheral vasodilatory therapy in chronic congestive heart failure: Prolonged effectiveness of isosorbide dinitrate. Am J Cardiol 39:84, 1977.

24. Russek HI: The therapeutic role of coronary vasodilators: glyceryl trinitrate, isosorbide dinitrate and pentaerythritol tetranitrate. Am J Med Sci 252:9, 1966.

25. Bussmann WD, Lohner J, Kaltenbach M: Orally administered isosorbide dinitrate in patients with and without left ventricular failure due to acute myocardial infarction. Am J Cardiol 39:91, 1977.

26. Sweatman T, Strauss G, Selzer A, Cohn KE: The long-acting hemodynamic effects of isosorbide dinitrate. Am J Cardiol 29:475, 1972.

27. Rackley CE, Mantle JA, Russel RO, Rogers WJ: Hemodynamic effects of sublingual and oral long-acting nitrates. In DT Mason ed. Advances in heart disease 1, Grune & Stratton, New York 1977, p. 59.

28. Crawford MH, Karliner JS, O'Rourke RA: Favorable effects of oral maintenance digoxin therapy on left ventricular performance in normal subjects: echocardiographic study. Am J Cardiol 38:843, 1976.

29. Frishman W, Smithen C, Befeler B, Kligfield P, Killip T: Noninvasive assessment of clinical response to oral propranolol therapy. Am J Cardiol 35:635, 1975.

30. Bibra H von, Gibson DG, Nityanandank: Effects of propranolol on left ventricular wall movement in patients with ischaemic heart disease. Br Heart J 43:293, 1980.

31. Bett JHN, Dryburgh L, Hetherington DE: Echocardiographic comparison of haemodynamic effects of metroprolol and propranolol. Br Heart J 43:541, 1980.

32. Bastiaans OL, Meltzer RS, McGhie J, Verbeek PW, Roelandt J: Quantification from two-dimensional echocardiographic images. In: Echocardiology (Rijsterborgh H ed.), Martinus Nijhoff, The Hague, 1981, p. 131.

33. Hecht HS, Taylor R, Weng M, Shah PN: Comparative evaluation of segmental asynergy in remote myocardial infarction by two-dimensional echocardiography. Am J Cardiol 47:1020, 1981.

34. Schiller NB, Acquatella H, Ports TA, Drew D, Goerke, J, Ringertz H, Silverman NH, Brundage R, Botvinick EH, Boswell R, Carlsson E, Parmley WW: Left ventricular volume from paired biplane two-dimensional echocardiography. Circulation 60:547, 1979.

35. Starling MR, Crawford MH, Sorensen SG, Levi B, Richards KL, O'Rourke RA: Comparative accuracy of apical biplane cross-sectional echocardiography and gated equilibrium radionuclide angiography for estimating left ventricular size and performance. Circulation 63:1075, 1981.

36. Erbel R, Schweizer P, Meyer J, Grenner H, Krebs W, Effert S: Bestimmung der Volumina und der Ejektionsfraktion des linken Ventrikels aus dem zweidimensionalen Echokardiogramm bei Patienten mit koronarer Herzerkrankung. Z Kardiol 69:52, 1980.

37. Wyatt HL, Meerbaum S, Heng MK, Rit J, Gueret P, Corday: Experimental evaluation of the extent of myocardial dyssynergy and infarct size by two-dimensional echocardiography. Circulation 63:597, 1981.

38. Meltzer RS, Woythaler CN, Buda AJ, Griffin GC, Harrison WD, Martin RP, Harrison DC, Popp RL: Two-dimensional echocardiographic quantification of infarct size alteration by pharmacologic agents.

39. Gueret P, Meerbaum S, Corday E, Uchiyama T, Wyatt HL, Broffman J: Differential effects of nitroprusside on ischemic and nonischemic myocardial segments demonstrated by computer-assisted two-dimensional echocardiography. Am J Cardiol 48:59, 1981.

30. Beeder C, Charuzi Y, Loh, IK, Staniloff H, Swann HJC: Relationship between segmental abnormalities and global left ventricular function in coronary artery disease: Validation of a theoretical model. Am Heart J 102:330, 1981.

41. Eaton LW, Weiss JL, Bulkley BH, Garrison JB, Weisfeldt: Regional cardiac dilatation after acute myocardial infarction. N Engl J Med 46:832, 1980.

SUBJECT INDEX

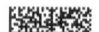